LIPID-LOWERING THERAPY AND PROGRESSION OF CORONARY ATHEROSCLEROSIS

Developments in
Cardiovascular Medicine

VOLUME 180

The titles published in this series are listed at the end of this volume.

Lipid-lowering Therapy and Progression of Coronary Atherosclerosis

edited by

A.V.G. BRUSCHKE
Department of Cardiology, University Hospital Leiden,
The Netherlands

J.H.C. REIBER
Department of Diagnostic Radiology and Nuclear Medicine,
University Hospital Leiden, The Netherlands

K.I. LIE
University of Amsterdam,
The Netherlands

and

H.J.J. WELLENS
Interuniversity Cardiology Institute of The Netherlands,
Utrecht, The Netherlands

KLUWER ACADEMIC PUBLISHERS

DORDRECHT / BOSTON / LONDON

Distributors

for the United States and Canada: Kluwer Academic Publishers, PO Box 358, Accord Station, Hingham, MA 02018-0358, USA
for all other countries: Kluwer Academic Publishers Group, Distribution Center, PO Box 322, 3300 AH Dordrecht, The Netherlands

A catalogue record for this book is available from the British Library
ISBN-13: 978-94-010-6551-1   e-ISBN-13: 978-94-009-0143-8
DOI: 10.1007/978-94-009-0143-8

Copyright

Published in the United Kingdom by Kluwer Academic Publishers,
PO Box 55, Lancaster, UK.

Kluwer Academic Publishers BV incorporates the publishing programmes of
D. Reidel, Martinus Nijhoff, Dr W. Junk and MTP Press.

Typeset by Speedlith Photo Litho Ltd., Stretford, Manchester, UK

Table of contents

List of contributors

EDWIN L. ALDERMAN
Division of Cardiovascular Medicine
Cardiovascular Research Building
Stanford University School of Medicine
Stanford
CA 94305
USA

THEO J.C. VAN BERKEL
Division of Biopharmaceutics
Leiden-Amsterdam
Center for Drug Research
Sylvius Laboratories
University of Leiden
P.O. Box 9503
2300 RA Leiden
The Netherlands

ALBERT V.G. BRUSCHKE
Department of Cardiology
University Hospital Leiden
P.O. Box 9600
2300 RC Leiden
The Netherlands
Co-authors: J. Wouter Jukema, Ad J. van Boven, Egbert T. Bal,
Johan H.C. Reiber, Aeilko H. Zwinderman

H. BUCHWALD
University of Minnesota
Department of Surgery
Box 290 UMHC
420 Delaware Street SE
Minneapolis
MN 55455
USA
Co-author: C.T. Campos

LUCIEN CAMPEAU
Institut de Cardiologie de Montréal
5000 Est
rue Bélanger
Montréal
Quebec
H1T 1C8
Canada
Co-authors: Michael Domanski, Nancy L. Geller, Genell Knatterud,
Jacques Lespérance, Yves Rosenberg, David Waters, Carl White

L. CASHIN-HEMPHILL
Boston Heart Foundation
139 Main Street
Cambridge
MA 02124
USA

PIM J. DE FEYTER
Catheterization Laboratory
Thoraxcenter Bd 416
University Hospital Dijkzigt
Dr. Molewaterplein 40
3015 GD Rotterdam
The Netherlands

C. MICHAEL GIBSON
West Roxbury Veterans Administration Hospital
1400 VFW Parkway
West Roxbury
MA 02132
USA
Co-authors: Peter H. Stone, Richard C. Pasternak, Frank M. Sacks

J. WOUTER JUKEMA
Department of Cardiology
University Hospital Leiden
P.O. Box 9600
2300 RC Leiden
The Netherlands
Co-authors: Ad J. van Boven, Johan H.C. Reiber, Aeilko H. Zwinderman,
Kong I. Lie, Albert V.G. Bruschke

D.M. KRAMSCH
Vascular Research
Division of Cardiology
University of Southern California
Los Angeles, CA
USA

A.A. KROON
Department of Medicine
Division of General Internal Medicine
University Hospital Nijmegen
P.O. Box 9101
6500 HB Nijmegen
The Netherlands
Co-author: Anton F.H. Stalenhoef

VINCENT M.G. MAHER
Division of Cardiology
University School of Medicine RG-22
Seattle
Washington 98195
USA

G.B. JOHN MANCINI
Eric W. Hamber Prof and Head
Department of Medicine
The University of British Columbia and University Hospital
2211 Wesbrook Mall
Vancouver
Canada V6T 2B5
USA

JOHAN H.C. REIBER
Department of Diagnostic Radiology and Nuclear Medicine
University Hospital Leiden
P.O. Box 9600
2300 RC Leiden
The Netherlands
Co-authors: J. Wouter Jukema, Gerhard Koning, Albert V.G. Bruschke

G.F. WATTS
Department of Medicine
University of Western Australia
Royal Perth Hospital
Box X2213 GPO
Perth
Western Australia 6001

HEIN J.J. WELLENS
Interuniversity Cardiology Institute of The Netherlands
P.O. Box 19258
3501 DG Utrecht
The Netherlands
Co-author: Albert V.G. Bruschke

Introduction

The introduction of a highly effective lipid lowering class of drugs, the HMG-CoA reductase inhibitors, has given a strong impulse to new research designed to determine the clinical and pathological–anatomical effects of lipid lowering in patients with coronary atherosclerosis. New developments in computer-assisted quantitative analysis of coronary arteriograms have made it possible to determine with great precision the morphology of atherosclerotic lesions and time-related changes in the coronary arteries assessed by sequential coronary arteriographic examinations.

Recently, several large lipid intervention studies using repeated quantitative coronary arteriography have been reported. These studies have provided essential information about the anatomical–pathological consequences of lipid lowering in man and have led to a better understanding of the clinical effects.

Almost all studies have shown a beneficial effect of lipid lowering therapy; however, differences in patient selection, study design and arteriographic methods make it difficult and, to a certain extent, impossible to compare the outcomes of different studies. Yet, by careful comparison of all arteriographic trials it may be possible to determine more accurately what currently may be considered proven, which hypotheses should be rejected, and which aspects merit further investigation. To make an in-depth comparison of studies possible the 'Koninklijke Nederlandse Academie van Wetenschappen' (Royal Netherlands Academy of Sciences) together with the Netherlands Heart Foundation has given the Interuniversity Cardiology Institute, the Netherlands (ICIN) the opportunity to organize a meeting of the principal investigators of all lipid intervention trials using anatomical changes demonstrated by coronary arteriography as the primary endpoint. Sponsorship was also obtained from the Wijnand M. Pon Foundation and an educational grant from Bristol Meyers Squibb.

The meeting was held October 3–4, 1994, at the KNAW headquarters in Amsterdam. A brief overview of each trial was presented, emphasizing the specific merits and limitations of each study. Possible mechanisms by which lipid lowering may influence progression or regression of atherosclerosis were discussed and methodological aspects, especially those relating to quantitative coronary arteriography and biochemical aspects, were critically reviewed.

We wish to thank the participants for submitting their manuscripts, which contain new information and express personal views that cannot be found in regular publications. They contribute significantly to a better understanding of the role of lipid lowering therapy and indicate new directions for future research.

A.V.G. Bruschke, MD
K.I. Lie, MD
J.H.C. Reiber, PhD
H.J.J. Wellens, MD

PART ONE

Mechanisms of normal progression and regression

1. Role of lipoproteins in progression of coronary arteriosclerosis

T. J. C. VAN BERKEL

Summary

Lipoproteins are responsible for the transport of cholesterol (esters) and triglycerides. Chylomicron-(remnants), VLDL-remnants (β-VLDL) and (modified) LDL are considered to be atherogenic while high levels of HDL do protect against arteriosclerosis. The liver plays a decisive role in the regulation of the plasma levels of atherogenic lipoproteins. The primary liver interaction site of chylomicron remnants and VLDL remnants (β-VLDL) is still unidentified, whereas the subsequent cellular uptake is likely to be mediated in concert by the LDL-receptor-related protein and the LDL receptor. The nature of the primary interaction site of remnants (remnant receptor) might be a liver-specific proteoglycan or a liver-specific protein. Atherogenic modified LDL can be recognized by a family of scavenger receptors. A newly identified 95-kDa protein forms the most likely candidate for mediating the in-vivo uptake of oxidized LDL from the circulation and may, therefore, protect the body against the presence of oxidized LDL in the blood compartment. HDL do pick up peripheral cholesterol and deliver cholesterol (esters) to the liver. The anti-atherogenic action of HDL may reside in specific subfractions containing specific apolipoproteins.

Introduction

The identification of the atherogenic nature of specific (sub)classes of lipoproteins has stimulated research into the molecular nature of the mechanisms that regulate the levels of these lipoproteins in the blood. During the last decade[1], it has become generally accepted that the liver plays a decisive role in controlling the plasma levels of atherogenic lipoproteins. The liver is the only organ that can irreversibly convert cholesterol to degradation products (bile acids) and excrete them from the body. Receptor-mediated uptake of atherogenic lipoproteins in the liver plays a crucial role in this process. During the last few years, major research has focused on the mechanisms by which chylomicron and VLDL remnants (β-VLDL) interact with the liver cells and how they are removed subsequently from the circulation.

The literature on the atherogenic nature of modified LDL is expanding rapidly. Modified LDL interacts avidly with the scavenger receptors on macrophages,

A.V.G. Bruschke et al. (eds): Lipid-lowering therapy and progression of atherosclerosis, 3–16.
© 1996 Kluwer Academic Publishers.

including tissue-macrophages in the liver and spleen. The characterization and identification of these receptors forms an important research issue because scavenger-receptor-mediated uptake may be an initial event in the formation of foam cells.

Metabolism of chylomicrons and β-VLDL

Chylomicrons and VLDL interact with lipoprotein lipase (LPL) after entering the blood circulation. This interaction leads to hydrolysis of most of their triglycerides. The size of chylomicrons (80–1000 nm) decreases to a mean size of approximately 90 nm for their remnants[2]. During this process, the apolipoprotein (apo) pattern of remnants shows a relative increase in apoE and a relative decrease in apoA and apoC, compared with chylomicrons[3]. In addition to its enzymatic role, evidence is accumulating that LPL can form a bridge between lipoproteins and cells by its ability to bind to both proteoglycans and lipoproteins[4]. The amount of circulating LPL in vivo is maintained generally at a low level because of the rapid removal of LPL by the liver[5]. No direct evidence is available to prove that the interaction of chylomicron remnants or β-VLDL with the liver in vivo involves LPL. Moreover, it has been found[6] that circulating LPL is associated mainly with LDL and HDL.

It has been established that the chylomicron and VLDL remnants, when injected intravenously into animals, are rapidly cleared from the circulation by the liver[3,7]. The liver cell type that contributes most to the uptake of these remnants is the parenchymal cell[7]. The primary interaction site for remnants in the liver is under active discussion[8-13]. The presence of apoE on the lipoprotein remnants is essential, suggesting that a binding site recognizing apoE must be present on the surface of the parenchymal cell. The effect of apoE on remnant binding is antagonized by apoC-III[14]. It was suggested[14] that apoC-III binds preferentially to the remnant recognition site on parenchymal cells. After binding, apoC-III loses its affinity for the remnants, thus preventing the uptake of the particles.

The in-vivo clearance of remnants can be completely blocked by lactoferrin[7]. Lactoferrin is a Fe^{3+}-carrying protein and contains a high concentration of positively charged amino acids at its N-terminus (amino acid residues 2–31). This domain contains a cluster of four arginine residues (residues 2–5) and an arginine/lysine-rich sequence at the amino acid positions 25–31 (Arg-X-X-Arg-Lys-X-Arg). X-ray crystallographic data and molecular modelling studies indicate that the latter structure resembles the amino acid positions 142–148 (Arg-X-X-Arg-Lys-Arg-X) of apoE present in the LDL-receptor-binding sequence. Following injection of lactoferrin in vivo, it associates rapidly with the liver parenchymal cells. If, however, the lactoferrin arginine residues are modified by 1,2-cyclohexanedione, the inhibitory effect on remnant clearance in vivo is blocked completely[15]. Modification of the arginine residues also strongly reduces the liver association of lactoferrin. The four arginine residues at positions 2–5 of lactoferrin can be removed by aminopeptidase-M (APM) treatment (actually 14 N-terminal amino acids are removed). Ziere et al.[15] found that APM-treated lactoferrin (APM-lactoferrin) associated with the liver at the same rate as native lactoferrin, whereas its internalization rate was increased markedly in comparison with native lactoferrin. APM-lactoferrin bound to parenchymal liver cells with a higher affinity and lower capacity than native lactoferrin, and is a more potent inhibitor of β-VLDL binding. Selective derivatization of APM-lactoferrin with 1,2-cyclohexanedione resulted in a loss of its capacity to inhibit the uptake of β-VLDL, indicating that arginine residues are involved. The Arg/Lys-enriched sequence at position 25–31 of lactoferrin resembles the binding site of apoE and may, therefore, prevent β-VLDL binding to the remnant receptor[15].

The in-vivo contribution of the LDL receptor to the removal of chylomicron remnants is the subject of active research. Choi and Cooper[10] found that an anti-LDL-receptor antibody reduced the uptake of iodinated chylomicron remnants by the liver to about 50%. In contrast, Kita et al.[16] found no abnormal remnant uptake in the Watanabe heritable hyperlipidaemic (WHHL) rabbit, an animal with dysfunctional LDL receptors. Similarly in humans, the lack of LDL receptors does not lead to a pathological change in the metabolism of dietary fat[17]. A more recent study by Demacker et al.[18] indicates that apoB$_{48}$ removal in WHHL rabbits is normal. Bowler et al.[19] voiced doubts about the original finding of Kita et al[16]; however, these doubts were caused by the exchange of retinylpalmitate to the increased lipoprotein pool in WHHL rabbits, as correctly pointed out by Demacker et al.[18]. The complete inhibition of remnant removal by lactoferrin[7], which does not block the LDL receptor, also indicates that a LDL-receptor-independent pathway is responsible mainly for the initial recognition of remnants.

Recognition of lipoprotein remnants by liver

The receptors and potential binding sites involved in lipoprotein remnant metabolism are illustrated in Figure 1.1. There is no doubt that the LDL-receptor-related protein (LRP) is able to interact with apoE-enriched β-VLDL[20], the 39-kDa receptor-associated protein[20–22], activated α_2-macroglobulin[23], recombinant tissue-type plasminogen activator[24–26], tissue-type plasminogen activator/plasminogen activator inhibitor complexes, urokinase-type plasminogen activator/plasminogen activator inhibitor complexes[27,28], pseudomonas exotoxin (A)[29], chicken vitellogenin[30], LPL[31,32] and lactoferrin[20]. Although in-vitro studies with cultured cells or isolated LRP allow the characterization of such an interaction, the in-vivo evidence for its multifunctionality is still limited. Overexpression of the selective 39-kDa protein inhibitor or in-vivo infusion may lead to a better understanding of the relative importance of some alternative routes for the uptake of any of the aforementioned ligands. In relation to this, it must be emphasized that, in fibroblasts with normal LDL receptors, apoE-enriched β-VLDL prefers the LDL-receptor-mediated route rather than LRP[33]. At present, I like to suggest that LRP forms a multifunctional back-up system that operates when the primary more-specific interaction sites do not function adequately.

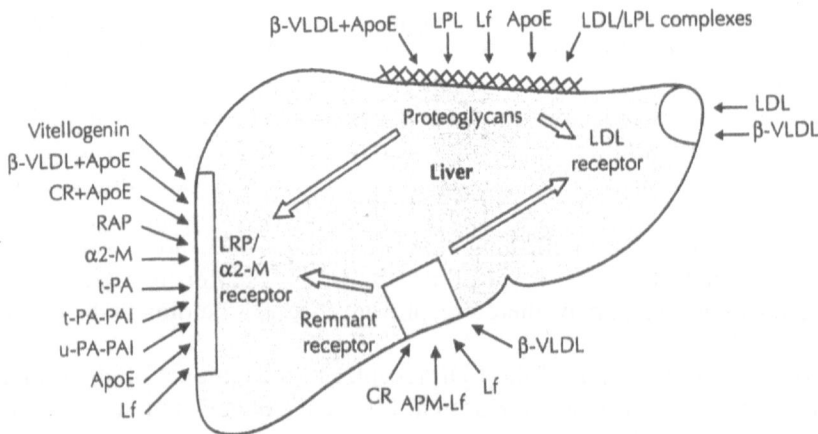

Figure 1.1. Receptor and binding sites involved in the binding of lipoprotein remnants and (aminopeptidase-M-treated) lactoferrin. APM-Lf, aminopeptidase-M-treated lactoferrin; ApoE, apolipoprotein E; CR, chylomicron remnants; Lf, lactoferrin; LPL, lipoprotein lipase; LRP, LDL-receptor-related protein; α_2M, α_2-macroglobulin; PAI, plasminogen activator inhibitor; RAP: 39-kDa receptor-associated protein: t-PA: tissue-type plasminogen activator:; u-PA, urokinase-type plasminogen activator.

In liver cells, apoE-enriched β-VLDL may also bind to proteoglycans[34], whereas the LDL receptor and a LDL-receptor-independent pathway (remnant receptor) form binding sites for circulating (not artificially apoE-enriched) β-VLDL. A specific remnant-recognition site, mentioned as the remnant receptor (Figure 1), represents a primary interaction site when the LDL receptor is down-regulated, for example when high concentrations of circulating LDL are present. This may be relevant even in the presence of LDL receptors because the normal amount of circulating LDL in humans may prevent remnant interaction with LDL receptors. In rats, the numbers of LDL receptors in liver parenchymal cells are rather low, leaving the remnant receptor as the only available uptake site. Candidate receptor proteins, such as LRP and the lipolysis-stimulated receptor[9,35], should also be studied in vivo to reinforce the theory that they can function as the primary recognition site or as the endocytotic uptake site. It is clear that further characterization of the specific molecule responsible for the liver-specific uptake of chylomicron-remnants and β-VLDL may lead to new pharmaceutical tools to lower the blood concentration of these atherogenic lipoproteins.

Modified lipoproteins as atherogenic particles

Macrophage-derived foam cells are an important feature of early atherosclerotic lesions[36]. Native LDL does not provoke foam cell formation because effective accumulation of cholesterol (esters) from LDL is prevented by down-regulation of the native LDL receptor[37]. Various modifications of LDL produce lipoprotein particles that interact with the scavenger receptors and thus lead to foam cell formation in cultured macrophages. Some years ago, it was established[38] that acetylated LDL (Ac-LDL), when injected into rats, was cleared rapidly from the circulation by the liver. Subsequently, it was determined[39] that, within the liver, the parenchymal and endothelial cells were responsible mainly for this uptake. In recent years, the hypothesis concerning the pathophysiological importance of modified LDL as an atherogenic particle has been strengthened mainly as a result of the work performed by Steinberg et al.[40]. The evidence suggested that oxidatively modified LDL, rather than Ac-LDL, was the physiological representative of modified LDL. Upon in-vivo injection of oxidized LDL (Ox-LDL), it was rapidly removed from the circulation by the liver, like Ac-LDL. In contrast to Ac-LDL, however, Kupffer cells were the main site for Ox-LDL uptake in the liver[41].

Besides LDL, cholesterol-ester-rich lipoproteins like lipoprotein (a) (Lp(a)), and β-VLDL, also constitute a risk factor for atherosclerosis. Probucol prevented the progression of atherosclerosis in cholesterol-fed rabbits (in which β-VLDL is the main atherogenic particle)[42]. This suggested that oxidation of β-VLDL was involved in atherogenesis. Oxidized β-VLDL was taken up from the circulation by the liver at the same rate as native β-VLDL. In contrast to native β-VLDL, which interacts primarily with parenchymal liver cells, the main site of uptake of oxidized β-VLDL was the Kupffer cell[43].

Lp(a) cannot be efficiently removed from the blood because LDL-receptor recognition of Lp(a) is hampered by little (a). The prolonged circulation time may, therefore, allow oxidative modification of Lp(a). Certain higher-molecular-weight forms of Lp(a) have been correlated with a greater risk for coronary heart diseases[44]. The manner in which oxidized Lp(a) interacts with the liver depends on the degree of Lp(a) oxidation and the size of the Lp(a) isoforms. Both of these aspects have been studied[45]. Again the Kupffer cell was the major site for liver uptake of the mildly oxidized 610-kDa form of Lp(a), whereas the endothelial cell appeared to interact more avidly with the oxidized 440-kDa form. It may be of interest to investigate whether the macrophages of the arterial wall interact differently with mildly oxidized Lp(a) of differing molecular weights.

When [³H]cholesteryl-oleate-labelled Ox-LDL was injected into rats[46], the radiolabelled cholesteryl esters were almost completely hydrolyzed within 1 h after injection. During this time interval, the Kupffer-cell-associated radio-activity declined to 32% of the maximal uptake value[46]. In serum, the highest specific radioactivity of resecreted [³H]cholesteryl esters was associated with HDL, indicating a role for HDL as the active cholesterol acceptor in vivo. Subsequently, radioactivity was secreted into the bile as bile acids at a rate threefold higher than that observed after the administration of [³H]cholesteryl-oleate-labelled Ac-LDL. The rapid processing of cholesteryl esters derived from Ox-LDL to bile acids indicates that Kupffer cells form an efficient protection system against the presence of atherogenic Ox-LDL particles in the blood compartment[46] (Figure 1.2).

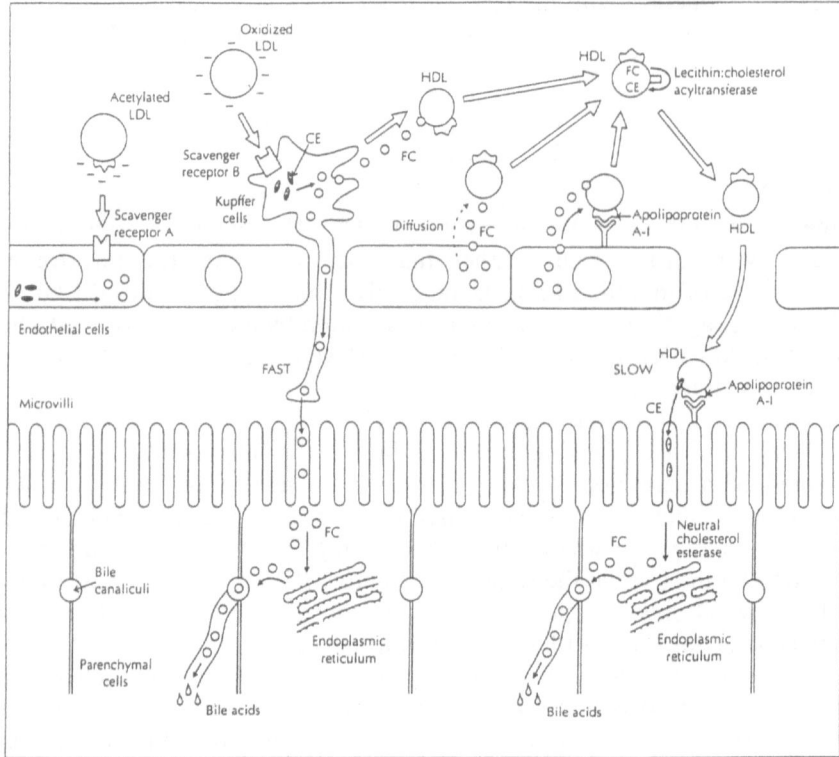

Figure 1.2. The transport of cholesterol from liver endothelial and Kupffer cells to parenchymal cells and bile. Oxidized LDL (randomly negatively charged) is taken up mainly by the Kupffer cells through binding to the scavenger receptor B (95-kDa oxidized LDL-receptor protein). Internalization of oxidized LDL is accomplished predominantly by membrane foldings and worm-like structures. Hydrolysis of cholesteryl esters (CE) occurs in the lysosomes. Free cholesterol (FC) is subsequently transported from the Kupffer cells to the parenchymal cells via two different routes. The major route, which occurs very fast, depends on direct cell–cell contact between the Kupffer and parenchymal cells. FC enters the parenchymal cell and is directly converted into bile acids and secreted into the bile. In addition, Kupffer cells may release FC to HDL. Cholesterol is esterified in HDL and transported to the parenchymal liver cells as described above. The latter route occurs at a slower rate. Acetylated LDL is taken up mainly by liver endothelial cells mediated by scavenger receptor A. After hydrolysis of the CE to FC, subsequent transport to the parenchymal cells is mediated mainly by HDL. This occurs at a slower rate than the indicated direct route for oxidized LDL.

Scavenger receptors

Non-reciprocal cross-competition between Ac-LDL and Ox-LDL was reported in murine peritoneal macrophages[47,48] and liver cells[38]. Non-reciprocal cross-competition occurs when one ligand competes efficiently for the binding of a second ligand, whereas the second ligand does not, or only partially, compete for the binding of the first. The presence of multiple binding sites on a single receptor or the existence of multiple receptors, may explain these observations.

The different cellular specificity of Ox-LDL vs Ac-LDL in the liver indicates that different receptors probably do exist[41]. Ligand blots indicate that the Ac-LDL interaction with liver endothelial cells is exerted by the 220-kDa protein[49] as characterized originally by Kodama et al.[50]. However, in both murine peritoneal macrophages, in foam cells from the atherosclerotic plaque[51], and in Kupffer cells[49], a 95-kDa protein was identified as the specific interaction site for Ox-LDL. For the following reasons, it is suggested[49] that the 95-kDa binding protein forms the most likely candidate for mediating the in-vivo uptake of Ox-LDL from the circulation:

1. The 95-kDa binding protein is present specifically on the Kupffer cell, which forms the major site for hepatic uptake of Ox-LDL;
2. The binding specificity of the 95-kDa protein for Ox-LDL whereby Ac-LDL and LDL are ineffective;
3. The saturable Ca^{2+}-independent kinetics of Ox-LDL binding to the 95-kDa protein ($Kd = 15\,\mu g/ml$) are comparable to those found with Kupffer cells in suspension ($Kd = 14\,\mu g/ml$); and
4. The 95-kDa protein already recognizes moderately Ox-LDL.

Two macrophage proteins, the Fc RII-B$_2$ receptor and CD36, have been identified as possible interaction sites for Ox-LDL by expression cloning. The Fc RII-B$_2$ receptor had a molecular weight of 50 kDa and recognized Ox-LDL, although recognition was not coupled with uptake[52]. In contrast, the 88-kDa protein, CD36, recognized and internalized Ox-LDL[53]. On the basis of its molecular mass, CD36 seems to be within the molecular-weight range of the 95-kDa protein. Further characterization of CD36 and the 95-kDa protein is necessary before the presence or absence of a relationship between the two molecules can be established.

Function of scavenger receptors

Modified lipoproteins are recognized by unusual receptors (scavenger receptors) that exhibit a broad ligand-binding specificity. In a recent review, Krieger et al.[54] mentioned the following as substrates for scavenger receptors:

1. Chemically modified lipoproteins, such as Ac-LDL, Ox-LDL and maleylated and formaldehyde-treated albumin;
2. Polyribonucleotides, including poly I and poly G;
3. Natural and modified polysaccharides, such as carrageenan and dextran sulphate;
4. Anionic phospholipids, including phosphatidylserine; and
5. Other molecules, such as polyvinyl sulphate, asbestos and endotoxin.

The common feature of all these substrates is their polyanionic nature, although many polyanions (poly C and poly A) do not form a ligand for the scavenger receptor. Pearson et al.[55] showed that a base-quartet-stabilized four-stranded helix appeared to be a necessary structural determinant for oligonucleotide and polynucleotide binding to scavenger receptors. The spatial distribution of the negatively charged phosphates in polynucleotide quadraplexes provided a charged surface complementary to the collagenous ligand-binding domain of the receptor. Furthermore, Zhang et al.[56] showed that a relatively simple domain, consisting of a cluster of derivatized lysine residues, is sufficient for recognition by scavenger receptors.

Structural studies on various domains within the scavenger receptors (type I and II)[57], and the Ox-LDL-specific receptor[49], are needed to define their substrate specificity more precisely[57-59]. In addition, different species express scavenger receptors with varying specificity[60-63]. Elegant studies by Doi et al.[64] have shown that the 'charged collagen' structure containing a lysine cluster forms a positively charged groove, which interacts specifically with negatively charged ligands[64]. The generation of scavenger-receptor knock-out mice will, however, be necessary to obtain further direct information on the (patho)physiological function of the various types of scavenger receptors.

HDL as protection factor for arteriosclerosis

HDL play an important role in maintaining whole-body cholesterol homeostasis. The inverse correlation of HDL cholesterol levels with the incidence and prevalence of coronary artery disease[65] can be explained by the role of HDL in reverse cholesterol transport, a term originally introduced by Glomset in 1968[66]. Reverse cholesterol transport identifies a series of metabolic events resulting in the transport of peripheral cholesterol to the liver. The removal of peripheral free cholesterol by HDL is followed by the esterification of free cholesterol by the enzyme lecithin:cholesterol acyltransferase (LCAT) which utilizes apoA-I present on HDL as cofactor. By converting cholesterol to its insoluble esterified form, LCAT forms the driving force for a concentration gradient from the plasma membrane to HDL. The newly formed cholesteryl esters can be transferred from HDL to other lipoproteins by the cholesteryl ester transfer protein (CETP) and delivered to the liver for secretion in the bile either by HDL itself or via VLDL or LDL.

Though the concept of reverse cholesterol transport is generally accepted, the exact mechanism by which reverse cholesterol transport is regulated is still not elucidated. Also, in-vivo evidence for reverse cholesterol transport remains scarce.

Studies in humans or intact animals are very complex and difficult to interpret. Studies in patients with HDL-metabolism-related disorders show conflicting effects of HDL cholesterol levels on atherosclerosis. Experimental evidence supporting the beneficial role of HDL in atherosclerosis has been obtained with cholesterol-fed rabbits. Weekly injections of HDL induced regression of fatty streak lesions[67,68]. With transgenic mice, the introduction of a human apoA-I gene into mice resulted in elevated levels of plasma apoA-I, due to the expression of the human gene. The high levels of apoA-I were found to be associated with high levels of HDL[69,70] and led to the presence of HDL_{2b} and HDL_{3a}. The FCR of apoA-I was high[71]. The variation in gene loci affecting the apoA-I expression and HDL concentration has been found to have a major protective effect on diet-induced atherosclerosis in these mice[72]. Recently, it has been reported that transgenic mice expressing both human A-I and A-II are not protected, supporting the theory that apoA-I particles are specifically anti-atherogenic[73].

Since the liver is the major cholesterol-processing organ, the secretion of cholesterol into the bile, in its unesterified form or processed into bile acids, is an important route for the body to dispose of excess cholesterol. In man, it has been shown that free cholesterol from HDL is the major substrate for biliary cholesterol[74]. In rats, we have shown that liver parenchymal cells secrete bile acids derived from HDL cholesteryl esters at a higher rate than LDL-derived cholesteryl esters[75]. These studies all indicate that HDL cholesterol (esters) are a preferential substrate for bile-acid synthesis and secretion.

In our group, we used an in-vivo model for studying reverse cholesterol transport. In this model, liver endothelial cells were rapidly labelled with [^{3}H]cholesteryl esters by injecting labelled acetylated LDL. The hydrolysis of cholesteryl esters and subsequent transport of [^{3}H]cholesterol through the serum compartment to the liver parenchymal cells and secretion into the bile were followed[76]. By using unrestrained bile-cannulated rats, the time-dependent appearance of radiolabelled cholesterol and bile acids can be quantified. When liver endothelial cells were loaded with [^{3}H]cholesteryl esters by injecting radiolabelled acetylated LDL, we found that resecreted radiolabelled free cholesterol used HDL as a transport vehicle. The specific activity of radio-labelled cholesterol was found to be highest in the HDL fraction (Figure 2). In the serum, [^{3}H]cholesterol was converted into cholesterol esters which is consistent with the action of LCAT. Serum lowing of the HDL levels by pretreatment of the rats with ethinyl estradiol resulted in a less-efficient transport of radiolabelled bile acids to the parenchymal cells and bile, thus supporting in vivo the essential role of HDL in mediating reverse cholesterol transport.

Conclusion

A still unidentified recognition site for remnants is responsible for the specific primary interaction of remnants with the liver. It is conceivable that the subsequent uptake can be mediated by LRP, the LDL receptor, or both (see arrow in Figure 1). The multifunctionality of LRP allows it to function as the uptake system. The primary interaction site of remnants (indicated as the remnant receptor) might be a liver-specific proteoglycan or a liver-specific protein (i.e. hepatic lipase, apoE, or a still unidentified protein).

The modified forms of LDL can be recognized by a family of scavenger receptors. The (patho)physiological functions of the individual scavenger receptors are under active investigation, including a role as adhesion molecules. The liver uptake of Ox-LDL is likely to be mediated by a newly identified 95-kDa protein[49] that is expressed by peritoneal macrophages and foam cells from atherosclerotic plaques[51]. It has been shown[49] that mildly Ox-LDL interacts with the 95-kDa protein. It can be concluded, therefore, that this liver protein acts to protect against circulating (mildly) Ox-LDL, and it may also mediate foam-cell formation in atherosclerotic plaques.

Evidence for in-vivo reverse cholesterol transport is still limited. The obtained results, however, do sustain the overall view of the role of HDL in transporting cholesterol in the body. HDL do pick up peripheral cholesterol and deliver cholesterol (esters) to the liver[76]. The efficient secretion of bile acids derived from HDL cholesterol esters[75] confirms the supposed essential role of HDL in reverse cholesterol transport.

References

1. Dietschy JM, Turley SD, Spady DK. Role of liver in the maintenance of cholesterol and low density lipoprotein homeostasis in different animal species, including humans. J Lipid Res. 1993;34:1637–59.
2. Redgrave TG, Small DM. Quantitation of the transfer of surface phospholipid of chylomicrons to the high density lipoprotein fraction during the catabolism of chylomicrons in the rat. J Clin Invest. 1979;64:162–71.
3. Windler E, Chao Y, Havel RJ. Determinants of hepatic uptake of triglyceride-rich lipoproteins and their remnants in the rat. J Biol Chem. 1980;255:5475–80.
4. Mulder M, Lombardi P, Jansen H, van Berkel TJC, Frants RR, Havekes LM. Low density lipoprotein receptor internalizes low density and very low density lipoproteins that are bound to heparan sulfate proteoglycans via lipoprotein lipase. J Biol Chem. 1993;268:9369–75.
5. Olivecrona T, Bengtsson-Olivecrona G. Lipases involved in lipoprotein metabolism. Curr Opin Lipidol. 1990;1:116–21.
6. Vilella E, Joven J. Lipoprotein lipase binding to plasma lipoproteins. Med Sci Res. 1991;19: 111–12.
7. van Dijk MC, Ziere GJ, Boers W, Linthorst C, Bijsterbosch MK, van Berkel TJC. Recognition of chylomicron remnants and beta-migrating very-low-density lipoproteins by the remnant receptor of parenchymal liver cells is distinct from the liver alpha 2-macroglobulin-recognition site. Biochem J. 1991;279:863–70.
8. Gudmundsen O, Berg T, Roos N, Nenseter MS. Hepatic uptake of beta-VLDL in cholesterol-fed rabbits. J Lipid Res. 1993;34:589–600.
9. Yen FT, Mann CJ, Guermani LM, et al. Identification of a lipolysis-stimulated receptor that is distinct from the LDL receptor and the LDL receptor-related protein. Biochemistry. 1994;33: 1172–80.
10. Choi SY, Cooper AD. A comparison of the roles of the low density lipoprotein (LDL) receptor and the LDL receptor-related protein/alpha 2-macroglobulin receptor in chylomicron remnant removal in the mouse in vivo. J Biol Chem. 1993;268:15804–11.
11. Nykjaer A, Bengtsson-Olivecrona G, Lookene A, et al. The alpha 2-macroglobulin receptor/low density lipoprotein receptor-related protein binds lipoprotein lipase and beta-migrating very low density lipoprotein associated with the lipase. J Biol Chem. 1993;268: 15048–55.
12. Jäckle S, Huber C, Moestrup S, Gliemann J, Beisiegel U. In vivo removal of beta-VLDL, chylomicron remnants, and alpha 2-macroglobulin in the rat. J Lipid Res. 1993;34:309–15.
13. van Dijk MC, Kruijt JK, Boers W, Linthorst C, van Berkel TJC. Distinct properties of the recognition sites for beta-very low density lipoprotein (remnant receptor) and alpha 2-macroglobulin (low density lipoprotein receptor-related protein) on rat parenchymal cells. J Biol Chem. 1992;267:17732–7.
14. van Berkel TJC, Kruijt JK, Scheek LM, Groot PH. Effect of apolipoproteins E and C-III on the interaction of chylomicrons with parenchymal and non-parenchymal cells from rat liver. Biochem J. 1983;216:71–80.

15. Ziere GJ, Bijsterbosch MK, van Berkel TJC. Removal of 14 N-terminal amino acids of lactoferrin enhances its affinity for parenchymal liver cells and potentiates the inhibition of beta-very low density lipoprotein binding. J Biol Chem. 1993;268:27069–75.
16. Kita T, Goldstein JL, Brown MS, Watanabe Y, Hornick CA, Havel RJ. Hepatic uptake of chylomicron remnants in WHHL rabbits: a mechanism genetically distinct from the low density lipoprotein receptor. Proc Natl Acad Sci USA. 1982;79:3623–7.
17. Rubinsztein DC, Cohen JC, Berger GM, van der Westhuyzen DR, Coetzee GA, Gevers W. Chylomicron remnant clearance from the plasma is normal in familial hypercholesterolemic homozygotes with defined receptor defects. J Clin Invest. 1990;86:1306–12.
18. Demacker PN, van Heijst PJ, Stalenhoef AF. A study of the chylomicron metabolism in WHHL rabbits after fat loading. Discrepancy between results based on measurement of apoprotein B-48 or retinyl palmitate. Biochem J. 1992;285:641–6.
19. Bowler A, Redgrave TG, Mamo JC. Chylomicron-remnant clearance in homozygote and heterozygote Watanabe-heritable-hyperlipidaemic rabbits is defective. Lack of evidence for an independent chylomicron-remnant receptor. Biochem J. 1991;276:381–6.
20. Willnow TE, Goldstein JL, Orth K, Brown MS, Herz J. Low density lipoprotein receptor-related protein and gp330 bind similar ligands, including plasminogen activator-inhibitor complexes and lactoferrin, an inhibitor of chylomicron remnant clearance. J Biol Chem. 1992; 267:26172–80.
21. Warshawsky I, Bu G, Schwartz AL. Identification of domains on the 39-kDa protein that inhibit the binding of ligands to the low density lipoprotein receptor-related protein. J Biol Chem. 1993;268:22046–54.
22. Warshawsky I, Bu G, Schwartz AL. Binding analysis of amino-terminal and carboxyl-terminal regions of the 39-kDa protein to the low density lipoprotein receptor-related protein. J Biol Chem. 1994;269:3325–30.
23. Van Leuven F, Cassiman JJ, Van den Berghe H. Functional modifications of alpha 2-macroglobulin by primary amines. I. Characterization of alpha 2 M after derivatization by methylamine and by factor XIII. J Biol Chem. 1981;256:9016–22.
24. Bu G, Maksymovitch EA, Schwartz AL. Receptor-mediated endocytosis of tissue-type plasminogen activator by low density lipoprotein receptor-related protein on human hepatoma HepG2 cells. J Biol Chem. 1993;268:13002–9.
25. Bu G, Williams S, Strickland DK, Schwartz AL. Low density lipoprotein receptor-related protein/alpha 2-macroglobulin receptor is an hepatic receptor for tissue-type plasminogen activator. Proc Natl Acad Sci USA. 1992;89:7427–31.
26. Bu G, Morton PA, Schwartz AL. Identification and partial characterization by chemical cross-linking of a binding protein for tissue-type plasminogen activator (t-PA) on rat hepatoma cells. A plasminogen activator inhibitor type 1-independent t-PA receptor. J Biol Chem. 1992;267: 15595–602.
27. Kounnas MZ, Henkin J, Argraves WS, Strickland DK. Low density lipoprotein receptor-related protein/alpha 2-macroglobulin receptor mediates cellular uptake of pro-urokinase. J Biol Chem. 1993;268:21862–7.
28. Orth K, Madison EL, Gething MJ, Sambrook JF, Herz J. Complexes of tissue-type plasminogen activator and its serpin inhibitor plasminogen-activator inhibitor type 1 are internalized by means of the low density lipoprotein receptor-related protein/alpha 2-macroglobulin receptor. Proc Natl Acad Sci USA. 1992;89:7422–6.
29. Kounnas MZ, Morris RE, Thompson MR, FitzGerald DJ, Strickland DK, Saelinger CB. The alpha 2-macroglobulin receptor/low density lipoprotein receptor-related protein binds and internalizes Pseudomonas exotoxin A. J Biol Chem. 1992;267:12420–3.
30. Nimpf J, Stifani S, Bilous PT, Schneider WJ. The somatic cell-specific low density lipoprotein receptor-related protein of the chicken. Close kinship to mammalian low density lipoprotein receptor gene family members. J Biol Chem. 1994;269:212–9.
31. Chappell DA, Fry GL, Waknitz MA, et al. Lipoprotein lipase induces catabolism of normal triglyceride-rich lipoproteins via the low density lipoprotein receptor-related protein/alpha 2-macroglobulin receptor in vitro. A process facilitated by cell-surface proteoglycans. J Biol

Chem. 1993;268:14168–75.

32. Kounnas MZ, Chappell DA, Strickland DK, Argraves WS. Glycoprotein 330, a member of the low density lipoprotein receptor family, binds lipoprotein lipase in vitro. J Biol Chem. 1993;268:14176–81.

33. Kowal RC, Herz J, Goldstein JL, Esser V, Brown MS. Low density lipoprotein receptor-related protein mediates uptake of cholesteryl esters derived from apoprotein E-enriched lipoproteins. Proc Natl Acad Sci USA. 1989;86:5810–14.

34. Ji ZS, Brecht WJ, Miranda RD, Hussain MM, Innerarity TL, Mahley RW. Role of heparan sulfate proteoglycans in the binding and uptake of apolipoprotein E-enriched remnant lipo-proteins by cultured cells. J Biol Chem. 1993;268:10160–7.

35. Bihain BE, Yen FT. Free fatty acids activate a high-affinity saturable pathway for degradation of low-density lipoproteins in fibroblasts from a subject homozygous for familial hyper-cholesterolemia. Biochemistry. 1992;31:4628–36.

36. Ross R. The pathogenesis of atherosclerosis: a perspective for the 1990s. Nature. 1993;362:801–9.

37. Brown MS, Basu SK, Falck JR, Ho YK, Goldstein JL. The scavenger cell pathway for lipoprotein degradation: specificity of the binding site that mediates the uptake of negatively-charged LDL by macrophages. J Supramol Struct. 1980;13:67–81.

38. van Berkel TJC, Nagelkerke JF, Harkes L, Kruijt JK. Processing of acetylated human low-density lipoprotein by parenchymal and non-parenchymal liver cells. Involvement of calmodulin? Biochem J. 1982;208:493–503.

39. Nagelkerke JF, Barto KP, van Berkel TJ. In vivo and in vitro uptake and degradation of acetylated low density lipoprotein by rat liver endothelial, Kupffer, and parenchymal cells. J Biol Chem. 1983;258:12221–7.

40. Steinberg D, Parthasarathy S, Carew TE, Khoo JC, Witztum JL. Beyond cholesterol. Modifications of low-density lipoprotein that increase its atherogenicity. N Engl J Med. 1989;320:915–24.

41. van Berkel TJC, De Rijke YB, Kruijt JK. Different fate in vivo of oxidatively modified low density lipoprotein and acetylated low density lipoprotein in rats. Recognition by various receptors on Kupffer and endothelial liver cells. J Biol Chem. 1991;266:2282–9.

42. Tawara K, Ishihara M, Ogawa H, Tomikawa M. Effect of probucol, pantethine and their combinations on serum lipoprotein metabolism and on the incidence of atheromatous lesions in the rabbit. Jpn J Pharmcol. 1986;41:211–22.

43. de Rijke YB, Hessels EM, van Berkel TJC. Recognition sites on rat liver cells for oxidatively modified beta-very low density lipoproteins. Arterioscler Thromb. 1992;12:41–9.

44. Seed M, Hoppichler F, Reaveley D, et al. Relation of serum lipoprotein(a) concentration and apolipoprotein(a) phenotype to coronary heart disease in patients with familial hyper-cholesterolemia. N Engl J Med. 1990;322:1494–9.

45. de Rijke YB, Jurgens G, Hessels EM, Hermann A, van Berkel TJC. In vivo fate and scavenger receptor recognition of oxidized lipoprotein[a] isoforms in rats. J Lipid Res. 1992;33:1315–25.

46. Pieters MN, Esbach S, Schouten D, Brouwer A, Knook DL, Van Berkel TJC. Cholesteryl esters from oxidized low-density lipoproteins are in vivo rapidly hydrolyzed in rat Kupffer cells and transported to liver parenchymal cells and bile. Hepatology. 1994;19:1459–67.

47. Sparrow CP, Parthasarathy S, Steinberg D. A macrophage receptor that recognizes oxidized low density lipoprotein but not acetylated low density lipoprotein. J Biol Chem. 1989;264:2599–604.

48. Arai H, Kita T, Yokode M, Narumiya S, Kawai C. Multiple receptors for modified low density lipoproteins in mouse peritoneal macrophages: different uptake mechanisms for acetylated and oxidized low density lipoproteins. Biochem Biophys Res Commun. 1989;159:1375–82.

49. de Rijke YB, van Berkel TJC. Rat liver Kupffer and endothelial cells express different binding proteins for modified low density lipoproteins. Kupffer cells express a 95-kDa membrane protein as a specific binding site for oxidized low density lipoproteins. J Biol Chem. 1994;269:824–7.

50. Kodama T, Freeman M, Rohrer L, Zabrecky J, Matsudaira P, Krieger M. Type I macrophage

scavenger receptor contains alpha-helical and collagen-like coiled coils. Nature. 1990;343: 531–5.

51. Ottnad E, Via DP, Frubis J, et al. Differentiation of binding sites on reconstituted hepatic scavenger receptors using oxidized low-density lipoprotein. Biochem J. 1992;281:745–51.
52. Stanton LW, White RT, Bryant CM, Protter AA, Endemann G. A macrophage Fc receptor for IgG is also a receptor for oxidized low density lipoprotein. J Biol Chem. 1992;267:22446–51.
53. Endemann G, Stanton LW, Madden KS, Bryant CM, White RT, Protter AA. CD36 is a receptor for oxidized low density lipoprotein. J Biol Chem. 1993;268:11811–16.
54. Krieger M, Acton S, Ashkenas J, Pearson A, Penman M, Resnick D. Molecular flypaper, host defense, and atherosclerosis. Structure, binding properties, and functions of macrophage scavenger receptors. J Biol Chem. 1993;268:4569–72.
55. Pearson AM, Rich A, Krieger M. Polynucleotide binding to macrophage scavenger receptors depends on the formation of base-quartet-stabilized four-stranded helices. J Biol Chem. 1993; 268:3546–54.
56. Zhang H, Yang Y, Steinbrecher UP. Structural requirements for the binding of modified proteins to the scavenger receptor of macrophages. J Biol Chem. 1993;268:5535–42.
57. Resnick D, Freedman NJ, Xu S, Krieger M. Secreted extracellular domains of macrophage scavenger receptors form elongated trimers which specifically bind crocidolite asbestos. J Biol Chem. 1993;268:3538–45.
58. Acton S, Resnick D, Freeman M, Ekkel Y, Ashkenas J, Krieger M. The collagenous domains of macrophage scavenger receptors and complement component C1q mediate their similar, but not identical, binding specificities for polyanionic ligands. J Biol Chem. 1993;268:3530–7.
59. Ashkenas J, Penman M, Vasile E, Acton S, Freeman M, Krieger M. Structures and high and low affinity ligand binding properties of murine type I and type II macrophage scavenger receptors. J Lipid Res. 1993;34:983–1000.
60. Dejager S, Mietus-Synder M, Pitas RE. Oxidized low density lipoproteins bind to the scavenger receptor expressed by rabbit smooth muscle cells and macrophages. Arterioscler Thromb. 1993;13:371–8.
61. Ueda Y, Arai H, Kawashima A, et al. Different expression of modified low density lipoprotein receptors in rabbit peritoneal macrophages and Kupffer cells. Atherosclerosis. 1993;101: 25–35.
62. Suzaki K, Kobori S, Ide M, et al. Acetyl-low density lipoprotein receptors on rat mesangial cells. Atherosclerosis. 1993;101:177–84.
63. Miyazaki A, Sakai M, Yamaguchi E, Sakamoto Y, Shichiri M, Horiuchi S. Two independent macrophage receptors for acetylated high-density lipoprotein. Biochim Biophys Acta. 1993; 1170:143–50.
64. Doi T, Higashino K, Kurihara Y, et al. Charged collagen structure mediates the recognition of negatively charged macromolecules by macrophage scavenger receptors. J Biol Chem. 1993;268:2126–33.
65. Miller GJ, Miller NE. Plasma-high-density-lipoprotein concentration and development of ischaemic heart-disease. Lancet. 1975,1.16–19.
66. Glomset JA. The plasma lecithins: cholesterol acyltransferase reaction. J Lipid Res. 1968;9: 155–67.
67. Badimon JJ, Badimon L, Galvez A, Dische R, Fuster V. High density lipoprotein plasma fractions inhibit aortic fatty streaks in cholesterol-fed rabbits. Lab Invest. 1989;60:455–61.
68. Badimon JJ, Badimon L, Fuster V. Regression of atherosclerotic lesions by high density lipoprotein plasma fraction in the cholesterol-fed rabbit. J Clin Invest. 1990;85:1234–41.
69. Walsh A, Ito Y, Breslow JL. High levels of human apolipoprotein A-I in transgenic mice result in increased plasma levels of small high density lipoprotein (HDL) particles comparable to human HDL3. J Biol Chem. 1989;264:6488–94.
70. Rubin EM, Ishida BY, Clift SM, Krauss RM. Expression of human apolipoprotein A-I in transgenic mice results in reduced plasma levels of murine apolipoprotein A-I and the appearance of two new high density lipoprotein size subclasses. Proc Natl Acad Sci USA. 1991;88:434–8.

71. Brinton EA, Eisenberg S, Breslow JL. Elevated high density lipoprotein cholesterol levels correlate with decreased apolipoprotein A-I and A-II fractional catabolic rate in women. J Clin Invest. 1989;84:262–9.
72. Rubin EM, Krauss RM, Spangler EA, Verstuyft JG, Clift SM. Inhibition of early atherogenesis in transgenic mice by human apolipoprotein AI. Nature. 1991;353:265–7.
73. Aalto-Setälä K. European Vascular Biology Association Meeting, March 23–27 1993, Tampere, Finland.
74. Schwartz CC, Halloran LG, Vlahcevic ZR, Gregory DH, Swell L. Preferential utilization of free cholesterol from high-density lipoproteins for biliary cholesterol secretion in man. Science. 1978;200:62–4.
75. Pieters MN, Schouten D, Bakkeren HF, et al. Selective uptake of cholesteryl esters from apolipoprotein-E-free high-density lipoproteins by rat parenchymal cells in vivo is efficiently coupled to bile acid synthesis. Biochem J. 1991;280:359–65.
76. Bakkeren HF, Kuipers F, Vonk RJ, Van Berkel TJC. Evidence for reverse cholesterol transport in vivo from liver endothelial cells to parenchymal cells and bile by high-density lipoprotein. Biochem J. 1990;268:685–91.

2. Pathophysiological basis for lipid intervention trials

H. BUCHWALD and C. T. CAMPOS

Summary

The pathophysiology of the atherosclerotic plaque consists of the interaction of four cell types (T lymphocytes, macrophages, smooth muscle cells and endothelial cells), several processes (notably low density lipoprotein oxidation and inflammation), and numerous attractant, agonist and antagonist factors. The most recent conceptualization of the pathophysiology of atherosclerosis emphasizes that the clinically dangerous lesions are not necessarily the largest or most stenotic plaques but seem to be the smaller plaques, rich in lipids. Thus, lipid intervention trials test not only the benefits of risk factor modification, but assess the direct benefits of converting active plaques, with thin caps, rich in lipids, and susceptible to fissuring and acute thrombosis, into stable plaques with a reduced lipid content and a thicker more fibrous cap.

Introduction

Research into the mechanisms of atherogenesis has followed two interlocking pathways. Epidemiologists have used population data to define risk factors which predispose to the development of atherosclerosis. Cell biologists have sought to define the cellular and the subcellular events of atherosclerosis through the study of lesion development at the tissue level. Since the initial induction of atherosclerosis by cholesterol feeding in rabbits by Anitschkow in 1913[1], the causal relationship between cholesterol and experimental atherosclerosis has clearly been established. Epidemiological analyses, including the Seven Countries Study[2], the Framingham Study[3] and the Pooling Project[4], have confirmed this relationship in humans. The screening results of the Multiple Risk Factor Intervention Trial precisely related the total serum cholesterol level and the subsequent six-year coronary heart disease mortality rate in 361 662 asymptomatic men[5].

The experimental induction of atherogenesis and the subsequent pantheon of epidemiological evidence in support of the lipid/atherosclerosis theory are phenomena of the 20th century, and were preceded by the clinical observations of the stigmata of familial hypercholesterolaemia by Rayer[6] and Addison and Gull[7] in the 19th century. The pathophysiological evidence of the relationship of atherosclerotic plaques to clinical disease goes back still further to da Vinci[8],

A.V.G. Bruschke et al. (eds): Lipid-lowering therapy and progression of atherosclerosis, 17–28.
© 1996 Kluwer Academic Publishers.

who, in the 16th century prior to knowledge of the circulation of blood, accurately drew the lesions of atherosclerosis in the coronary arteries following dissection of a centenarian, stating that, 'the clinkers...choked the life force out of the heart.' The first known lipid-laden atherosclerosis plaque lesions can be dated back 32 centuries to the time of Menephtah and Rameses, pharaohs of Egypt, whose mummies were subjected to autopsy in the early 1900s[9–11].

This brief overview of the pathophysiological basis for lipid intervention trials will first discuss the standard pathophysiology of atherosclerotic plaques, followed by a synopsis of newer concepts in pathophysiology, and will conclude with a perspective of the role of lipid intervention trials within the pathophysiological framework.

Standard pathophysiology

The pathophysiology of the atherosclerotic plaque consists of the interaction of four cell types, several processes (notably low density lipoprotein (LDL) oxidation and inflammation) and numerous attractant, agonist and antagonist factors.

The cells

T lymphocytes

The presence of the T lymphocyte evokes consideration of an immune or rejection process. There are numerous T lymphocytes present in the early and later stages of atherosclerosis[12,13]. Obviously, these mediator cells are not spectators. Is atherosclerosis, at least in part, an autoimmune disease, another example of a defence mechanism gone astray? When my co-workers and I suppressed T lymphocytes with cyclosporine in a New Zealand white rabbit cholesterol-fed atherosclerosis model, we achieved a significant reduction in the thoracic aortic cholesterol content (TACC), an index of the severity of atherosclerotic lesions[14].

Macrophages

Circulating monocytes are attracted to arterial predilection sites of tissue damage, adhere to dysfunctional endothelium, penetrate the endothelial barrier and accumulate in the subendothelial space[15]. The monocytes/macrophages phagocytize lipids and, thereby, are transformed into the signature cell of the atherosclerotic plaque, the foam cell[16]. Macrophages are also the hallmark cell of chronic inflammation, and the atherosclerosis process, as will be discussed, involves all of the elements of an inflammatory process. Macrophages can overaccumulate lipids, primarily cholesterol, die and rupture, releasing a fatty gruel into the subendothelial space, which, in turn, engenders an engulfment response by modified smooth muscle cells[17,18].

We hypothesized that depletion of circulating monocytes/macrophages would reduce the entry of these cells into the arterial intima and greatly decrease the

Table 2.1. Effect of intraperitoneal silica on atherosclerosis (Bourdages et al., Reference 20 and unpublished observations).

	n	Time (weeks)	Thoracic aortic cholesterol content (mg/g)
Induction model			
Controls	6	7	5.7±0.8
Silica	6	7	1.2±0.1*
Controls	5	14	10.8±2.4
Silica	7	14	2.7±0.2*
Regression model			
Controls	6	7	10.2±0.8
Mock injection	9	14	11.9±1.7
Silica	8	14	3.1±0.5†

Results as mean±SEM, at sacrifice; *$p<0.001$, compared with the equivalent time control group; †$p<0.05$, compared with the control group and with the mock injection group.

severity of the atherosclerotic process. We tested this question in a cholesterol-fed New Zealand white rabbit preparation, inoculated with intraperitoneal silica. Macrophages are attracted to the foreign body silica particles and take up silica, which reacts with the membranes of the secondary lysosomes, causing the lysosome contents and the silica particles to escape into the cytoplasm of the cell, in turn leading to cell death and the release of the silica[19]. The process of silica fibrocytosis will repeat itself, serving as a continuing attractant for circulating monocytes.

In a controlled experiment, we injected silica (0.8 g in saline) into the peritoneal cavity of New Zealand white rabbits in a cholesterol-supplemented diet-induced model of atherosclerosis (Bourdages, unpublished observations). Without significant differences in the plasma cholesterol level between groups, there was a difference in early atherosclerosis at 7 weeks and in marked atherosclerosis at 14 weeks between the control animals and those receiving the silica injections. The TACC was highly statistically significantly different between the control and the silica-treated animals ($p<0.001$; Table 1). We repeated this experiment in a regression model and demonstrated, by gross pathology and Oil-red-0 staining, histology and TACC analysis, that silica treatment induces atherosclerotic plaque regression as well[20]. In association with these findings, there was a transient reduction in the percentage of monocytes in differential cell counts (Table 1).

It has been contended by Gerrity[21] that the monocytes/macrophages are attempting to clear the arterial wall of cholesterol deposits. Based on our findings, we would disagree with this conclusion, and we would postulate that the macrophages are responsible for plasma cholesterol uptake and subsequent deposition in the arterial wall. With the depletion of macrophages, an increase in cholesterol deposition would be expected if macrophages cleared intimal cholesterol; however, macrophage depletion resulted in decreased cholesterol deposition and a reduction in atherosclerotic lesions.

Smooth muscle cells

In atherosclerosis, the smooth muscle cells of the media migrate into the subendothelial space and can be found in both early and late lesions. They are present in varying amounts in early fatty streaks; however, they are the predominant cell in fibrous plaques. They are responsible for the cellular and elaborated collagen wall of the encapsulated plaque[22]. The clinical manifestations of atherosclerosis are due to the growth of the atherosclerotic plaque and the fissuring or rupture of the plaque. It is the collagen or matrix content of the plaque, in particular the thickness and the density of the cap or luminal surface of the plaque, which determines plaque stability.

Endothelial cells

It has long been considered that the endothelial cell has primarily a barrier function and that injury to this barrier precipitates the atherosclerotic process[23]. In addition, the endothelial cell determines the nature of the lipoproteins and other plasma constituents that reach the subendothelial space. These cells bind LDL through specific affinity receptors and modify LDL so that it can be recognized and ingested by macrophages[24]. Furthermore, these cells elaborate many factors involved, in one way or another, in the atherosclerotic process, including vasoactive agents[25,26] and growth factors[27-29]. The endothelial cell is also protective with respect to angiogenesis, elaborating endothelium-derived relaxing factor (EDRF) or nitric oxide (NO), which is responsible for the normal state of vascular relaxation, and inhibits platelet aggregation, leukocyte adhesion and vascular smooth muscle growth (Creager, unpublished observations).

LDL oxidation

The role of oxidation of the LDL moiety in macrophage lipid accumulation and foam cell formation has been well elucidated, in particular by Steinberg[30,31]. Indeed, there are several current atherosclerosis trials exploring the efficacy of antioxidants as anti-atherogenic agents. Vitamin E, the body's main chain-breaking antioxidant, has received considerable attention for its potential role in preventing the atherosclerotic process[32,33]. Prasad and Kalra[34] reported that diet-induced hypercholesterolaemic New Zealand white rabbits supplemented with vitamin E ($40\,mg\,kg^{-1}\,day^{-1}$) had atherosclerotic plaques that were significantly smaller than those found in unsupplemented hypercholesterolaemic rabbits. We studied New Zealand white rabbits on $30\,mg\,kg^{-1}\,day^{-1}$ of vitamin E and found a highly statistically significant decrease in TACC at 14 weeks in the vitamin E-supplemented rabbits (13.67 vs 47.01 mg cholesterol/g, $p = 0.0001$)[35]. There were no concomitant statistically significant changes in plasma total cholesterol or lipoprotein levels. The atherogenic lipoproteins of the vitamin E-supplemented animals had significantly increased protection against oxidation as evidenced by increased lag times to copper-induced oxidation (>720 vs $252.60\,min$, $p = 0.002$).

Table 2.2. Effect of prednisone and non-steroidal anti-inflammatory agents (indomethacin, phenylbutazone) on atherosclerosis (from References 41 and 42).

	n	Time (weeks)	Thoracic aortic cholesterol content (mg/g)
Prednisone			
Controls	9	9	3.4±0.5
1.0 mg/kg prednisone	10	9	2.3±0.4*
5.0 mg/kg prednisone	8	9	1.7±0.1*†
Non-steroidal anti-inflammatory drugs			
Controls	15	16	15.9±0.9
5 mg/kg indomethacin	14	16	11.4±0.9**
10 mg/kg phenylbutazone	14	16	10.1±0.6‡

Results as mean±SEM, at sacrifice; $*p<0.001$, compared with the prednisone control group; $†p<0.001$, compared with the 1.0 mg/kg prednisone group; $**p<0.02$, compared with the non-steroidal control group; $‡p<0.001$, compared with the non-steroidal control group.

In addition, there were fewer oxidation products in the aortic walls of the supplemented rabbits as shown by comparison of aortic lipid hydroperoxide levels (6.78 vs 13.65 μmol/L H_2O_2, $p=0.03$).

Inflammation

Many of the cells involved in the process of atherogenesis are cells that are characteristic of the inflammatory response[36]. Adhesion and penetration of cells into the atherosclerotic focus may be due to chemotactic agents released in the inflammatory arachidonic acid cascade[37]. Arachidonic acid is the precursor of the cyclooxygenase (prostacyclins, prostaglandins, thromboxane A_2, thromboxane B_2), and lipoxygenase (HPETEs, leukotrienes A–E) compounds. If the pathogenic changes of atherogenesis include inflammatory responses mediated by the cyclooxygenase and lipoxygenase pathways, then it can be hypothesized that inhibition of these pathways should arrest the development of atherosclerotic lesions. Prednisone exerts its inhibitory effect early in the arachidonic acid cascade by reducing the activity of phospholipase A_2 necessary for the release of the arachidonic acid substrate[38]. The non-steroidal anti-inflammatory drugs have long been known to bind cyclooxygenase reversibly, which in turn, inhibits the formation of prostacyclins, prostaglandins and thromboxanes[39,40]. There is recent evidence that the lipoxygenase pathway leading to the production of the leukotrienes is also inhibited by non-steroidal anti-inflammatory drugs[39,40]. This inhibition would block the synthesis of the lipoxygenase products, including leukotriene B_4, which is a macrophage chemoattractant, and 12-HPETE, which is highly chemotactic for vascular smooth muscle cells. We have shown in our laboratory that both prednisone[41] and non-steroidal anti-inflammatory drugs (indomethacin and phenylbutazone)[42] inhibit atherogenesis in a New Zealand white rabbit model (Table 2).

Chemotactic factors

This overview does not permit discussion of the numerous chemotactic factors elaborated by the four cardinal atherosclerotic cells, and the mechanisms of lipoprotein oxidation and inflammation involved in atherogenesis. These factors include the chemoattractants: GM-CSF, M-CSF, VEGF, βFGF, MCP-1, TGFβ and PDGF; the growth agonists: GM-CSF, M-CSF, H-EGF, IGF-1, VEGF, βFGF, IL-1, TNFα, TGFα, TGFβ, and PDGF; and the growth antagonists: IFN-γ, IL-1 and TGFβ. Certain of these factors can have totally opposing actions depending on the nature of the active cellular and chemical milieu.

Newer pathophysiology

The previous discussion focused on the development of the atherosclerotic plaque without consideration of the role of thrombosis. The plaque that gradually grows by accretion to total occlusion without thrombosis is uncommon. As a rule, plaques are involved in a dynamic and continuous process of intraluminal thrombosis and subendothelial haemorrhage and thrombus formation. The role of thrombosis in the atherogenic process was suggested by von Rokitansky in 1852[43], and coronary thrombotic occlusion as a cause of acute myocardial infarction was suspected by Herrick in 1912[44]. Acute intraluminal thrombosis usually occurs secondary to atherosclerotic plaque disruption and is responsible for the acute coronary syndromes of unstable angina and myocardial infarction[45]. The intraluminal thrombotic process is dynamic and can be repetitive[13,45,46]. In some patients, the thrombus is labile and is associated with intermittent or transient vessel occlusion and the ischaemic syndrome of unstable angina (Fuster, 1988). In others, fixed thrombus formation will lead to a more chronic occlusion, resulting in an acute myocardial infarction[47]. The same clinical syndromes can be precipitated by intraplaque haemorrhage and thrombosis[48]. In addition, plaques grow by repetitive organization of smaller mural thrombi and their incorporation into the evolving lesion[49]. Davies et al.[50] have demonstrated plaques with healed fissures in various stages of thrombosis and thrombus organization, suggesting that most fissures seal and incorporate thrombus, probably without clinical symptoms.

What distinguishes a stable plaque from an active plaque which will fissure or rupture? Davies and co-workers, employing elegant pathological dissections and staining techniques, showed that fissured plaques commonly contain an abundant lipid pool in the intima and that the fissure frequently occurs at the junction of the fibrous cap with the adjacent normal arterial wall[13,51], precipitating thrombus formation (Figures 1–4). Using computer modelling analysis of tensile stress across the vessel wall, these investigators found areas of high stress in the plaque cap overlying a rich lipid pool. In this area, they also found a lack of underlying collagen support of the cap and an increased macrophage content within the plaque. Thus, the active plaque susceptible to fissuring and thrombus formation has a thin cap and exhibits the characteristic pathological triad of high lipid, low collagen and high macrophage content.

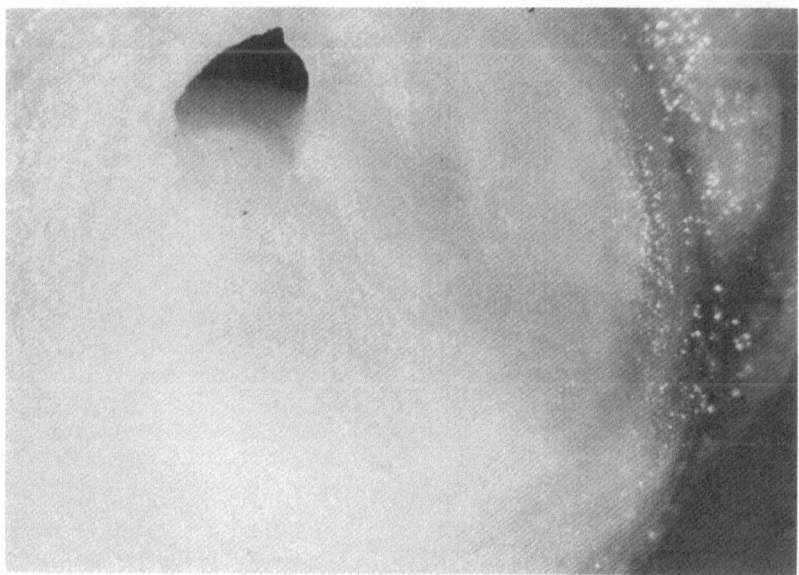

Figure 2.1. Stable atherosclerotic plaque with a fibrous cap and a patent lumen (courtesy of Dr M. Davies, London).

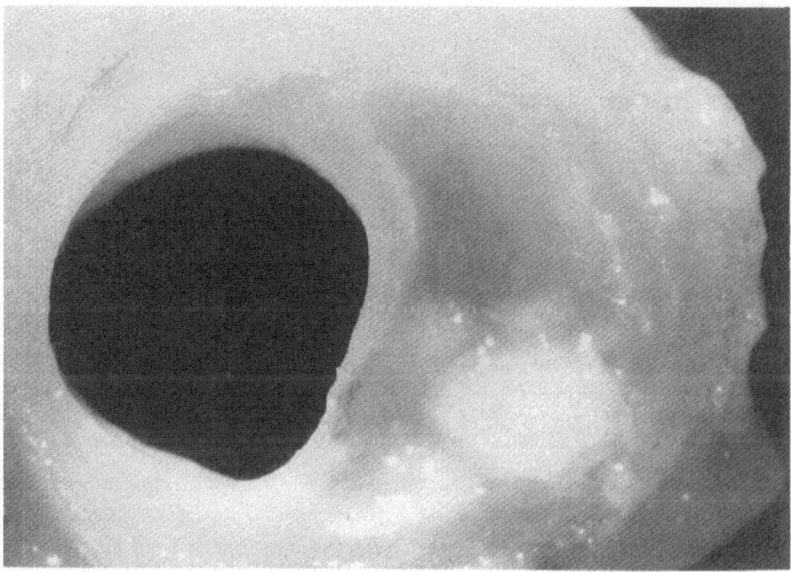

Figure 2.2. Unstable atherosclerotic plaque with a thin cap poor in collagen content overlying an abundant intimal lipid pool (courtesy of Dr M. Davies, London).

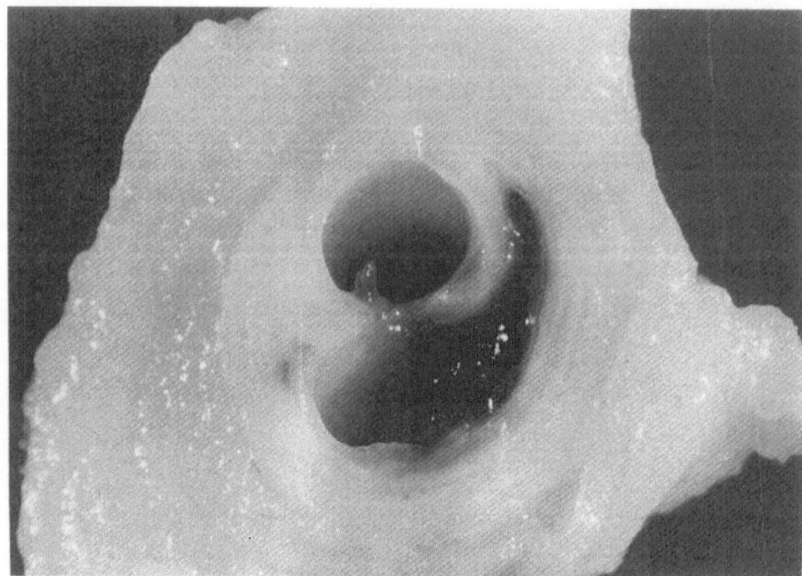

Figure 2.3.   Unstable fissured plaque with rupture of the thin fibrous cap at the junction of the cap with the adjacent wall, as well as thrombus within the plaque (courtesy of Dr M. Davies, London).

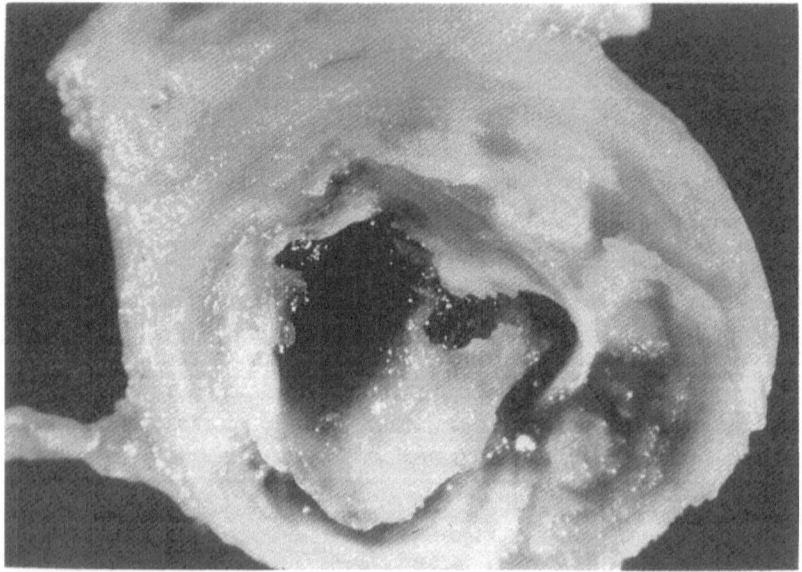

Figure 2.4.   Destroyed plaque with an extended fissure and thrombus within the plaque and in the lumen of the artery (courtesy of Dr M. Davies, London).

Standard contrast arteriograms will not allow determination of stable (fibrous) vs active (fatty) plaques. However, newer techniques, such as intravascular ultrasonography, may be able to provide a visual image of arterial wall morphology in the living patient[52].

The severity of coronary artery stenosis and the number of diseased vessels are markers for future cardiac morbidity and mortality[53]. The relative changes in atherosclerotic lesions on sequential arteriograms are predictive of the clinical events of overall and coronary heart disease mortality, and the combined endpoint of coronary heart disease mortality and confirmed non-fatal myocardial infarction[54]. In recent years, it has become apparent that less severe angiographic stenoses may account for up to two thirds of cases of unstable angina or acute myocardial infarction[55]. Ambrose et al.[56] reported a study of patients with unstable angina who had two sequential arteriograms, revealing that 72% of the lesions that had progressed had less than 50% stenosis on the first arteriogram. The lesions that progressed to less than total occlusion had in most cases eccentric shapes, characterized by a narrow neck and overhanging edges or scalloped borders. These are precisely the lesions of plaque disruption, with or without a partially occlusive thrombus[57]. A more recent arteriographic study by Ambrose et al.[58] in myocardial infarction patients with prior sequential angiograms showed that the culprit lesion in half the cases had less than a 50% stenosis and, in over two thirds of cases, less than a 70% stenosis. Further confirmation of these findings has been offered by Little and co-workers[59,60], Nobuyoshi et al.[61], and most recently in the Familial Atherosclerosis Treatment Study (FATS; unpublished observations). In FATS, 10–20% of the lesions were thought to be thin capped and lipid rich; however, 80–90% of acute events were related to these lesions.

Pathophysiological perspective of lipid intervention trials

The message of the newer pathophysiology of atherosclerosis is that the clinically dangerous lesions are not necessarily large severely stenotic plaques but seem to be smaller lipid-rich plaques. Thus, lipid intervention trials test not only the benefits of risk factor modification, but assess the direct benefits of converting active plaques, with thin caps, rich in lipids, and susceptible to fissuring and thrombosis, to stable plaques, with a reduced lipid content and a thicker more fibrous cap. In the Program on the Surgical Control of the Hyperlipidemias (POSCH), this pathophysiological basis for lipid intervention trials seems to have been confirmed[54,62]. For a given and identical change in sequential arteriograms, there was a significant difference in the clinical events of overall and coronary heart disease mortality, and the combined endpoint of coronary heart disease mortality and confirmed non-fatal myocardial infarction, between the control and the partial ileal bypass groups. This finding can be interpreted as demonstrating that, for a given arteriographic change in a lesion, the intervention group, but not the control group, benefited by a decrease in the lipid content of the plaque.

References

1. Anitschkow N, Chalatow S. Ueber experimentelle cholesterinsteatose und ihre bedeutung für die Entstehung einiger pathologischer prozesse. Centralbl Allg Pathol Anat. 1913;24:1–9.
2. Keys A. Coronary heart disease in seven countries. Circulation. 1970;41(Suppl.):I1–211.
3. Kannel WB, Castelli WP, Gordon T, McNamara PM. Serum cholesterol, lipoproteins, and the risk of coronary heart disease: the Framingham Study. Ann Intern Med. 1971;74:1–12.
4. The Pooling Project Research Group. Relationship of blood pressure, serum cholesterol, smoking habit, relative weight, and ECG abnormalities to incidence of major coronary events: final report of the Pooling Project Research Group. J Chron Dis. 1978;31:201–306.
5. Martin MJ, Hulley SB, Browner WS, et al. Serum cholesterol, blood pressure, and mortality: implications from a cohort of 361,662 men. Lancet. 1986;2:933–6.
6. Rayer PFO. Traité theorique et pratiques des maladies de la peau, fondé sur de nouvelles recherches d'anatomie et de physiologie pathologiques. Paris: JB Bailliére; 1826.
7. Addison T, Gull W. On a certain affection of the skin, vitiliogidea – (a) plana, (b) tuberosa; with remarks. Guys' Hosp Rep. 1851;7:265–76.
8. Heydenreich LH. Leonardo da Vinci. Basel: Holbein, 1954.
9. Smith GE. The development of our knowledge of arteriosclerosis. In: Codry EV, editor. Arteriosclerosis. New York: Macmillan Co; 1933:21.
10. Shattock SG. A report on the pathological condition of the aorta of King Menephtah, traditionally regarded as the pharaoh of the Exodus. Proc R Soc Med Lond. 1908;122–7.
11. Ruffer R. On arterial lesions found in Egyptian mummies. J Pathol Bact. 1911;15:453–62.
12. Jonasson L, Holm J, Skalli O, Bondjers G, Hansson GK. Regional accumulation of T cells, macrophages, and smooth muscle cells in the human atherosclerotic plaque. Arteriosclerosis. 1986;6:131–8.
13. Woolf N, Davies MJ. Interrelationship between atherosclerosis and thrombosis. In: Fuster V, Verstraete M, editors. Thrombosis in cardiovascular disorders. Philadelphia: WB Saunders; 1992:41–77.
14. Menchaca HJ, Campos CT, Michalek VN, Buchwald H. Effects of immunomodulation by cyclosporine on plasma lipoprotein levels and atherosclerosis development. Surg Forum. 1991;42:356–7.
15. Ross R. The pathogenesis of atherosclerosis – an update. N Engl J Med. 1986;314:488–500.
16. Brown MS, Goldstein JL. Lipoprotein metabolism in the macrophages: implications for cholesterol deposition in atherosclerosis. Annu Rev Biochem. 1983;52:223–61.
17. Stary HC. Evolution and progression of atherosclerotic lesions in coronary arteries of children and young adults. Arteriosclerosis. 1989;99(Suppl. I):I19–32.
18. Schwartz CJ, Valente AJ, Sprague EA, Kelley JL, Nerem RM. The pathogenesis of atherosclerosis. Clin Cardiol. 1991;14(Suppl. I):I1–16.
19. O'Rourke EJ, Halstead SB, Allison AC, Platts-Mills TAE. Specific lethality of silica for human peripheral blood mononuclear phagocytes, in vitro. J Immunol Meth. 1978;19:137–51.
20. Bourdages H, Menchaca H, Matthews AJ, et al. Administration of intraperitoneal silica enhances regression of atherosclerosis in a rabbit model. Surg Forum. 1994;45:378–80.
21. Gerrity RG. The role of the monocyte in atherogenesis. Am J Pathol. 1981;103:181–90.
22. Burke JM, Ross R. Synthesis of connective tissue macromolecules by smooth muscle. Int Rev Connect Tissue Res. 1979;8:119–57.
23. Ross R. Atherosclerosis – a problem of the biology of arterial wall cells and their interaction with blood components. Arteriosclerosis. 1981;1:293–311.
24. Steinberg D. Lipoproteins and atherosclerosis. A look back and a look ahead. Arteriosclerosis. 1983;3:283–301.
25. Moncada S, Herman AG, Higgs EA, Vane JR. Differential formation of prostacyclin (PGX or PGI$_2$) by layers of the arterial wall: an explanation for the antithrombotic properties of vascular endothelium. Thromb Res. 1977;11:323–44.
26. Furchgott RF. Role of endothelium in responses of vascular smooth muscle. Circ Res. 1983;53:557–73.

27. Gajdusik CM, DiCorleto P, Ross R, Schwartz SM. An endothelial cell-derived growth factor. J Cell Biol. 1980;85:467–72.
28. DiCorleto PE, Bowen-Pope DF. Cultured endothelial cells produce a platelet-derived growth factor-like protein. Proc Natl Acad Sci USA. 1983;80:1919–23.
29. DiCorleto PE, Gajdusek CM, Schwartz SM, Ross R. Biochemical properties of the endothelium-derived growth factor: comparison to other growth factors. J Cell Physiol. 1983; 114:339–45.
30. Steinberg D, Parthasarathy S, Carew TE, Khoo JC, Witzum JL. Beyond cholesterol. N Engl J Med. 1989;320:915–24.
31. Steinberg D. Antioxidants and atherosclerosis. Circulation. 1991;84:1420–5.
32. Janero DR. Therapeutic potential of vitamin E in the pathogenesis of spontaneous atherogenesis. Free Rad Biol Med. 1991;11:129–44.
33. Ferns GA, Konneh M, Anggard EE. Vitamin E: the evidence for an anti-atherogenic role. Artery. 1993;20:61–94.
34. Prasad K, Kalra J. Oxygen free radicals and hypercholesterolemic atherosclerosis: Effect of vitamin E. Am Heart J. 1993;125:958–73.
35. Matthews AJ, Belcher J, Balla J, et al. Vitamin E inhibits atherosclerosis in the diet-induced hypercholesterolemic rabbit model. Surg Forum. 1994;45:36–8.
36. Poston RN, Davies DF. Immunity and inflammation in the pathogenesis of atherosclerosis. Atherosclerosis. 1974;19:353–67.
37. Bailey JM, Butler J. Anti-inflammatory drugs in experimental atherosclerosis. Part 6. Combination therapy with steroid and non-steroid agents. Atherosclerosis. 1985;54:205–12.
38. Bailey JM, Watson R, Bombard AT, Randazzo R. Anti-inflammatory drugs in experimental atherosclerosis. Part 5. Influence of cortisone acetate on short-term and long-term cholesterol fluxes in atherosclerotic aorta. Atherosclerosis. 1984;51:299–306.
39. Hochberg MC. NSAIDs: Patterns of usage and side effects. Hosp Pract. 1989;15:167–74.
40. Hochberg MC. NSAIDs: Mechanisms and pathways of action. Hosp Pract. 1989;15:185–98.
41. Stoller DK, Campos CT, Grorud CB, Michalek V, Buchwald H. Prednisone reduction of atherosclerosis in diet-induced hypercholesterolemic rabbits: does immunomodulation play a role? Surg Forum. 1990;41:351–4.
42. Stoller DK, Grorud CB, Michalek V, Buchwald H. Reduction of atherosclerosis with nonsteroidal anti-inflammatory drugs. J Surg Res. 1993;54:7–11.
43. von Rokitansky C. A manual of pathological anatomy: volume 4. London: Sydenham Society; 1852:261.
44. Herrick JB. Clinical features of sudden obstruction of the coronary arteries. JAMA. 1912; 59:2015–20.
45. Falk E. Morphologic features of unstable atherothrombotic plaques underlying acute coronary syndromes. Am J Cardiol. 1989;63:114E–20E.
46. Willerson JT, Golino P, Eidt J, Campbell WB, Buja M. Specific platelet mediators and unstable coronary artery lesions: experimental evidence and potential clinical implications. Circulation. 1989;80.198–205.
47. Fuster V, Badimon L, Cohen M, Ambrose JA, Badimon JJ, Chesebro J. Insights into the pathogenesis of acute ischemic syndromes. Circulation. 1988;77:1213–20.
48. Roberts WC, Buja LM. The frequency and significance of coronary arterial thrombi and other observations in fatal acute myocardial infarction: a study of 107 necropsy patients. Am J Med. 1972;52.425–43.
49. Falk E. Unstable angina with fatal outcome: dynamic coronary thrombosis leading to infarction and/or sudden death: autopsy evidence of recurrent mural thrombosis with peripheral embolization culminating in total vascular occlusion. Circulation. 1985;71:699–708.
50. Davies MJ, Bland MJ, Hangartner WR, Angelini A, Thomas AC. Factors influencing the presence or absence of acute coronary thrombi in sudden ischemic death. Eur Heart J. 1989;10: 203–8.
51. Richardson PD, Davies MJ, Born GVR. Influence of plaque configuration and stress distribution on fissuring of coronary atherosclerotic plaques. Lancet. 1989;2:941–4.

52. Nissen SE, Gurley JC, Grines CL, et al. Intravascular ultrasound assessment of lumen size and wall morphology in normal subjects and patients with coronary artery disease. Circulation. 1991;84:1087–99.

53. Moise A, Lesperance J, Theroux P, Taeymans Y, Goulet C, Bourassa MG. Clinical and angiographic predictors of new total coronary occlusion in coronary artery disease: analysis of 313 nonoperated patients. Am J Cardiol. 1984;54:1176–81.

54. Buchwald H, Matts JP, Fitch LL, et al. Changes in sequential coronary arteriograms and subsequent coronary events. JAMA. 1992;268:1429–33.

55. Fuster V, Stein B, Ambrose JA, Badimon L, Badimon JJ, Chesebro JH. Atherosclerotic plaque rupture and thrombosis: evolving concepts. Circulation. 1990;82(3 Suppl.):II47–59.

56. Ambrose JA, Winters SL, Arora RR, et al. Angiographic evolution of coronary artery morphology in unstable angina. J Am Coll Cardiol. 1986;7:472–8.

57. Ambrose JA, Winters SL, Stern A, et al. Angiographic morphology and the pathogenesis of unstable angina pectoris. J Am Coll Cardiol. 1985;5:609–16.

58. Ambrose JA, Tannenbaum MA, Alexopoulos D, et al. Angiographic progression of coronary artery disease and the development of myocardial infarction. J Am Coll Cardiol. 1988;12:56–62.

59. Little WC, Constantinescu M, Applegate RJ, et al. Can coronary angiography predict the site of a subsequent myocardial infarction in patients with mild-to-moderate coronary artery disease? Circulation. 1988;78:1157–66.

60. Little WC. Angiographic assessment of the culprit coronary artery lesions before acute myocardial infarction. Am J Cardiol. 1990;66:44G–7G.

61. Nobuyoshi M, Tanaka M, Nosaka H, et al. Progression of coronary artherosclerosis: is coronary spasm related to progression? J Am Coll Cardiol. 1991;18:904–10.

62. Buchwald H, Varco RL, Matts JP, et al. Effect of partial ileal bypass surgery on mortality and morbidity from coronary heart disease in patients with hypercholesterolemia. Report of the Program on the Surgical Control of the Hyperlipidemias (POSCH). N Engl J Med. 1990; 323:946–55.

PART TWO

Methodological aspects of angiographic trials

3. The use of metabolic measurements in angiographic regression trials

G. F. WATTS

Summary

The principal reasons for undertaking metabolic measurements in angiographic trials are to test the experimental hypothesis, to monitor the safety of therapeutic interventions and to generate new hypotheses concerning the determinants of coronary atherosclerosis. All analytical and biological sources of variation should be minimized, with consistent use of quality control material and, ideally, a reference laboratory. Potential confounders in studies testing the lipid hypothesis include genetic, nutritional, free radical, thrombotic and endocrine variables. Hitherto, the results of angiographic regression trials have consistently confirmed that apolipoprotein B containing lipoproteins, in particular low density lipoproteins (LDL) and intermediate density lipoproteins (IDL), accelerate progression of coronary atherosclerosis; inverse associations with high density lipoprotein (HDL) cholesterol have also been demonstrated. New hypotheses include a role for triglyceride-rich lipoproteins in the development of early coronary lesions and for hepatic lipase, tri-iodothyronine, HDL_3 and dietary stearic acid in determining progression of established coronary atherosclerosis. There is at present no recognized biochemical marker of atherosclerotic change for use in clinical practice, but preliminary evidence suggests a role for serial measurements of total plasma sialic acid concentration.

Introduction

Angiographic regression trials allow a more rigorous test of the lipid hypothesis of atherosclerosis than conventional clinic trials[1]. There are several purposes for undertaking metabolic measurements in regression trials: to test the experimental hypothesis and to generate new hypotheses, to define the sample population, to test for confounding variables, and to monitor patient compliance and the safety of interventions. In planning and designing regression trials, it is therefore important to define carefully the protocol of metabolic measurements. This article discusses the use of these measurements in regression trials and summarizes the evidence that has accrued concerning the metabolic determinants of the progression of coronary artery disease (CAD).

A.V.G. Bruschke et al. *(eds): Lipid-lowering therapy and progression of atherosclerosis, 31–43*
© 1996 *Kluwer Academic Publishers.*

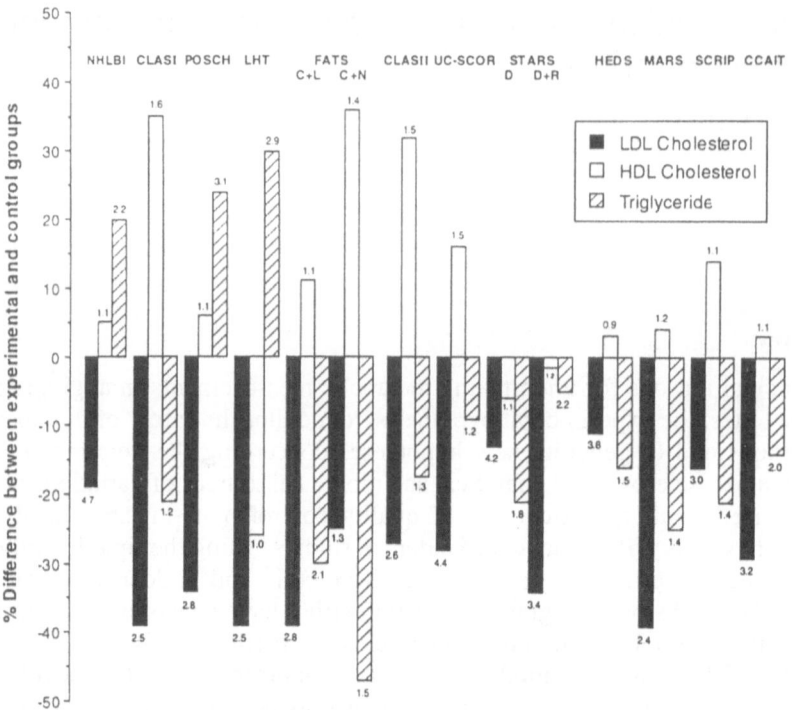

Figure 3.1. Percentage (%) difference between experimental and control groups for in-trial plasma concentrations of low density lipoprotein (LDL) cholesterol, high density lipoprotein (HDL) cholesterol and triglycerides in 12 randomized, controlled trials of lipid-lowering therapy. Numbers given at end of bars refer to in-trial plasma lipid concentrations (mmol/L). NHLBI, National Heart, Lung and Blood Institute Study[2]; CLAS, Cholesterol Lowering Atherosclerosis Study[3,7]; POSCH, Program of Surgical Control of Hyperlipidaemia[4]; LHT, Lifestyle Heart Trial[5]; FATS, Familial Atherosclerosis Treatment Study[6]; UC-SCOR, University of California Special Centre of Research Trial[8]; STARS, St Thomas' Atherosclerosis Regression Study[9]; HEDS, Heidelberg Exercise Diet Study[10]; MARS, Monitored Atherosclerosis Regression Study[11]; SCRIP, Stanford Coronary Risk Intervention Project[12,13]; CCAIT, Canadian Coronary Atherosclerosis Intervention Trial[14]. C+L, colestipol and lovastatin; C+N, colestipol and niacin; D, diet; D+R, diet and cholestyramine.

Testing and generating hypotheses

In trials aiming to test the effect of lipid-lowering interventions on the progression of CAD, the basic tests of the experimental hypotheses will involve measuring plasma cholesterol, triglyceride and HDL concentration, and, where appropriate, calculating LDL-cholesterol by the Friedewald formula. Figure 3.1 shows the relative changes in plasma LDL-cholesterol, triglyceride and HDL-cholesterol concentrations in randomized angiographic regression trials[2-14]. It is noteworthy that the most consistent change studied is the reduction in plasma LDL-cholesterol and that the degree of reduction is greater than that in conventional clinical trials of lipid lowering[1]. Additional analyses will be required depending on the specific aims of the study and may involve immunochemical assays for apolipoproteins and the separation of lipoproteins by ultra-centrifugation or gradient gel electrophoresis[15-17]. Trials testing manipulations of alimentary lipaemia, free radical activity and insulin resistance will also involve more clinically and technically demanding measurements. Besides examining metabolic variables that may be causally related to CAD, complete validation of the experimental hypotheses requires measuring variables that reflect changes in coronary lesions and this is discussed later.

To fully test the experimental hypotheses, confounding variables must be examined. Possible confounders in angiographic trials of lipid lowering treatment include genetic, nutritional, free radical, thrombotic and endocrine factors[10,18-22]. Besides being useful for adjusting for confounding, these measurements may be employed to generate new hypotheses concerning the determinants of the progression of CAD. The additional analyses may, however, involve sophisticated laboratory procedures and, obviously, extra expenditure. Of the genetic variables, apolipoprotein E genotyping may be useful in adjusting for independent effects on progression of CAD and for variability in response to therapeutic interventions[23,24]. Confounding due to nutrient intake may be assessed by detailed dietary interview, and by analysing the polyunsaturated fatty acid composition of erythrocyte membranes and/or microbiopsies of subcutaneous fat[25]. The role of free radicals in atherosclerosis is increasingly being recognized[21], but full assessment is complex and there is no reliable method, at present, for determining lipoprotein oxidation in vivo[26]. Of the tests available, the most popular is the continuous monitoring of the formation of conjugated dienes during copper-ion-mediated oxidation of LDL[27]. Thrombotic factors, such as plasma fibrinogen, factor VIIc and plasminogen activator inhibitor I, should also be recorded[28,29] since these may confound lipoprotein-mediated risk of CAD. Endocrine changes may alter lipoprotein metabolism and, as in the case of thyroid[22], growth[30] and sex hormones[31] may independently influence the course of CAD. The success in employing some or all of the above measurements to generate new hypotheses will be determined, not only by the sample size of the study, but also by the extent of the distribution of measured variables among subjects.

Analytical considerations

Attention must be given to minimizing both analytical and pre-analytical sources of measurement variation and bias. These may present problems with the indices of lipoprotein metabolism[32,33]. For plasma cholesterol, the total measurement coefficient of variation should be $<5\%$[34], requiring an interassay coefficient of variation of $<3\%$. Ideally, similar analytical precision is required for triglyceride and HDL-cholesterol analyses. Whilst reproducibility may not be problematic, poor standardization of assays will compromise comparisons among studies and future meta-analyses of outcome variables. Bias in lipid and apolipoprotein assays is generally due to the 'matrix effect' on calibrants, and a useful recommendation is that, for all lipid-related analyses, a reputable laboratory linked to the CDC Network be employed[32]. Lipoproteins are commonly quantified by measuring their cholesterol content. Calculation of LDL-cholesterol by the Friedewald formula includes a contribution due to IDL, but, if necessary, these components should be separated using ultracentrifugation[16]. The separation of lipoprotein particles by stepwise ultracentrifugation is subject to poor analytical recovery in non-expert hands. Measurement of apolipoprotein (apo) and lipoprotein(a) (Lp(a)) is still hampered by poor assay specificity, difficulties with standardization and lack of a reference method[35,36]. Immunoturbidimetry and nephelometry are appropriate for apoB and apo-AI, but enzyme-linked or radio-immunoassays should be employed to quantify apoE and apoC[35]. The complex and polymorphic nature of Lp(a) and its crossreactivity with plasminogen continue to present analytical problems[36]. It is noteworthy that pre-analytical sources of variation in lipid and apolipoprotein assays can account for more than 60% of total measurement variation[33]. These can be minimized by standardizing the sampling technique, the time of sampling and storing material when appropriate at −70°C. Pre-analytical variation will also be offset by standardizing behavioural conditions and by increasing the number of replicate measurements during the trial[37].

Biochemical markers of atherosclerosis

Whatever experimental manipulations are being tested in angiographic regression trials, it is highly desirable to employ a biochemical marker(s) of atherosclerotic change. The cellular components of atherosclerosis involve the interactions between endothelial cells, macrophages and smooth muscle cells. This interaction results in the formation of the atherosclerotic plaque and relies on the release of chemoattractant factors, adhesion molecules, cytokines and growth factors, all of which may potentially be assayed in plasma[38]. These markers of the cellular processes of atherogenesis need to be tested in future clinical trials. In the St Thomas' Atherosclerosis Regression Study (STARS), we did not find that changes in platelet-derived growth factor were correlated with changes in coronary luminal dimensions[39]. Markers of endothelial damage, or of altered metabolism of the extracellular matrix of the arterial wall, may be particularly useful in monitoring regression in vivo. Von Willebrand factor is a specific, stable and circulating product of the endothelial cell that may be both causally and casually related to atherosclerosis[40]. Although in STARS we found significant differences between the intervention and the control groups, we were unable to find a significant correlation between angiographic change and plasma von Willebrand factor concentrations[41]. Sialic acid generically refers to a group of acetylated derivatives of neuraminic acid that are constituents of glyco-proteins and are also highly concentrated on the surface of vascular endothelia[42,43]; elevated plasma levels have been shown to predict cardiovascular mortality[44]. In STARS, we found that changes in total serum sialic acid were correlated with changes in coronary luminal dimensions (Figure 2): this may reflect alterations in acute inflammatory response, damage to endothelial cell surfaces, or perturbed glycoprotein synthesis in the extracellular matrix[45]. Since the association of serum sialic acid with coronary luminal change was only

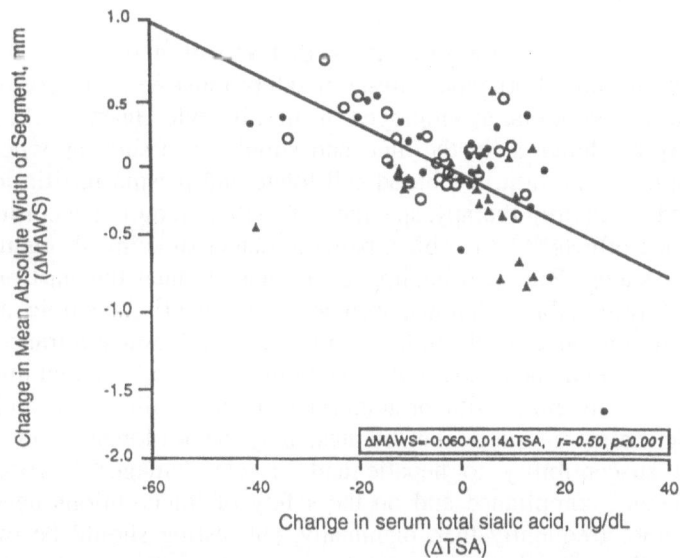

Figure 3.2. Association between change in mean absolute width of coronary segments (ΔMAWS) and change in plasma total sialic acid concentration (ΔTSA) in STARS[9,45]. Usual care groups (▲); diet group (●); diet and cholestyramine group (○).

partially mediated by the plasma concentrations of LDL-cholesterol and apoB, we have hypothesized that it may reflect both the atherotic and sclerotic components of the lesional changes[45].

Monitoring compliance

The monitoring of compliance with the intervention to which subjects have been randomized is essential to rigorously test the experimental hypotheses of the study. This is another approach to checking on confounding variables. Use of rapidly automated assays or desk-top analysers employing 'dry' chemistry allows assessment of compliance at the time patients attend for clinical review. This permits the most efficient administration of therapeutic intervention[9]. To ascertain compliance with drugs, plasma or urine concentrations may be measured[46]. Plasma mevalonic acid or lathosterol concentrations reflect in-vivo cholesterol synthesis and may be used specifically to monitor compliance with statins[47]. Plasma alkaline phosphatase activity may rise with resins and fall with fibrates. The most direct method for assessing adherence to a fat-modified diet is to assay the polyunsaturated fatty acid composition of erythrocyte membranes or adipose tissue microbiopsies[25]. This technique does not, however, provide reliable information for measuring compliance with dietary saturated fat or cholesterol. Independent checks on abstention from cigarette smoking or alcohol may be carried out by monitoring urinary nicotine and alcohol levels, respectively.

Monitoring safety

In addition to monitoring the efficacy of diet and drug therapies for hyper-lipidaemia, both their short- and long-term safety must be regularly reviewed. With very restrictive diets, as employed in the Lifestyle Heart Trial[5], essential elements may be deficient in the diet, and simple tests such as whole blood haemoglobin concentration, red blood cell folate and plasma ferritin levels are recommended. With drug therapy, specific tests will be required according to the recognized side effects[48,49], the object being to detect subclinical organ damage or deficiency states. Bile-acid-binding resins may reduce the gastrointestinal absorption of fat-soluble vitamins, iron and folic acid[2]. Nicotinic acid may impair glucose tolerance, result in hyperuricaemia, and induce a transaminitis[3]. Liver and muscle enzymes should also be monitored in patients taking fibrates and statins[3,7,11,14]. In those with proteinuria and renal failure, the half-life of water-soluble drugs, in particular fibrates, may be prolonged and this will increase the susceptibility to hepatic and muscle damage[48,49]. Biochemical checks on patient compliance and on the safety of interventions need not be carried out more frequently than biannually, but testing should be intensified when abnormalities are identified.

Metabolic determinants of CAD in angiographic trials

Besides testing the efficacy of therapeutic reduction in a risk factor, coronary regression trials can shed light on the determinants of the course of CAD. This section describes the methods of data analysis, the results of trials to date and some new hypotheses that have been generated.

Data analysis

The association between coronary luminal change and a metabolic variable may be analysed using linear or logistic regression analysis, with a multivariable approach to adjust for confounders. The outcome variable may be calculated on a per-patient or per-lesion basis[1], but the segmental approach will require correction for intraclass correlation[50] and this may involve multilevel modelling. Predictor variables may be expressed as a relative change or as a mean in-trial value[9]. Analysis may be restricted to the placebo group or to the intervention group[15], but, if the data are pooled, a test for co-linearity will be required. In pooled data, treatment group assignment needs to be entered as a co-variate in the regression model[16]. As employed in the MARS trial[51], lesional analysis allows correlations with early and late stages of coronary atherosclerosis to be examined. From a practical viewpoint, one of the objectives of the correlational analyses is to determine values for metabolic or nutritional variables below which stabilization or regression of coronary lesions is most likely, since these targets may be useful in recommending therapy.

Table 3.1. Metabolic variables found to be significantly correlated with progression of coronary artery disease in angiographic trials of lipid-lowering therapy[2-16,22,51-56]. See text for discussion.

Positive correlates	Negative correlates
• Total cholesterol	• HDL-cholesterol
• LDL-cholesterol	• HDL$_3$-cholesterol
• LDL$_3$-cholesterol	• Apolipoprotein A-I
• Apolipoprotein B	• HDL ApoC-III
• Triglyceride	
• IDL-cholesterol	
• non-HDL-cholesterol	
• non-HDL ApoC-III	
• Lipoprotein(a)	

Summary of findings

Table 3.1 summarizes the significant positive and negative associations of angiographic change reported in lipid-lowering trials to date[6,8,9,14-16,22,41,51-54]. These findings were generally based on multivariate regression analysis with appropriate adjustments for confounding variables. The most uniform result testifies to the key role of apoB-containing lipoproteins in CAD. Both the in-trial and change in plasma concentrations have been associated with coronary luminal change, with results being more consistent with the former. In the most recently published angiographic trial, change in LDL-cholesterol was not correlated with change in minimum lumen diameter[54].

Differences amongst studies reflect differences in the selection of patients, angiographic measurements and interventions employed[1]. The use of a particular lipid-lowering treatment is important as this may confound the contribution made by certain species of lipoproteins. Conversely, treatment may unmask important metabolic relationships. This is exemplified in both the Cholesterol Lowering Atherosclerosis Study (CLAS) and Monitored Atherosclerosis Regression Study (MARS) trials in which the role of triglyceride-rich lipoproteins, measured by apoC-III concentration, was revealed after plasma LDL-cholesterol concentration fell substantially with drug intervention[15,51]. STARS examined the correlations of angiographic change with a wide spectrum of metabolic variables[41]. The best predictor of both diffuse and focal estimates of atherosclerosis was the in-trial plasma concentration of LDL-cholesterol (Figure 3.3). Slightly less-significant correlations were found with both apoB and Lp(a), and no associations were found with triglyceride, HDL-cholesterol, apoA-I, thyroid hormones, vitamin E, fibrinogen, von Willebrand factor antigen and post-load plasma glucose[41]. Table 3.2 compares the mean absolute levels of LDL-cholesterol, apoB and Lp(a) in patients defined as showing regression, no change and progression of CAD; it can be seen that the levels for intervention should be an LDL-cholesterol concentration <3.5 mmol/L or an apoB concentration

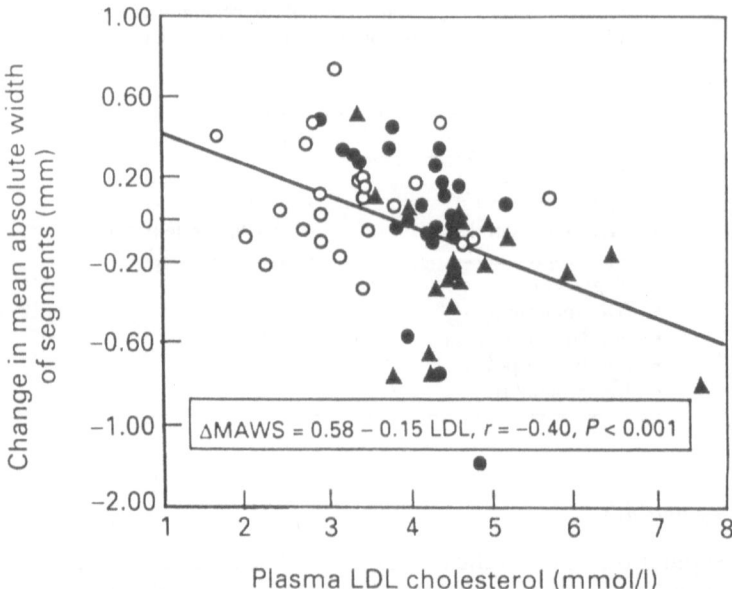

Figure 3.3.   Association between change in mean absolute width of coronary segments (ΔMAWS) and in-trial plasma concentration of LDL-cholesterol in STARS[9]. Usual care groups (▲); diet group (●); diet and cholestyramine group (○).

Table 3.2.   In-trial plasma concentration of LDL-cholesterol, apolipoprotein B and lipoprotein(a) in patients showing progression, no change or regression of coronary artery disease in STARS[9,41].

	Course of angiographic coronary artery disease			
	Progression ($n=16$)	No change ($n=39$)	Regression ($n=19$)	p value
LDL-cholesterol (mmol/L)	4.83 (0.27)	4.14 (0.13)	3.33 (0.15)	<0.001
Apolipoprotein B (g/L)	1.41 (0.06)	1.24 (0.03)	1.15 (0.05)	0.002
Lipoprotein(a) (g/L)	0.32 (0.03, 3.26)	0.20 (0.03, 1.98)	0.21 (0.02, 1.94)	0.326

Mean (SEM)

< 1.2 g/L. In univariate analysis, change in mean absolute width of coronary segments was also reciprocally correlated with the in-trial concentration of both IDL- and LDL_3-cholesterol, as well as positively correlated with HDL_3-cholesterol concentration[16] (Figure 4). Multivariate analysis adjusting for other risk factors showed that the strongest association of progression was with LDL_3, the small dense subclass of LDL, consistent with its recognized causative role in coronary artery disease and myocardial infarction[17]. Two other studies have shown that remnant particles may be the best predictors of progression of coronary artery disease[55,56], but the discrepancies again may be due to differences in the selection of patients and interventions employed. It should be noted that

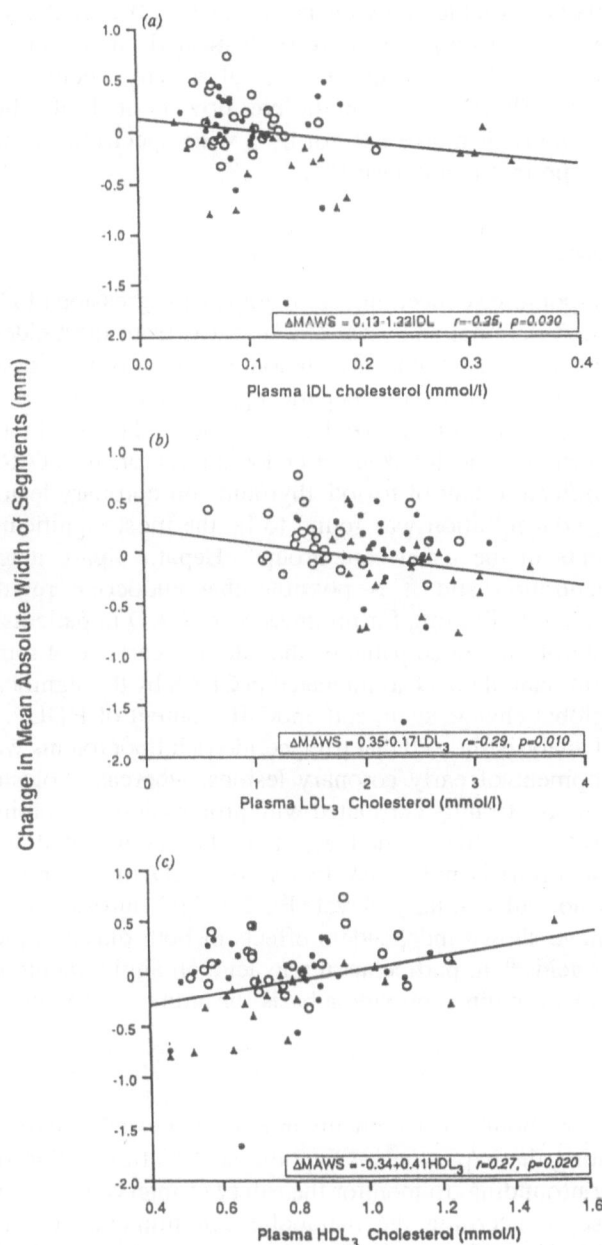

Figure 3.4. Association between change in mean absolute width of coronary segments (ΔMAWS) and in-trial cholesterol concentration of IDL (*a*), LDL₃ (*b*) and HDL₃ (*c*) subfractions[16]. Usual care group (▲); diet group (●); diet and cholestyramine group (○).

lipoprotein-related variables only, at best, explain 30% of the variance in the change in CAD, suggesting that more sophisticated parameters, such as those related to alimentary lipaemia or free radical activity, should be examined in future trials. In STARS, the predictive power of LDL-cholesterol was confounded by nutrient intake but not by a wide spectrum of candidate genes involved in lipoprotein metabolism[19,20].

New hypotheses

Several new hypotheses concerning angiographic progression of CAD have been generated by correlational analyses. The first was from the Leiden Intervention Trial showing an independent association between progression of coronary lesions and plasma post-heparin hepatic lipase activity, tri-iodothyronine and HDL-cholesterol[22]. This emphasized a key role of hepatic lipase in 'reverse cholesterol transport' and invoked an endocrine factor. In STARS, we did not confirm a significant effect of tri-iodothyronine on coronary lesion growth, but plasma HDL_3 concentration was found to be the most significant predictor of CAD in patients in the usual care group[16]. Hepatic lipase determines HDL_3 particle concentration and it is possible that endocrine regulation of this metabolic step is rate limiting for progression of CAD in patients with elevated plasma cholesterol. In treated patients, the rate of clearance of remnant particles may be a determinant of CAD, as indicated in CLAS by the significant association between the global change score and apoC-III content of HDL[15]. In the MARS study, lesional analysis showed that triglyceride-rich lipoproteins were risk factors for the development of early coronary lesions, whereas cholesterol-rich lipo-proteins were more strongly correlated with progression of established lesions[51]. A recent report from the Heidelberg study has contributed to the growing hypothesis that Lp(a) is not a risk factor for CAD in patients whose plasma cholesterol is not substantially elevated[57]. Detailed nutritional analyses in the STARS trial have shown independent effects of both plasma lipids and dietary saturated fatty acids[20], in particular stearic acid, on angiographic progression of CAD. These novel findings provide a basis for future experimental studies.

Conclusion

The principal metabolic measurements in regression trials should be targeted at rigorously testing the experimental hypothesis. Additional tests should be used to check for confounding, to monitor the safety of interventions, and to generate new hypotheses concerning the metabolic determinants of coronary athero-sclerosis. Estimation of factors that may be causally related to the progression of CAD should ideally be coupled with a simple biochemical test of atherosclerotic change. Analytical and biological errors must be minimized for all measurements and links with a lipid reference laboratory are recommended; standardization remains a problem with all apolipoprotein assays. The current body of evidence suggests that apoB-containing lipoproteins, in particular IDL and LDL, are the major metabolic aggravators of progression of CAD, with some protection afforded by elevated plasma levels of HDL. New hypotheses suggest that hepatic lipase, apolipoprotein C-III and dietary stearic acid may be important determinants of the progression of CAD, and a specific role for triglyceride-rich lipoproteins in initiating new coronary lesions has also been proposed. Serial measurement of plasma total sialic acid may be the most convenient biochemical marker to monitor angiographic change at present. Correlational analyses of metabolic variables with angiographic indices may provide target levels for optimizing interventional strategies to mitigate progression of coronary atherosclerosis and, by extension, the development of new coronary lesions. Therapeutic targets need to take account of pretreatment plasma risk factor levels[58].

Acknowledgements

I acknowledge my principal co-investigators in STARS: Professor Barry Lewis (University of London), Dr J.N.H. Brunt (University of Manchester) and Dr D.J. Coltart (St Thomas' Hospital, UMDS).

References

1. Watts GF. Lipid-lowering therapy and regression of atherosclerosis. Endocrinol Metab. 1994;1:71–87.
2. Brensike JF, Levy RI, Kelsey SF, et al. Effects of therapy with cholestyramine on progression of coronary atherosclerosis: results of the NHLBI Type II Coronary Intervention Study. Circulation. 1984;69:313–24.
3. Blankenhorn DH, Nessim SA, Johnson RL, et al. Beneficial effects of combined colestipol–niacin therapy on coronary atherosclerosis and coronary venous bypass grafts. JAMA. 1987; 257:3233–40.
4. Buchwald H, Varco RL, Matts JP, et al. Effect of partial ileal bypass surgery on mortality and morbidity from coronary heart disease in patients with hypercholesterolaemia. Report of the Program on the Surgical Control of the Hyperlipidaemias (POSCH). N Engl J Med. 1990; 323:946–55.
5. Ornish D, Brown SE, Scherwitz L, et al. Can lifestyle changes reverse coronary heart disease? The Lifestyle Heart Trial. Lancet. 1990;336:129–33.
6. Brown BG, Albers JJ, Fisher LD, et al. Regression of coronary artery disease as a result of intensive lipid-lowering in men with high levels of apolipoprotein B. N Engl J Med. 1990; 323:1289–98.
7. Cashin-Hemphill L, Mack WJ, Pogoda J, et al. Beneficial effects of colestipol–niacin on coronary atherosclerosis: a 4 year follow-up. JAMA. 1990;264:3013–7.
8. Kane JP, Malloy MJ, Ports TA, et al. Regression of coronary atherosclerosis during treatment of familial hypercholesterolaemia with combined drug regimens. JAMA. 1990;264:3007–12.
9. Watts GF, Lewis B, Brunt NJH, et al. Effects on coronary artery disease of lipid-lowering diet, or diet plus cholestyramine, in the St Thomas' Atherosclerosis Regression Study (STARS). Lancet. 1992;339:536–69.
10. Schuler G, Hambrecht R, Schlierf G, et al. Regular physical exercise and low-fat diet. Effects on progression of coronary artery disease. Circulation. 1992;86:1–11.
11. Blankenhorn DH, Azen SP, Kramsch DM, et al. Coronary angiographic changes with lovastatin therapy. The Monitor Atherosclerosis Regression Study (MARS). Ann Intern Med. 1993; 119:969–76.
12. Alderman EL, Haskell WL, Fair JM, et al. Effects of intensive multiple risk factor reduction on coronary atherosclerosis and clinical cardiac events in men and women with coronary artery

disease. The Stanford Coronary Risk Intervention Project (SCRIP). Circulation. 1994;89: 975–1000.

13. Quinn TG, Alderman E, McMillan A, et al. Development of new atherosclerotic lesions during the Stanford Coronary Risk Intervention Project (SCRIP). J Am Coll Cardiol. 1994;24:900–8.

14. Waters D, Higginson L, Gladston P, et al. Effects of monotherapy with an HMG-CoA reductase inhibitor on the progression of coronary atherosclerosis as assessed by serial quantitative arteriography. The Canadian Coronary Atherosclerosis Intervention Trial. Circulation. 1994; 89:959–68.

15. Blankenhorn DH, Alaupovic P, Wickham E, et al. Prediction of angiographic change in native human coronary arteries and aortocoronary bypass grafts: lipid and non-lipid risk factors. Circulation. 1990;81:470–6.

16. Watts GF, Mandalia S, Brunt JNH, et al. Independent associations between plasma lipoprotein subfraction levels and the course of coronary artery disease in the St Thomas' Atherosclerosis Regression Study (STARS). Metabolism. 1993;42:1461–7.

17. Austin HA, Breslow JL, Hennekens CH, et al. Low-density lipoprotein subclass patterns and risk of myocardial infarction. JAMA. 1988;260:1917–21.

18. Swales JD. The ACE gene: A cardiovascular risk factor. J R Coll Phys Lond. 1993;27:106–8.

19. Peacock R, Watts GF, Mandalia S, et al. Associations between genotypes of the apolipoprotein E, B, AI-CIII-AIV and lipoprotein lipase genes and coronary artery disease in the St Thomas' Atherosclerosis Regression Study (STARS). Nutr Metab Cardiovasc Dis. 1994;44:128–36.

20. Watts GF, Jackson P, Mandalia S, et al. Nutrient intake and progression of coronary artery disease. Am J Cardiol.1994;73:328–32.

21. Regnström J, Nilsson J, Tornvall H, et al. Susceptibility to low-density lipoprotein oxidation and coronary atherosclerosis in man. Lancet. 1992;339:1183–6.

22. Barth JD, Jansen H, Kromhout D, et al. Diet and the role of lipoproteins, lipases, and thyroid hormones in coronary lesion growth. J Cardiovasc Pharmacol. 1987;10(Suppl 8):S42–6.

23. Walden CC, Hegele RA. Apolipoprotein E in hyperlipidaemia. Ann Intern Med. 1994;120: 1026–36.

24. Hixson E. Apolipoprotein E polymorphisms affect atherosclerosis in young males. Arterioscler Thromb. 1991;11:1237–44.

25. Katan HM, Birgelen AV, Deslypere JP, et al. Biological markers of dietary intake, with emphasis on fatty acids. Ann Nutr Metab. 1991;35:249–52.

26. Chait A. Methods for assessing lipid and lipoprotein oxidation. Curr Opin Lipidol. 1992;3: 389–94.

27. Esterbauer H, Striegl G, Puhl H, Rotheneder M. Continuous monitoring of in vitro oxidation of human LDL. Free Radic Res Commun. 1989;6:67–75.

28. Thompson WD, Smith EB. Atherosclerosis and the coagulation system. J Pathol. 1989;159: 97–106.

29. Jukan-Vague I, Alessi MC. Plasminogen activator inhibitor I and atherosclerosis. Thromb Haemost. 1993;70:138–43.

30. Bengtsson BA. The consequences of growth hormone deficiency in adults. Acta Endocrinol. 1993;128(Suppl 2):2–5.

31. Bush TL, Fried LP, Barrett-Connor E. Cholesterol, lipoproteins and coronary heart disease in women. Clin Chem. 1988;34:B60–B70.

32. Miller WG. Matrix effects in the measurement and standardization of lipids and lipoproteins. Curr Opin Lipidol. 1992;3:361–4.

33. Cooper GR, Myers GL, Smith SJ, Schlant RC. Blood lipid measurements. Variations and practical utility. JAMA. 1992;267:1652–60.

34. National Cholesterol Education Programme, Laboratory Standardization Panel, National Heart, Lung and Blood Institute. Recommendations for improving cholesterol measurement. Bethesda: National Cholesterol Education Program, February 1990; 1–81: NIH Publication 90-2964.

35. Rader DJ, Hoeg JM, Brewer HB. Quantitation of plasma apolipoproteins in the primary and secondary prevention of coronary artery disease. Ann Intern Med. 1994;120:1012–25.

36. Labeur C, Rosseneu M. Methods for the measurement of lipoprotein(a) in the clinical laboratory. Curr Opin Lipidol. 1992;3:372–6.

37. Cooper GR, Sampson EJ, Smith SJ. Preanalytical, including biological, variation in lipid and apolipoprotein measurements. Curr Opin Lipidol. 1992;6:365–71.
38. Schmitz G, Lackner KJ. The value of cellular markers for the assessment of cardiovascular risk. Curr Opin Lipidol. 1993;4:461–70.
39. Bath PM, Blann AD, Watts GF. No association between serum platelet-derived growth factor, platelet size, and regression of angiographically-defined coronary artery disease. Platelets. 1994;5:135–8.
40. Blann AD, McCollum CN. Von Willebrand factor, endothelial cell damage and atherosclerosis. Eur J Vasc Surg. 1994;8:10–5.
41. Watts GF, Mandalia S, Brunt JNH, et al. Metabolic determinants of the course of coronary artery disease in men. Clin Chem. 1995;40:2240–6.
42. Schauer R. Sialic acids and their role as biological markers. Trends Biochem Sci. 1985;10:357–60.
43. Born GV, Palinski W. Unusually high concentrations of sialic acid on the surface of vascular endothelium. Br J Exp Pathol. 1985;66:543–9.
44. Lindberg G, Eklund G, Gullberg B, Rastam L. Serum sialic acid concentration and cardiovascular mortality. Br Med J. 1991;302:143–6.
45. Watts GF, Crook MA, Haq S, Mandalia S. Serum sialic acid as an indicator of change in coronary artery disease. Metabolism. 1995;44:147–8.
46. Azen S, Blankenhorn DH, Nessim S. Planning and evaluation of studies on atherosclerosis in controlled clinical trials. In: Malinow MR, Blaton VH, editors. Regression of atherosclerotic lesions: experimental studies and observations in humans. New York: Plenum Press; 1984:263–75.
47. Parker TS, McNamara DJ, Brown CD, et al. Plasma mevalonate as a measure of cholesterol synthesis in man. J Clin Invest. 1984;74:795–804.
48. Johnston JD, Watts GF. Lipid-lowering drugs in the management of atherosclerosis. Curr Pract Surg. 1994;6:45–51.
49. Hunninghake DB. Drug treatment of dyslipoproteinaemia. Endocrinol Metab Clin N Am. 1990;19:345–60.
50. Gibson CM, Sandor T, Stone PH, et al. Quantitative angiographic and statistical methods to assess serial changes in coronary luminal diameter and implications for regression trials. Am J Cardiol. 1992;69:1286–90.
51. Hodis HN, Mack WJ, Azen SP, et al. Triglyceride- and cholesterol-rich lipoproteins have a differential effect on mild/moderate and severe lesion progression as assessed by quantitative coronary angiography in a controlled trial of lovastatin. Circulation. 1994;90:42–9.
52. Levy RI, Brensike JP, Epstein SE, et al. The influence of changes in lipid values induced by cholestyramine and diet on progression of coronary artery disease: results of the NHLBI Type II Coronary Intervention Study. Circulation. 1984;69:325–37.
53. Bunte T, Hahmann HW, Hellwig N, et al. Effects of fenofibrate on angiographically examined coronary atherosclerosis and left ventricular function in hypercholesterolaemic patients. Atherosclerosis. 1993;98:127–38.
54. MAAS Investigators. Effect of simvastatin on coronary atheroma: the Multicentre Anti-Atheroma Study (MAAS). [Published erratum appears in Lancet. 994;344:762] Lancet. 1994;344:633–8.
55. Krauss RM, Lindgren FT, Williams PT, et al. Intermediate-density lipoproteins and progression of coronary artery disease in hypercholesterolaemic men. Lancet. 1987;2:62–6.
56. Phillips NR, Waters D, Havel RJ. Plasma lipoproteins and progression of coronary artery disease evaluated by angiography and clinical events. Circulation. 1993;88:2762–70.
57. Marburger C, Hambrecht R, Niebauer J, et al. Association between lipoprotein(a) and progression of coronary artery disease in middle-aged men. Am J Cardiol. 1994;73:742–6.
58 Sacks FM, Gibson CM, Rosner B, et al. The influence of pretreatment low density lipoprotein cholesterol concentrations on the effect of hypocholesterolaemic therapy on coronary atherosclerosis in angiographic trials. Am J Cardiol. 1995;76:78C–85C.

4. Quality control in quantitative coronary arteriography

J. H. C. REIBER, J. W. JUKEMA, G. KONING and
A. V. G. BRUSCHKE

Summary

The assessment of changes in coronary morphology in lipid intervention trials was carried out initially by visual interpretation on a consensus basis and later by quantitative coronary arteriography (QCA), sometimes supported by visual interpretation. The higher accuracy and precision of the computer-aided approach, however, can only be achieved under highly standardized circumstances. An overview is given on the necessary precautions to be taken regarding:

1. The X-ray and imaging system;
2. The arteriographic image acquisition procedure; and
3. The quantitative image analysis procedure.

For sixteen lipid-intervention trials which were carried out since 1987, it has been checked to what extent nine quality-control issues were applied in these trials. It could be concluded that, as time progressed, trials have conformed increasingly to these standards. However, there is still room for further improvements. Therefore, for new studies, maximal attention should be given to these and other items, not only at the start of the study, but also during the course of the trial.

Introduction

Despite its known limitations, quantitative coronary arteriography (QCA) has established itself over the past ten years as the gold standard to assess changes in coronary morphology, in regression/progression type studies as well as in coronary intervention studies, in an objective and reproducible manner[1-4]. Medium- and long-term variability in the assessment of absolute coronary dimensions has been shown to be of the order of 0.20 mm (1 SD) under standardized conditions and with state-of-the-art QCA equipment[5]. However, it should be realized that the changes to be observed are much smaller, particularly in regression/progression studies. Assuming a natural progression rate of 2.5% per year of the vessel diameter, this would result in a decrease of approximately 0.05 mm per year for an average vessel diameter of 2 mm[6]. These data are in accordance with the recently published data from the REGRESS (Regression Growth Evaluation Statin Study) trial in which, over a period of two years, the mean segment diameter in the placebo group narrowed by 0.10 mm and the median value of the obstruction diameter by 0.09 mm[7].

A.V.G. Bruschke et al. *(eds): Lipid-lowering therapy and progression of atherosclerosis, 45–63.*
© 1996 *Kluwer Academic Publishers.*

These numbers demonstrate that this powerful and widely available tool has definite limitations in measuring these small changes, mainly due to the fact that angiography is a two-dimensional projection technique with a limited spatial resolution and signal-to-noise ratio. However, alternative measurement techniques have not been developed yet. Since the introduction of intracoronary ultrasound (ICUS), much scientific evidence has been obtained about the progressive nature of coronary artery disease. Intravascular ultrasound (IVUS) is basically a three-dimensional technique which allows a precise assessment of the coronary vessel shape and its wall thickness[8]. However, many technical problems still need to be solved before IVUS could possibly be used in regression/progression studies in which the entire coronary tree needs to be studied[9] in a manner which causes little or no harm to the patient. It is likely that these disadvantages will be much greater than the potential benefits.

It has been shown that the number of patients that needs to be investigated to demonstrate a certain effect of a proposed drug is proportional to the variability of the measurement technique divided by the number of years between the arteriograms squared[10]. From the view-point of population size, duration and cost-effectiveness of a study, it is therefore of great importance to minimize the variations in arteriographic data acquisition and computer analysis procedures. In the entire process, from image acquisition in the catheterization laboratory through the quantitative analysis on a particular QCA system, there are many potential error sources. Each of these individual error sources should be minimized as much as possible to obtain the best results overall. Recognition of which precautions need to be taken can best be achieved by separating the entire procedure into three entities, which will be described in the following sections in more detail. These entities are:

1. The quality of the X-ray and imaging system;
2. The arteriographic image acquisition procedure; and
3. The quantitative image analysis procedure.

The quality of the X-ray and imaging system

Obviously, the quality of quantitative coronary analyses depends not only upon the quality of the QCA systems, but even more so upon the quality of the underlying arteriographic image data. Images with little image contrast result in a lower reliability of the detected contours; images may be so poor in quality that they cannot be analyzed at all. Significant changes in the film development process may have an effect on the contour detection. If the geometry of the X-ray system changes over time, the vessels will no longer be projected identically in the same angiographic views; this may be particularly troublesome in stenosed vessels with eccentric lesions. These effects are even more problematic when they occur slowly over time so that they may go unnoticed or may be detected only after the study has been completed.

Over the past ten years, there has been significant progress in X-ray imaging technology. Image quality is continually improving due to the availability of higher quality X-ray sources, image intensifiers, TV chains, the use of pulsed fluoroscopy, and real-time image enhancement. All modern X-ray systems from the different vendors satisfy the basic requirements for adequate coronary arteriography. On the one hand, the image carrier for the regression/progression studies is still the 35-mm cinefilm, mainly because it is a unit patient record that can be readily exchanged between the angiographic centres and the QCA core laboratory and because of its high spatial resolution[11].

However, not every catheterization laboratory participating in a clinical research trial is of the latest vintage. Whether a system is old or new, it can slowly or abruptly run out of its specifications. Therefore, quality assurance (QA) is of utmost importance. In addition to the actual image quality of a particular X-ray system, the stability of the image generation process over the study period plays an even greater role. Even if a system shows a certain systematic error in the measurements, small changes in vessel morphology can still be detected as long as this systematic error does not change over time. In other words, stability is more important than absolute accuracy. To ensure that this image quality is guaranteed over time, the following items are of major concern and should be measured on a regular basis with the appropriate tools and compared with previous measurements for trend analysis.

1. **X-ray system geometry**

   To be able to repeat angiographic imaging procedures reproducibly, accurate registration of the following X-ray system settings are required:

   Essential:
   a. Rotation angles (right anterior oblique, left anterior oblique)
   b. Angulation angles (caudal, cranial)
   c. Image intensifier mode (5″/6″/7″)

   Preferred:
   d. Tower or image intensifier height
   e. Table height
   f. Isocentre height (only for systems with movable isocentre)

   These data should be filled in on the appropriate case record forms during the catheterization procedure with the corresponding sequential run numbers. Important items are: (1) ease and reproducibility with which an X-ray stand can be positioned into a certain angiographic view; and (2) stability and agreement between mechanical and/or electronic rotation/angulation read-outs, etc. The only remaining uncertainty is the position of the patient on the table.

2. **Pincushion distortion**

   Older image intensifiers show significant geometric distortion at the edges of the images – particularly in the largest image mode – the so-called pincushion distortion. This results in a selective magnification of an object near the edges of the image, compared with its size in the centre of the field[12]. Further improvements in the quality of image intensifiers have resulted in a much lower degree of image distortion, although still not negligible. The geometric distortion can be assessed by recording a cm-grid held against the input screen of the image intensifier, usually in the AP-position. It is advisable to repeat this at regular intervals of 3–6 months and certainly after a major service procedure on the X-ray system has been carried out[13]. By doing so, changes in distribution of the magnitude and direction of the distortion can be assessed over time.

If the spatial distribution and extent of the distortion over the image can be fixed, it can be corrected for. However, Onnasch et al. and Solzbach et al. demonstrated that the distortion is rotation dependent due to the earth's magnetic field[14,15]. Further research in this field by our laboratory has shown that any measurement errors are due not only to the magnitude of the distortion in the region of interest (ROI) but even more to the change or the gradient of the distortion vectors in such a ROI[16]. This study also confirmed that the rotation and angulation of the X-ray gantry have a significant effect on the distribution of the sizes and directions of the correction vectors and their gradients. Even the presence of additional electromagnetic fields from other sources, e.g. video monitors in the catheterization laboratory, may have an effect on this geometric distortion. This means that if the correction data acquired in the standard AP-view is applied to another arteriographic view, more artefacts may be introduced rather than correction for any distortion present. Given the enormous complexity of this possible error source, our advice must be not to correct for pincushion distortion in intervention studies in which the arterial dimensions are to be compared in identical views. Even with only a small error at baseline, approximately the same error would be made at follow-up given the similarities of the corresponding angiographic views.

3. Transfer function of the X-ray system

Although X-ray systems are characterized by a relatively high resolving power of small objects (a modern 6–7″ image intensifier should resolve 3.8 linepairs/mm), an infinitely small object would still be displayed with finite dimensions. For example, if the grey levels along a scanline perpendicular to a thin copper wire of a cm-grid were plotted, an approximately Gaussian-shaped function would appear with a base much wider than the actual wire (Figure 4.1). As a result, many quantitative coronary arteriographic systems with automated edge detection techniques either cannot measure arterial sizes reliably below 0.7–0.8 mm or severely overestimate the vessel sizes below approximately 1.2 mm[17]. However, in QCA studies, the entire range of diameters, from roughly 0.5 mm upwards, should be measured reliably without size-dependent systematic or random errors.

Some researchers have tried to correct for this non-linearity by determining, for each X-ray system and image intensifier mode, the relationship between the true size of a vessel phantom and its measured size[18]. A

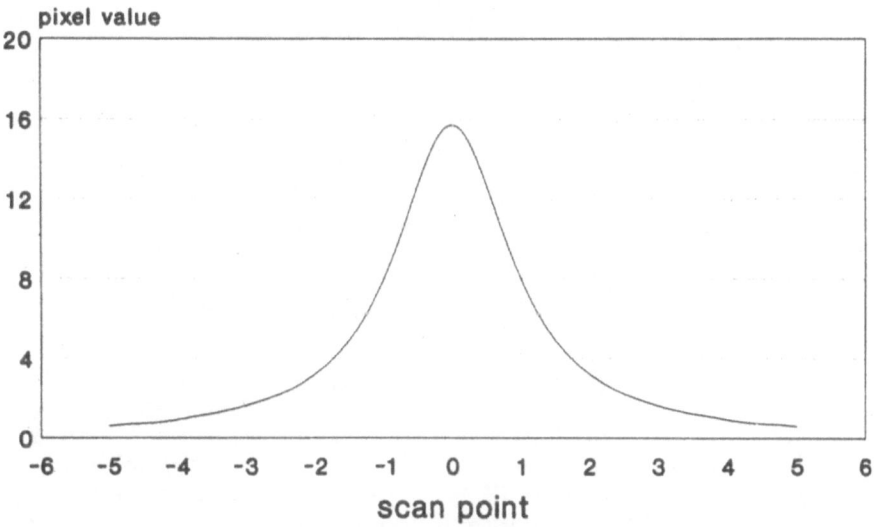

Figure 4.1. Typical example of the line-spread function measured for a particular X-ray system.

particular measured value in this range would then be corrected on the basis of this relationship. A definite disadvantage of this approach is that it introduces noise into the measurements. Due to the shallow slope of this function in the range below 1.2 mm, a small difference in the measured value will result in a large difference in the corrected value (Figure 4.2). Therefore, the best approach is to measure the actual modulation transfer function (MTF) of a particular X-ray imaging chain and correct for these effects in the calculations of the edge strength values in the actual contour detection module by means of deconvolution techniques[19]. Again, this means that, in practice, such MTF-curves must be measured and that these should be stable over time.

4. **Cinefilm development process**

The 35-mm cinefilm is the end product of the cardiac catheterization procedure. Therefore, a great deal of attention must be given to its quality and the consistency of its quality. The density (D) versus log (E = exposure) curve, or H and D curve (after Hurter and Driffield) should be measured using commercially available sensitometers and densitometers at regular scheduled times and whenever there is reason to suspect that there is a problem with the film processor or solution. If necessary, the temperature, developer time, etc. should be adjusted to obtain a consistent and optimal product. Generally, if a processed strip is within control limits at the beginning of the day, this satisfies the basic need to know that processing was proper at that time. Along the same lines, the photographers and angiographers should also check on a daily basis for scratches and dirty

Improper Vessel Size correction

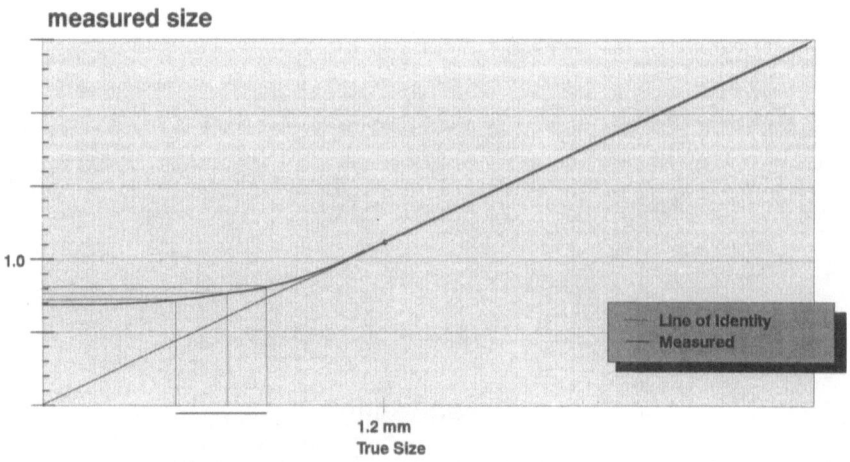

Figure 4.2.   Correction for limited resolution of X-ray chain.

spots on the film. Scratches, in particular, can be a major problem for QCA because of the associated sudden changes in grey levels in the images; contour detection techniques tend to follow the scratches.

5. **Quality Acceptance/Assurance reports**
    It is clear that proper 'calibration' of the participating catheterization laboratories, carried out on a regular basis (e.g. once every 3–4 months), improves the consistency and reliability of the image data. Only if these conditions are met can corresponding segments from multiple views be compared with a high degree of confidence. To determine the quality of the X-ray imaging chain and the possible changes therein over a study period, appropriate quality assurance (QA)* or calibration programmes have been developed for catheterization laboratories[11]. Items which are measured include, among others:
    a. Accuracy and precision of the rotation and angulation read-out devices on the X-ray gantry;
    b. Accuracy and precision of tower height and table read-out devices;
    c. Resolution of the X-ray system based on a modulation transfer function (MTF) analysis and on the basis of line-pair phantoms with an appropriate phantom, such as the MEDIS X-ray phantom;
    d. Determination of the large-detail detectability (LDD) of the X-ray system using an appropriate phantom, such as the MEDIS X-ray phantom;

*MEDIS Medical Imaging Systems, Nuenen, The Netherlands

Table 4.1. Grading of QA analysis of a catheterization laboratory.

Signal-to-noise ratio	7
Contrast	7
Detail	7
Geometric distortion	8
Reproducibility geometry X-ray system	7
Stability film development	8
Overall impression	7.3

e. Signal-to-noise ratio in the phantom images;
f. Spatial distribution and degree of pincushion distortion.
g. The quality of the cinefilm development process.

The derived data from these measurements are stored in a QA-database, allowing trend analysis from follow-up calibration procedures which are carried out at regular time intervals. As soon as it becomes evident that one of the parameters falls outside the normal ranges or may be drifting towards the threshold values, preventive maintenance procedures can be initiated. In addition to these regular calibration procedures, the quality of cardiac catheterization laboratories can be measured using the same techniques prior to inclusion in a clinical trial (Quality Acceptance programme). In this way, the principal investigator of such a trial and the sponsor will obtain objective criteria from which to choose those centres which are most suitable for participation in the trial as far as image quality is concerned. These results can be translated into a set of grades by comparing these individual results with a normal QA database in which the QA results from a large number of different X-ray systems have been stored. The average values and the standard deviations of the most important parameters have been used to generate grades from one to ten, so that the performance of another catheterization laboratory can be assessed objectively. The average values have been set to a grade of seven, and each increase or decrease by one standard deviation corresponds to an increase or decrease of the grade by one point, respectively. An example is given in Table 4.1.

QA measurements of a large number of catheterization laboratories in different regression/progression studies have demonstrated that the following technical problems were reported most frequently, listed in order of decreasing frequency:

1. Differences in X-ray gantries of catheterization laboratories in the same institute, leading to the proposal that patients must have their follow-up angiogram in the same room.

2. Unreliability of the electronic read-out devices of the rotation and angulation angles. This resulted in the strong advice to use only the mechanical read-out devices; at the same time, the electronic read-out devices had to be tuned.

3.   Changes in the large-detail detectability (LDD) or contrast resolution of the images and in the signal-to-noise ratios such that intermediate servicing was required.

4.   At the beginning of one of these studies, one particular catheterization laboratory was not included on the basis of a measured poor signal-to-noise ratio (grade 5) and poor reproducibility of the rotation/angulation settings (grade 5). As a result, this catheterization laboratory was replaced by another centre.

5.   In another example, the LDD on cinefilm was acceptable but not on the video monitors in the catheterization laboratory. This was taken care of by the service engineer.

6.   As a result of this QA programme, image quality of the catheterization laboratories involved in this study has gradually improved.

From the above, it is clear that the technical quality of the X-ray systems and the image generating processes can be controlled adequately. The final factor in the entire process is a human one, being the angiographer who actually performs the catheterization. The image quality is very much dependent upon the skills and dedication of this person in carrying out the procedures.

The arteriographic image acquisition procedure

In the actual arteriographic image acquisition procedure a number of items need to be standardized in order to obtain comparable data. Most of these precautions have been described in detail elsewhere and, therefore, will only be described here briefly[1,20].

1.   **Administration of vasodilative drug immediately prior to the arterio-graphic investigation**
     One of the most important variables in the quantitative assessment of coronary arterial dimensions is the vasomotor tone. If no precautions are taken, the vasomotor tone may differ even during consecutive coronary angiographic runs. An optimal vasodilative drug for controlling the vasomotor tone of the epicardial vessel should produce a quick (within 30 s to 1 min) and maximal response without influencing the haemodynamic state of the patient. Only nitrates and calcium antagonists satisfy these requirements. Jost et al. have demonstrated that the administration of 10 mg isosorbide dinitrate (ISDN) sublingually 10 min prior to arteriography satisfies these requirements with a maximum vasodilation for approximately 30 min[21]. Otherwise, a dose of 3 mg ISDN administered intracoronary has been shown to be well tolerated in clinical practice. This dose of 3 mg ISDN is equivalent to intracoronary administration of 0.3 mg of the nitrate nitroglycerin[22]. In practice, either ISDN or nitroglycerin have been used. What is important, is to establish a standardized and maximal vasodilation. The issue of standardized coronary vasodilation has arisen recently following

a publication by K Lance Gould MD et al., suggesting that lipid profile manipulation results in a restoration of endothelium-dependent vasodilation[23].

2. **Use of non-ionic and iso-osmolar contrast media**
   Collective studies offer experimental and clinical evidence of the advantages of the low-osmolality agents in cardiac radiology[24,25]. Jost and associates have clearly demonstrated that the vasodilative changes in vessel dimensions due to the administration of contrast medium are significantly smaller with use of a non-ionic contrast medium (<5.8%) than with use of an ionic contrast medium (< 18.9%)[26]. Therefore, in quantitative coronary angiographic studies, non-ionic contrast media with iso-osmolality are advocated; in addition, adequate injection intervals should be taken. However, the expense of these non-ionic contrast media may be prohibitive for certain studies. It has been felt by several investigators, although this has never, to our knowledge, been validated in an objective manner, that once a maximal vasodilator has been given the choice of contrast medium is no longer important.

3. **Selection of catheter material**
   To obtain absolute sizes of the vessel dimensions, calibration of the selected cineframes is necessary; almost exclusively, this has been performed on the basis of the contrast or guiding catheters. The radio-opacity of the materials of which the catheters are produced determine how well these are visible in the images. For an automated edge detection of the catheter shaft or tip to be reliable and reproducible, it is necessary for the image contrast of the catheter to be sufficiently high, as well as the sharpness of the edges of the displayed catheter; this last characteristic is denoted the edge strength. Over the last several years, we have tested several types of catheters for QCA purposes[11]. In these in-vitro and in-vivo acceptability studies, several requirements were set for a catheter to be acceptable. Among others, in the in-vivo studies, double the pooled standard deviation of the derived calibration factors should be smaller than 5% of the average calibration factor. In other words, double the coefficient of variation should be less than 5%. In practice, this means that, in 95% of cases, the error in the calibration factor would be limited to 5%. Similar but slightly more stringent requirements were set for the in-vitro studies. Based on these criteria, the following catheters were tested in our laboratory and accepted for QCA:

   Mallinckrodt Softouch 6F and 7F[27]
   Cordis, 6F Super Torque[11]
   Cordis, 7F High Flow[11]

Our experience has demonstrated that 5F catheters are not acceptable for calibration purposes! There are just too few pixels available for the measurements. Therefore, an absolute requirement is: always use catheters of sufficient size (6F or greater) and only those approved for QCA!

An issue has also been whether the selected frames for calibration should show the contrast- or saline-filled catheters. In our experience with the catheters approved for QCA, it did not make any difference whether calibration was performed on 'empty' or 'full' catheters[11,27]. Since the true outer diameters of these catheters are smaller than the French sizes listed by the manufacturer, it has been advocated that the actual sizes are measured with a precision micrometer. However, this represents a significant effort in the organizations of the QCA Angiographic Core Laboratories and of the participating cardiac catheterization laboratories. In the Dutch REGRESS-trial on regression/progression of coronary artery disease, a total of 2104 catheters from four different manufacturers were measured. It turned out that, in 2048 of the 2104 catheters, the variability in the measurements was 0.02–0.03 mm, which represents an error of only 1% of the average catheter sizes. In the remaining 56 catheter measurements, the variability was 0.04 mm. From these data we concluded that the stated mean values can be used for calibration purposes and that the requirement for sending these catheters to the QCA core laboratory could be eliminated in future trials. This has important practical consequences for running clinical trials and QCA core laboratory operations[28].

4. **Image acquisition protocol**

Several precautions in the actual image acquisition protocol are necessary to obtain optimal results:

a. Instruct the patient about the inspiration procedure.

b. Under fluoroscopy and deep inspiration by the patient:
    — Position X-ray system such that both a non-tapering part of the catheter and the coronary segment(s) of interest are well visible, preferably with minimal foreshortening and overlap;
    — Have a wedge-filter positioned by an X-ray technician to optimize image quality.

c. Administer contrast agent either manually or by power injector:
    — Left coronary system: 7 ml at rate of 5 ml/s
    — Right coronary system: 5 ml at rate of 3 ml/s;
    If backflow of contrast into the aorta does not occur, increase settings. If severe main stem stenosis is present, always administer contrast manually.

d. During arteriography:
    — Request a deep and reproducible inspiration from the patient;
    — Do not move the table.

e. Film speed must be set at a minimum of 25 frames/s. Lower speed (e.g. 12.5 f/s) does not allow the appropriate frame selection.

Quantitative image analysis procedure

In this last phase, a number of steps can be distinguished: acceptance/rejection of cinefilm for QCA, frame selection, calibration procedure, and vessel segment analysis.

1. **Acceptance/rejection of cinefilm**
   When a cinefilm arrives at the QCA core laboratory, it must be checked first for whether its quality is sufficient for QCA. In our Heart Core Laboratory, the following items are checked:

   a. Is the case record form for the angiographic views filled in completely?
   b. Does the angiographic view data correspond with the cinefilm sequences?
   c. Is the catheter size acceptable for QCA (6F or bigger)?
   d. Is the information on the catheters employed (size, brand, sequence numbers) complete?
   e. What is the image quality of the cinefilm as assessed visually (good, just acceptable, poor, unacceptable)?
   f. If the quality is not optimal, what are the reasons (poor filling of vessels with contrast, wedge filter insufficiently used, insufficient part of catheter visible, other)?
   g. What is the coronary vessel score (CVS) on a scale from 0 to 18?

   On the basis of all these items, an overall conclusion is reached, being: acceptable; to be completed; or unacceptable. Immediately after review of the film, the film acceptance form is sent to the participating hospital.
   The calculation of the CVS requires some further explanation. This score is based on the fact that a minimum of 9 coronary segments (RCA (prox, mid, distal), main, LCX (prox, dist) and LAD (prox, mid, dist)) are to be analysed from at least two views. If each of these 9 segments is visualized in two appropriate views, this will lead to a maximum score or grade of $9 \times 2 = 18$; other secondary or tertiary vessels are not included in this grading procedure. While previewing the cinefilm, the QCA technician selects, for each coronary segment, those frames that are suitable for QCA and assigns to each acceptable view a grade of 1 provided the second view for that segment is at least 60° apart. Segments that are occluded and the corresponding distal segments are also assigned a grade of 1, since this is beyond the control of the angiographer. Segments that are not visualized in a particular view with sufficient quality (image contrast too low, streaming, foreshortening, severe overlap, etc.) are assigned a grade of 0. By adding up these grades, the coronary vessel score is obtained in the range of 0–18. We have decided that a film should have a score of 14 or higher to be acceptable for QCA and to be included in a regression/progression study.

2. **Frame selection**
   Final frame selection is performed by a cardiologist or fellow, or by a highly trained QCA technician under the supervision of this cardiologist or fellow. We have developed the following guidelines:

   a. Select a frame in the 2nd or 3rd cardiac cycle following contrast injection.
   b. Make sure that the segment of interest is fully opacified; if not, go to another cardiac cycle.

c.   Select the frame at the end-diastole or in the diastasis period so that the effect of motion blur is minimal.
d.   If the angiographic view shows the segment minimally foreshortened, the frame with the largest luminal size at the obstruction is chosen.
e.   On the other hand, if foreshortening occurs at the obstruction, the frame with maximal narrowing (smallest luminal size) is chosen.
f.   If no appropriate frame can be found at end-diastole or in the diastasis period, for example due to vessel or catheter overlap, go to another part in the cardiac cycle, e.g. end-systole.

3. **Calibration procedure**
    After a film has been prepared following the guidelines described in points 1 and 2, the film can be handed over to the QCA technician for quantitative analysis on the QCA workstation. As mentioned earlier, calibration of the individual frames is of utmost importance. We have developed the following guidelines for the calibration procedure:

a.   Choose a frame that shows the catheter clearly visible with minimal overlap of contrast agent in the aorta, etc.
b.   For catheters approved for QCA, a frame may be selected with the catheter filled with either contrast agent or saline.
c.   The frame should show the catheter in a 'stable' position, i.e. minimal motion should occur with respect to preceding or following frames. Motion results in blurring of the projected object and therefore in an underestimated calibration factor.
d.   For calibration purposes, select a segment with sufficient length in a non-tapering portion of the catheter.
e.   If there is any doubt about the accuracy of the detected catheter contours, repeat the procedure in the same frame or select another frame.
f.   Variability in the calibration factor from repeated measurements should be less than 0.005 mm/pixel.

4. **Vessel segment analysis**
    Analysis of the coronary vessel segment on qualified state-of-the-art equipment, such as the CMS, is rather straightforward and has been well documented[1,11,19]. Briefly, a number of important guidelines are to be followed, among others:

—   Proper definition of beginning and end points of the arterial segment to be analysed according to the guidelines of the AHA[29].
—   The automated selection of the reference diameter has been found to be very practical and reproducible. However, user-selection of the reference diameter position is indicated if the reference diameter function tapers significantly either in the antegrade or retrograde direction.
—   Multiple lesions may occur in one and the same segment. Each of these lesions can be characterized individually from the overall diameter

function calculated for the entire segment and assigned an appropriate sequence code from proximal to distal, e.g. A, B, C or 1, 2, 3 etc.

Overview of quality control in lipid-intervention studies

Since 1987, a total of at least sixteen lipid-intervention trials have been carried out with the vast majority of these already published or submitted[7,30–43]. For each of these studies, we have obtained from the relevant literature and through direct contact with the principal investigators nine quality control issues and presented these in Table 4.2. The contents of this Table are straightforward but will, nevertheless, be discussed briefly in the following paragraphs.

In each of the studies listed, the viewing angles during the baseline (B) angiography were recorded on paper and repeated as accurately as possible at follow-up (FU). In the majority of these studies, the gantry table height was not standardized. The regular catheterization laboratory calibration procedure (Quality Assurance) was carried out in an extensive manner by a third party in three of the studies (Lifestyle, FATS and REGRESS); a rigorous internal check was carried out in the CCAIT study by the individual centres. The administration of a coronary vasodilator immediately prior to the angiographic acquisition is accepted nowadays; the most widely used technique is the sublingual administration of nitroglycerin.

In by far the majority of the studies, no special requirements were demanded on the use of contrast catheters; in some studies, the only requirement was that, at follow-up, the same catheter would be used as at baseline. In more recent years, when 6F catheters became popular, it was decided that the catheter size had to be 6F, 7F or bigger. In two studies special catheters with tantalum rings were used; the metal rings result in better definition of the edges in the angiograms. In the remaining studies, the outlines of the projected contrast catheters were used for calibration purposes. Only in a small minority of the studies (Lifestyle, STARS, MARS, MAAS and REGRESS) was the tip of the catheters measured with a precision micrometer to obtain a value for its true dimension instead of the nominal value as listed by the manufacturer. We have noted that there is a difference of approximately 0.1 mm between these values[28].

As far as QCA equipment is concerned, most of the studies published in 1990 and before were based on either visual interpretation or manual tracing by the Brown technique[44]. Later on, various systems with automated edge-detection techniques were employed. We have recently demonstrated that the systematic and random errors in measurements by the various QCA systems may differ significantly, and thereby hamper any meta-analyses[16]. It should be recognized that, theoretically, two systems with different systematic error responses may still yield similar differences between follow-up and baseline; under such circumstances, the results from different studies could be combined. This needs to be confirmed in practice. Personally, we are not very optimistic about the results. Using additional arguments, Brown et al. have also warned that 'meta-analyses' of these trials is likely to result in erroneous conclusions[45]. Their arguments were:

Table 4.2.   Quality control in lipid intervention trials.

Trial	Viewing angles recorded	Table height	Catheterization laboratory calibration	Vasodilator	Catheter requirements	Catheter measured	QCA equipment	Number of frames analysed	Pincushion correction
CLAS-I (1987)	Yes	Yes	No	Not in all patients; FU same as B	No	No	Visual+edge detection (Selzer)	3	Yes
NHLBI Type II (1989)	Yes	No	No	Nitro sublingually in most patients	No	No	Manual tracing (Brown)	2 cine or cut film	No
POSCH (1990)	?	No	No	?	No	No	Visual	—	No
SCOR (1990)	Yes	Yes	No	Nitro sublingually	USCI 7F with tantalum markers	No	Manual tracing (Brown)	3 adjacent frames	No
Lifestyle (1990)	Yes	Yes	Yes, every 6 mo	Not routinely, FU same as B	FU same as B	Yes	Edge detection (Kirkeeide)	1	Yes
FATS (1990)	Yes	Isocentre	Yes, monthly by third party	Nitrates+other vasoactive drugs; FU same as B	FU same as B	No	Visual+manual tracing (Brown)	3 frames for possibly changed lesions	Yes
CLAS-II (1990)	Yes	Yes	No	Not in all patients FU same as B	No	No	Visual	—	NA
STARS (1992)	Yes	Yes	No	No	Cordis 8F (90% cases)	Yes	Edge detection (Brunt)	3 adjacent frames	Yes
HARP (1992)	Yes	No	No	Nitro sublingually	FU same as B	No	Edge detection (Sandor)	5 consecutive ED frames	Yes

continued

Table 4.2. continued.

Trial	Viewing angles recorded	Table height	Catheterization laboratory calibration	Vasodilator	Catheter requirements	Catheter measured	QCA equipment	Number of frames analysed	Pincushion correction
Schuler (1992)	Yes	No	No	No	No	?	Edge detection (Kontron)	1	No
MARS (1993)	Yes	No	No	Nitro in most patients	No	Yes	Visual+edge detection (Selzer)	3 adjacent frames	Yes
CCAIT (1994)	Yes	No	Internally	Nitro sublingually	No	No	CMS	1	No
SCRIP (1994)	Yes	No	No	Nitro sublingually	7F or bigger with tantalum markers	No	Edge detection (Sanders)	1	No
MAAS (1994)	Yes	Fixed table systems	No	ISDN sublingually	6F or bigger	Yes	CAAS	1	Yes
REGRESS (1994)	Yes	Yes	Yes, third party	Nitro sublingually	Yes	Yes	CMS	1	No
PLAC-I (1994)	Yes	No	No	Nitro sublingually	6F or bigger	No	Image Comm	1	No

For explanations see text

1. The interventions were not all of a single class;
2. Patient selection criteria and study durations varied widely;
3. The number of lesions measured per patient also varied widely; and
4. The angiographic assessment ranged from visual scoring to QCA (as mentioned above).

Depending on which system was used, one or more frames per lesion were analysed. Some investigators/developers of these QCA systems felt that averaging the results from either adjacent frames or consecutive ED frames would improve the accuracy and precision of these measurements[46]. Theoretically, one could expect that the random errors decrease by the square root of the number of frames averaged, e.g. $\sqrt{3}$ or $\sqrt{5}$ for 3- or 5-frame averaging, respectively. However, since the vessel is not stationary, the actual improvement will be less. Work by Lippolt et al. has demonstrated that the random error in the measurements can be decreased by averaging the results from multiple frames[47]. They measured the mean vessel diameter of coronary segments using the CMS analysis in 6 frames from one angiographic run as follows: (1) in 3 consecutive frames (ED frame of one cycle, one frame before and one frame after), and (2) in the 3 corresponding frames of the next cycle. Comparing the diameters measured in the ED frames (single), the mean values of 2 (double) and 3 (triple) consecutive frames, the following random error values were found between the first and the second cycle: 0.112, 0.095 and 0.085 mm, respectively. They concluded that averaging of measurements in consecutive images can result in a reduction of the random error, and therefore increase the statistical power of clinical trials. On the other hand, Syvänne et al. found that averaging 3 or 5 consecutive cineframes did not improve the random error of repeated acquisitions for the mean segment diameter or the minimum obstruction diameter on the CMS[48]. The major difference between these two studies is that Lippolt compared results from different cardiac cycles from one and the same angiographic run, while Syvänne compared results from two different angiographic runs (also called short-term variability), thereby introducing more error sources. Apparently, the additional error sources negated the gain achieved by the multiple frame averaging. Reasons for the generally small or negligible improvements is that the edge detection software in the CMS is already very robust and that the minimum cost contour detection algorithm has been shown to perform better than other algorithms under low signal-to-noise conditions[49].

The final item concerns the question of whether pincushion correction was applied to the images. Of the 16 studies presented in Table 4.2, the correction was not applied in 8 studies, not applicable in 1 (visual interpretation) and therefore was applied in 6 studies. According to the earlier information on this subject in this chapter, it is our feeling that current pincushion correction algorithms may introduce more artefacts than they solve.

Conclusions

Standardization of image acquisition and analysis procedures and the proper catheterization laboratory calibration procedures play a major role in QCA. From this overview, it is apparent that lipid intervention trials have conformed increasingly to these standards as time has progressed. However, there is still room for further improvement. As a result, maximum attention should be given to these items in new studies, not only at the beginning of the study, but even more so during the course of the trial.

References

1. Reiber JHC, Serruys PW. Quantitative coronary arteriography. In: Marcus ML, Skorton DJ, Schelbert HR, Wolf GL, editors. Cardiac imaging. Philadelphia: W.B. Saunders Company; 1991:221–81.
2. Thompson GR. Progression and regression of coronary artery disease. Curr Opin Lipidol. 1992;3:263–7.
3. Lespérance J, Waters D. Measuring progression and regression of coronary atherosclerosis in clinical trials: problems and progress. Int J Cardiac Imaging. 1992;8:165–73.
4. Vos J, Feyter PJ de, Simoons ML, Tijssen JGP, Deckers JW. Retardation and arrest of progression or regression of coronary artery disease: a review. Progr Cardiovasc Dis. 1993;35: 435–54.
5. Reiber JHC, Koning G, Land CD von, Zwet PMJ van der. Why and how should QCA systems be validated? In:Reiber JHC, Serruys PW, editors. Progress in quantitative coronary arteriography. Dordrecht: Kluwer Academic Publishers; 1994:33–48.
6. Eggen DA, Solberg LA. Variation of atherosclerosis with age. Lab Inv. 1968;18:571–9.
7. Jukema JW, Bruschke AVG, Boven AJ van, et al. Effects of lipid lowering by pravastatin on progression and regression of coronary artery disease in symptomatic men with normal to moderately elevated serum cholesterol levels. The 'Regression Growth Evaluation Statin Study' (REGRESS). Circulation. 1995;91:2528–40.
8. Lowry RW, Kleiman NS, Raizner AE, Young JB. Is intravascular ultrasound better than quantitative coronary arteriography to assess cardiac allograft arteriopathy? Cath Cardiovasc Diagn. 1994;31:110–15.
9. Feyter PJ de, Di Mario C, Slager CJ, Serruys PW, Roelandt JRTC. Towards complete assessment of progression/regression of coronary atherosclerosis: implications for intervention trials. In: Reiber JHC, Serruys PW, editors. Progress in quantitative coronary arteriography. Dordrecht: Kluwer Academic Publishers; 1994:295–305.
10. Blankenhorn DH, Brooks SH. Angiographic trials of lipid-lowering therapy. Arteriosclerosis. 1981;1:242–9.
11. Reiber JHC, Land CD von, Koning G, et al. Comparison of accuracy and precision of quantitative coronary arterial analysis between cinefilm and digital systems. In: Reiber JHC, Serruys PW, editors. Progress in quantitative coronary arteriography. Dordrecht: Kluwer Academic Publishers; 1994:67–85.
12. Reiber JHC. An overview of coronary quantitation techniques as of 1989. In: Reiber JHC, Serruys PW, editors. Quantitative coronary arteriography. Dordrecht: Kluwer Academic Publishers; 1991:55–132.
13. Meijer DJH, van der Zwet PMJ, Reiber JHC. Fully automated PC-based assessment of pincushion distortion. Presented at the 4th International Symposium on Coronary Arteriography, Rotterdam, June 23–25. Abstract book. 1991:180.
14. Buschmeyer L, Onnasch DGW, Heintzen PH. Korrektur magnetfeldbedingter Bildverzeichnungen in bewegten Röntgen-Bildverstärker-Fernseh-Systemen. Biomed Tech. 1989;34: 209–10.

15. Solzbach U, Wollschläger H, Zeiher A, Just H. Optical distortion due to geomagnetism in quantitative angiography. Comput Cardiol. 1989;355–7.
16. Zwet PMJ van der, Meyer DJH, Reiber JHC. Automated and accurate assessment of the distribution, magnitude and direction of pincushion distortion in angiographic images. Invest Radiol. 1995;30:204–13.
17. Beauman GJ, Reiber JHC, Koning G, Houdt RCM van, Vogel RA. Angiographic core laboratory analyses of arterial phantom images: comparative evaluations of accuracy and precision. In: Reiber JHC, Serruys PW, editors. Progress in quantitative coronary arteriography. Dordrecht: Kluwer Academic Publishers; 1994:87–104.
18. Wong W-H, Kirkeeide RL, Gould KL. Computer application in angiography. In: Collins SM, Skorton DJ, editors. Cardiac imaging and image processing. New York: McGraw-Hill Book Company; 1986:106–238.
19. Reiber JHC, Zwet PMJ van der, Koning G, et al. Accuracy and precision of quantitative digital coronary arteriography: observer-, short- and medium-term variabilities. Cath Cardiovasc Diagn. 1993;28:187–98.
20. Reiber JHC, Boer A den, Serruys PW. Quality control in performing quantitative coronary arteriography. Am J Cardiac Imaging. 1989;3:172–9.
21. Jost S, Rafflenbeul W, Knop I, et al. Drug plasma levels and coronary vasodilation after isosorbide dinitrate chewing capsules. Eur Heart J. 1989;10(Suppl F):137–41.
22. Feldman RL, Marx JD, Pepine CJ, Conti CR. Analysis of coronary responses to various doses of intracoronary nitroglycerin. Circulation. 1982;66:321–7.
23. Gould KL, Martucci JP, Goldberg DI, et al. Short-term cholesterol lowering decreases size and severity of perfusion abnormalities by positron emission tomography after dipyridamole in patients with coronary artery disease. A potential noninvasive marker of healing coronary endothelium. Circulation. 1994;89:1530–8.
24. Cumberland DC. Low-osmolality contrast media in cardiac radiology. Invest Radiol. 1984; 19:S301–5.
25. Donadieu AM, Hartl C, Cardinal A, Bonnemain B. Incidence of ventricular fibrillation during coronary arteriography in the rabbit. A comparative study of isotonic Ioxaglate and Iohexol. Invest Radiol. 1987;22:106–10.
26. Jost S, Rafflenbeul W, Gerhardt U. Influence of ionic and non-ionic radiographic contrast media on the vasomotor tone of epicardial coronary arteries. Eur Heart J. 1989;10(Suppl F):60–5.
27. Koning G, Zwet PMJ van der, Land CD von, Reiber JHC. Angiographic assessment of dimensions of 6F and 7F Mallinckrodt Softouch® coronary contrast catheters from digital and cine arteriograms. Int J Card Imaging. 1992;8:153–61.
28. Reiber JHC, Jukema W, Boven A van, Houdt RM van, Lie KI, Bruschke AVG. Catheter sizes for quantitative coronary arteriography. Cath Cardiovasc Diagn. 1994;33:153–5.
29. Austen WG, Edwards JE, Frye RL, et al. A reporting system on patients evaluated for coronary artery disease. Report of the Ad Hoc Committee for Grading of Coronary Artery Disease, Council on Cardiovascular Surgery, American Heart Association, 1975. Circulation. 1975; 51–2:7–40.
30. Blankenhorn DH, Nessim SA, Johnson RL, Sanmarco ME, Azen SP, Cashin-Hemphill L. Beneficial effects of combined colestipol–niacin therapy on coronary atherosclerosis and coronary venous bypass grafts. JAMA. 1987;257:3233–40.
31. Brensike JF, Levy RI, Kelsey SF, et al. Effects of therapy with cholestyramine on progression of coronary arteriosclerosis: results of the NHLBI Type II coronary intervention study. Circulation. 1984;69:313–24.
32. Buchwald H, Matts JP, Fitch LL, et al. Program on the surgical control of the hyperlipidemias (POSCH): Design and methodology. J Clin Epidemiol. 1989;42:111–27.
33. Kane JP, Malloy MJ, Ports TA, Phillips NR, Diehl JC, Havel RJ. Regression of coronary atherosclerosis during treatment of familial hypercholesterolemia with combined drug regimens. JAMA. 1990;264:3007–12.
34. Ornish D, Brown SE, Scherwitz LW, et al. Can lifestyle changes reverse coronary heart disease? Lancet. 1990;336:129–33.

35. Brown BG, Albers JJ, Fisher LD, et al. Regression of coronary artery disease as a result of intensive lipid-lowering therapy in men with high levels of apolipoprotein B. N Engl J Med. 1990;323:1289–98.
36. Watts GF, Lewis B, Brunt JNH, et al. Effects on coronary artery disease of lipid-lowering diet, or diet plus cholestyramine, in the St. Thomas' Atherosclerosis Regression Study (STARS). Lancet. 1992;339:563–9.
37. Gibson CM, Sandor T, Stone PH, Pasternak RC, Rosner B, Sacks FM. Quantitative angiographic and statistical methods to assess serial changes in coronary luminal diameter and implications for atherosclerosis regression trials. Am J Cardiol. 1992;69:1286–90.
38. Schuler G, Hambrecht R, Schlierf G, et al. Regular physical exercise and low-fat diet. Effects on progression of coronary artery disease. Circulation. 1992;86:1–11.
39. Blankenhorn DH, Azen SP, Kramsch DM, et al. Coronary angiographic changes with lovastatin therapy. The Monitored Atherosclerosis Regression Study (MARS). Ann Intern Med. 1993;119:969–76.
40. Waters D, Higginson L, Gladstone P, et al. Effects of monotherapy with an HMG-CoA reductase inhibitor on the progression of coronary atherosclerosis as assessed by serial quantitative arteriography. The Canadian Coronary Atherosclerosis Intervention Trial. Circulation. 1994;89:959–68.
41. Haskell WL, Alderman EL, Fair JM, et al. Effects of intensive multiple risk factor reduction on coronary atherosclerosis and clinical cardiac events in men and women with coronary artery disease. The Stanford Coronary Risk Intervention Project (SCRIP). Circulation. 1994;89:975–90.
42. Dumont J-M. Effects of cholesterol reduction by simvastatin on progression of coronary atherosclerosis: design, baseline characteristics, and progress of the Multicentre Anti-Atheroma Study (MAAS). Cont Clin Trials. 1993;14:209–28.
43. Pitt B, Mancini GBJ, Ellis SG, Rosman HS, McGovern ME. Pravastatin limitation of atherosclerosis in the coronary arteries (PLACI). J Am Coll Cardiol. 1994;Feb:131A(Abstract).
44. Brown BG, Bolson E, Frimer M, Dodge HT. Quantitative coronary arteriography: estimation of dimensions, hemodynamic resistance, and atheroma mass of coronary artery lesions using the arteriogram and digital computation. Circulation. 1977;55:329–37.
45. Brown BG, Zhao X-Q, Sacco DE, Albers JJ. Lipid lowering and plaque regression. New insights into prevention of plaque disruption and clinical events in coronary disease. Circulation. 1993;87:1781–91.
46. Selzer RH, Shircore A, Lee PL, Hemphill L, Blankenhorn DH. A second look at quantitative coronary angiography: some unexpected problems. In: Reiber JHC, Serruys PW, editors. State of the art in quantitative coronary arteriography. Dordrecht: Kluwer Academic Publishers; 1986:125–43.
47. Lippolt P, Ehrhardt K, Riedel M, Rafflenbeul W, Lichtlen PR. Variability in quantitative coronary arteriography: higher precision by analysis in consecutive frames. J Am Coll Cardiol. 1994;Feb:209A(Abstract).
48. Syvänne M, Nieminen MS, Frick MH. Accuracy and precision of quantitative arteriography in the evaluation of coronary artery disease after coronary bypass surgery: a validation study. Int J Cardiac Imaging. 1994;10:243–52.
49. Gerbrands JJ. Segmentation of noisy images. Ph.D. Thesis, Delft University of Technology, 1988.

5. Is there a place for visual assessment?

L. CASHIN-HEMPHILL

Summary

This paper discusses prior criticism of human panel readings and presents the methodology of the Sanmarco/Blankenhorn 'GCS' along with its strengths and possible explanations of this strength.

Prior criticism of human panel readings

The ability of human panels to assess change in overall coronary atherosclerotic status over time has been much maligned. The most frequently cited reference is that of Detre et al. published in 1982[1]. It is useful, therefore, to examine this article closely. The human panelists were asked to assess whether change had taken place in individual lesions. They were asked whether change was definite, probable, or absent. They were also asked to determine the direction of change. Biostatisticians subsequently utilized an algorithm to compile these changes within a patient and determine the per-patient change status. This algorithm did not include either the location, the magnitude, or the 'meaning' of the changes taking place in the individual lesions. In essence, the humans were only allowed to perform as crude calipers, a function which, it is acknowledged, humans do not perform well. They were denied the opportunity to do that at which humans excel: to assign meaning to the changes taking place and to evaluate the overall clinical status of the patient. As an example, the progression of a lesion from 95% to 100% diameter stenosis is a definite change, but it is of little clinical significance. The biostatisticians in the Detre paper would assign equal weight to such a change as to a progression from 40% to 100% diameter stenosis. A human panel, if given the opportunity, would assign very different meanings to these two events. Another example is retrograde occlusion proximal to a total occlusion. Such a change is often quite dramatic, but is again recognized by the human 'neural net' as being of little clinical or prognostic significance.

The Sanmarco/Blankenhorn global change score (GCS)

It is more appropriate to look at the human panel GCS, developed by Drs. Sanmarco and Blankenhorn, to evaluate the reproducibility and usefulness of the human panel[2]. In the Sanmarco/Blankenhorn methodology, the human panelists not only reached consensus about the individual lesion changes, but also about

A.V.G. Bruschke et al. *(eds): Lipid-lowering therapy and progression of atherosclerosis, 65–70.*
© 1996 *Kluwer Academic Publishers.*

Table 5.1.   Interpanel agreement on GCS.

Level	Percent agreement
Perfect	71
≤1 Step	96
>1 Step	4

There was no instance of interpanel reverse direction of GCS.

the overall change score or GCS. The GCS incorporates the human interpretation or 'neural net' evaluation of the meaning of all the changes taking place. It is a seven-point score with three indicating maximal change, which, if in the direction of progression, would probably require revascularization. A score of one is a definite change, but of little clinical significance, and a score of two is intermediate. Thus the score ranges from −3 for maximal regression, through 0 to +3 for maximal progression. The reproducibility of the GCS has been tested and found to be far superior to that reported in the Detre paper[2]. Perfect inter-panel agreement on GCS occurred 71% of the time and agreement within one step 96% of the time. There was no instance of interpanel reversal of direction of GCS (regression becoming progression or vice versa) (Table 5.1). This compares with the statement in the Detre article that 'single-panel diagnosis can be said to be only 56% correct'. Other factors contributing to the improved reproducibility seen with the Sanmarco/Blankenhorn GCS are: improved film quality (the majority of films evaluated by readers in the Detre article were cut films) and the use of individualized drawings of the coronary tree (avoiding problems of nomenclature and 'realignment of lesions' necessary in the Detre article).

Strengths of the GCS

'The proof of the pudding is in the eating.' It is important to note that the GCS has provided highly statistically significant demonstration of treatment benefit in all three of the angiographic trials in which it has been employed: CLAS I[3], CLAS II[4], POSCH[5] and MARS[6]. Adding to its credibility, is the intuitively satisfying fact that there is progressive difference between treatment and control groups in CLAS I and II[4] and in POSCH at 3, 5, 7 and 10 years[5]. Finally, angiographic progression, as assessed by GCS, has been demonstrated to be a surrogate for future clinical cardiac events in both POSCH[7] and CLAS[8]. In the POSCH control group, 15% of no change/regressors by GCS experienced subsequent coronary death or non-fatal MI vs 33% of progressors ($p < 0.0001$). Interestingly, there was a residual treatment effect to ileal bypass which made GCS progression less predictive in the treated group but statistical significance was still reached. GCS was also predictive of CHD mortality (for trend $p = 0.003$) and even total mortality (for trend $p = 0.01$). Similarly, in the much smaller CLAS trial, there was a doubling in risk for future coronary events in progressors vs regressors by GCS (for trend $p < 0.01$). This ability to serve as a surrogate for future cardiac events is precisely the purpose of angiographic trials.

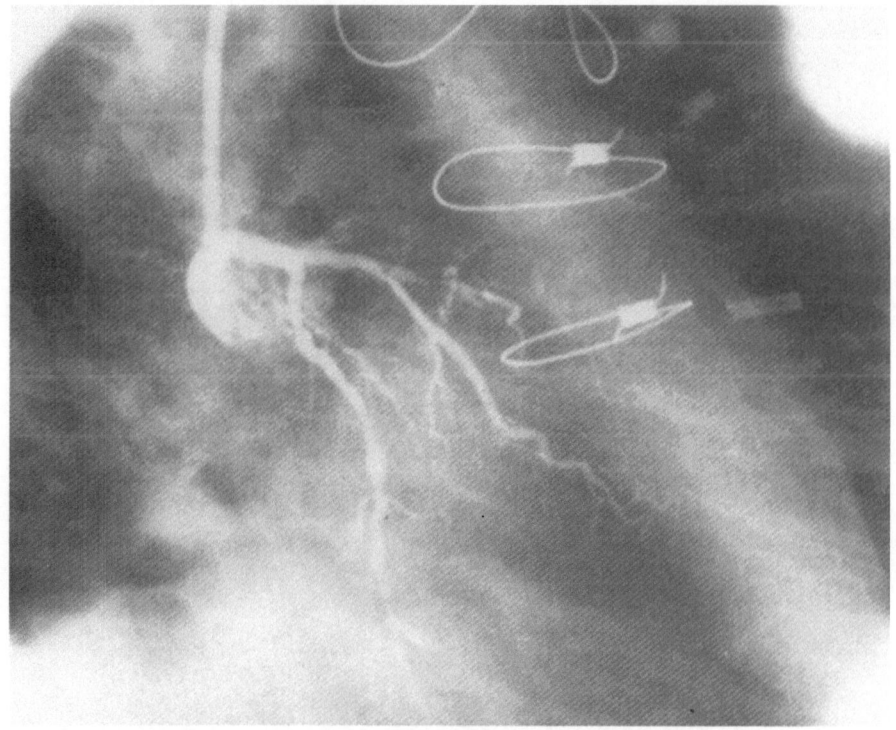

Figure 5.1. Subject DE in the MARS trial: diffuse disease in the circumflex with patent graft (not visualized here) at baseline.

Variables assessed by human readers but not by QCA

It is appropriate to ask what are the previously unquantified variables which the human 'neural net' evaluates and which quantitative coronary angiography (QCA) cannot. One possibility is the 'Glagov effect', the dilatation of coronary arteries which occurs with early atherosclerotic progression[9]. Such change would probably be disregarded by human readers but may be measured as 'regression' by QCA. Another possibility is demonstrated in a recent article by Kyriakidis et al. in Greece[10]. They looked at changes in flow and vessel size in the right coronary artery in subjects undergoing balloon angioplasty of the left anterior descending branch of the left coronary artery. During balloon inflation in the left anterior descending, they were able to demonstrate an increase in the diameter of the right coronary artery, acutely, of as much as 0.18 mm. In such cases, well-developed collaterals from the right coronary to the left anterior descending were present. Thus, an angiographic trial utilizing mean per-subject change in minimum lumen diameter as endpoint could be confounded. Progression in the left anterior descending could be negated by dilatation of segments in the right

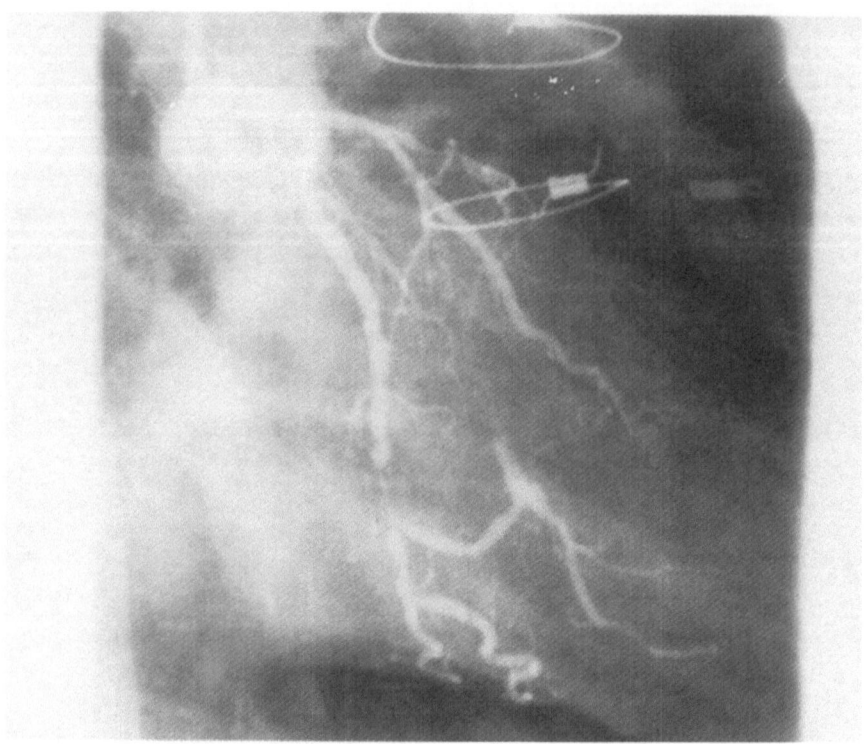

Figure 5.2.   Subject DE at two years: Circumflex – marginal graft has closed (note retrograde filling of pocket) and circumflex has regressed.

coronary artery. Again, in this situation, the dilatation of the right coronary artery, if noticed by the human panel, would be discounted as a compensatory change and the subject would be assigned a progression score.

A case in the MARS trial provides confirmation of the interaction between vessels that can occur as atherosclerosis progresses. Subject JD had a high-grade stenosis in the diagonal branch of the LAD at baseline. On follow-up angiogram, there was new total occlusion of the right coronary and circumflex. Collaterals had developed from the diagonal supplying both of these occluded vessels. Interestingly, the stenosis in the diagonal had regressed (human panel: 90% to 30%; QCA: 67% to 23% diameter stenosis). This raises the possibility of 'need-based' regression – regression induced by increased flow through a collateral supplying vessel. Again, human and QCA evaluation of the subjects overall status change could be discordant.

Another case, subject DE, had severe diffuse disease of the circumflex with a patent bypass to a marginal branch at baseline (Figure 5.1). On follow-up angiography (Figure 5.2), the graft had closed (note retrograde filling of graft pocket) and the circumflex demonstrated dramatic regression. Is the patient better or worse? Measurement alone, however accurate, does not answer this question.

Humans also excel at evaluating morphology of lesions. A recent abstract by Faxon and Detre[11] showed that visual assessments of PTCA sites were more predictive of long-term clinical success than quantitative coronary angiographic assessment. This was attributed to the ability of human readers to evaluate the meaning of morphological characteristics.

Conclusions

In conclusion, quantitative coronary angiography measures vessels accurately and reproducibly[12] but cannot make judgements about the meaning associated with those measures. Nor can quantitative coronary angiography 'see' the unexpected. The planned analysis of changes in collateral blood flow mentioned in the baseline paper of the nicardipine angiographic trial[13] is intriguing in this regard. Human panel analysis and quantitative coronary angiography should be seen as complementary or 'symbiotic' methodologies if we are to derive maximum information from serial angiographic trials.

References

1. Detre KM, Kelsey SF, Passamani ER, et al. Reliability of assessing change with sequential coronary angiography. Am Heart J. 1992;104:816–23.
2. Azen SP, Cashin-Hemphill L, Pogoda J, et al. Evaluation of human panelists in assessing coronary atherosclerosis. Arterioscler Thromb. 1991;11:385–94.
3. Blankenhorn DH, Nessim SA, Johnson RL, Sanmarco ME, Azen SP, Cashin-Hemphill L. Beneficial effects of combined colestipol–niacin therapy on coronary atherosclerosis and coronary venous bypass grafts [published erratum appears in JAMA. 1988;259:2698]. JAMA 1987;257:3233–40.
4. Cashin-Hemphill L, Mack WJ, Pogoda JM, Sanmarco ME, Azen SP, Blankenhorn DH. Beneficial effects of colestipol–niacin on coronary atherosclerosis. A 4-year follow-up. JAMA. 1990;264:3013–17.
5. Buchwald H, Varco RL, Matts JP, et al. Effect of partial ileal bypass surgery on mortality and morbidity from coronary heart disease in patients with hypercholesterolemia. Report of the Program on the Surgical Control of the Hyperlipidemias (POSCH). N Engl J Med. 1990;323:946–55.
6. Blankenhorn DH, Azen SP, Kramsch DM, et al. Coronary angiographic changes with lovastatin therapy. The Monitored Atherosclerosis Regression Study (MARS). The MARS Research Group. Ann Intern Med. 1993;119:969–76.
7. Buchwald H, Matts JP, Fitch LL, et al. Changes in sequential coronary arteriograms and subsequent coronary events. Surgical Control of the Hyperlipidemias (POSCH) Group. JAMA. 1992;268:1429–33.
8. Cashin-Hemphill L, Mack W, LaBree L, et al. Coronary progression predicts future cardiac events [abstract]. Circulation. 1993;88(4 Suppl):I363.
9. Glagov S, Weisenberg E, Zarins CK, Stankunavicius R, Kolettis GJ. Compensatory enlargement of human atherosclerotic coronary arteries. N Engl J Med. 1987;316:1371–5.
10. Kyriakidis MK, Petropoulakis PN, Tentolouris CA, et al. Relation between changes in blood flow of the contralateral coronary artery and the angiographic extent and function of recruitable collateral vessels arising from this artery during balloon coronary occlusion. J Am Coll Cardiol. 1994;23:869–78.

11. Faxon DP, Vogel R, Yeh W, Jacobs AK, Detre K. Visual angiographic readings are more predictive of a successful one year outcome than quanatitative angiographic readings (NHLBI PTCA Registry) [abstract]. J Am Coll Cardiol. 1993;21(2 Suppl A):339A.
12. Reiber JH, Serruys PW, Kooijman CJ, et al. Assessment of short-, medium-, and long-term variations in arterial dimensions from computer-assisted quantitation of coronary cineangiograms. Circulation. 1985;71:280–8.
13. Waters D, Freedman D, Lesperance J, et al. Design features of a controlled clinical trial to assess the effect of a calcium entry blocker upon the progression of coronary artery disease. Control Clin Trials. 1987;8:216–42.

6. Angiographic endpoints in progression trials

A. V. G. BRUSCHKE, J. W. JUKEMA, A. J. VAN BOVEN, E. T. BAL
J. H. C. REIBER, A. H. ZWINDERMAN

Summary

The use of different angiographic criteria represents one of the reasons why the results of angiographic trials are difficult to compare. In principle, this is an avoidable problem and therefore a serious attempt at standardization should be made. This chapter reviews the criteria which have been used in trials using quantitative coronary angiography and presents a proposal for standardization.

Introduction

All angiographic lipid intervention trials published after 1990 have used measurements derived from computer-assisted quantitative analysis as the primary endpoint[1-11]. However, due to a variety of factors, comparison of the outcomes of various studies remains cumbersome and, to a certain extent, impossible. These factors include variables which are difficult to influence, such as patient selection and baseline characteristics, duration of interval between studies, and choice of quantitative angiographic equipment. In addition, there are significant differences in angiographic criteria which have been used to assess progression and regression which, in principle, is an avoidable problem.

It is the purpose of this paper to examine the merits and limitations of different angiographic endpoints and to formulate recommendations for future studies.

General principles regarding the selection of angiographic endpoints

Categorically stated, progression or regression of coronary atherosclerosis may affect the vessel wall in either a focal or a global manner (Figure 6.1). If the changes are of a focal nature, then either existing lesions increase or decrease in severity or new localized narrowings develop. Most studies have used such focal changes as the sole primary endpoint which is not surprising because, traditionally, the severity of coronary atherosclerosis is depicted by the number and severity of narrowing lesions (often indicated as percentage reduction of lumen diameter). This is also related to the fact that only focal changes may be assessed fairly accurately by visual interpretation or with the help of electronic calipers and, if obstructive lesions are expressed in relative values (percentage narrowing), no calibration of the angiogram is required.

A.V.G. Bruschke et al. *(eds): Lipid-lowering therapy and progression of atherosclerosis, 71–77*
© 1996 *Kluwer Academic Publishers.*

Mean Segm. Diam. vs Min. Obstr. Diameter

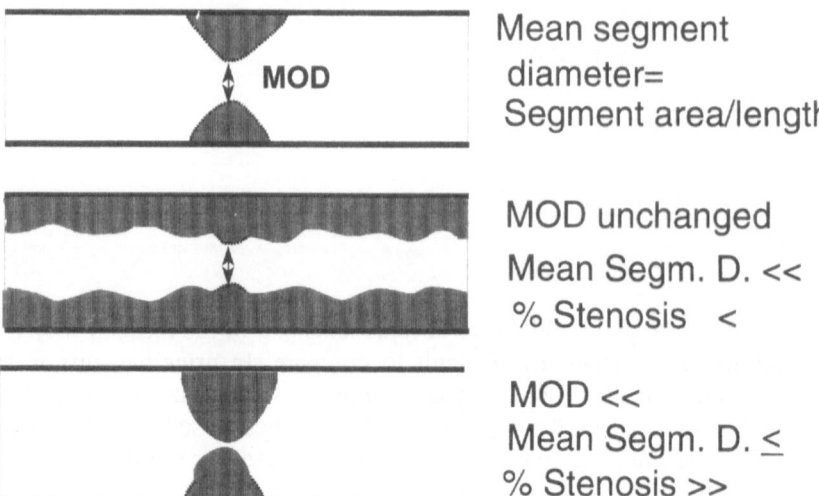

Mean segment
diameter=
Segment area/length

MOD unchanged
Mean Segm. D. <<
% Stenosis <

MOD <<
Mean Segm. D. ≤
% Stenosis >>

Figure 6.1. Diagrammatic representation of different forms of progression of coronary atherosclerosis. If progression is of a diffuse nature (middle panel), the mean segment diameter will decrease whereas the minimum obstruction diameter may remain unchanged. If progression is of a focal nature (lower panel) it is mainly the minimum obstruction diameter which changes. Usually, but not always, the two manifestations occur in combination.

However, if progression or regression affects the vessel wall in a diffuse or global manner, it is possible that the severity of existing lesions remains unchanged. In such cases, it is even possible that the percentage narrowing decreases because the diameter of the reference segment (the assumed normal portion of the vessel wall) also decreases. This distinction between focal and global changes has more than purely theoretical significance because it is conceivable that a certain drug has little influence on established atherosclerotic lesions but does influence the overall atherosclerotic involvement or vice versa.

Therefore, the primary angiographic endpoint or endpoints should account for both manifestations of progression. Focal changes may be adequately characterized by changes in the narrowest diameter within a lesion which we will call the minimum obstruction diameter (MOD). To avoid the problem induced by changes in the reference diameter, MOD should preferably be given in absolute values. Global changes, by virtue of their diffuse nature, primarily affect the mean diameter of a coronary artery or segment thereof. Like some other investigators, we have used the mean segment diameter (MSD) as a parameter to describe such changes. Obviously, MSD can only be adequately expressed in absolute numbers. Because global changes may not affect MOD and, conversely, focal changes may not change MSD appreciably, two primary angiographic endpoints, reflecting both aspects of progression, are needed to analyse adequately progression and regression. From a statistical standpoint, this may be cumbersome; however, at present, there appears to be no easier, yet adequate, solution.

Development of new lesions

In several studies, the development of new lesions has been used as a (usually secondary) criterion for progression[3,6,12]. However, this is hardly an adequate description of what is demonstrated by angiography. First, the fact that, in most studies, only patients with significant coronary atherosclerosis are included makes it difficult to be certain that angiographically normal-looking segments are indeed free from disease. In the second place, minor lesions may easily escape angiographic recognition. This technical aspect plays a role particularly in QCA because quantitative analyses are based upon single frames in which the influence of background noise, among other things caused by quantum noise, is more marked than in the moving cine angiogram[13], which makes it difficult to distinguish between a smooth vessel wall and minor irregularities. Consequently, in QCA studies, vessel wall irregularities causing less than 20% narrowing are often disregarded. To overcome this problem, some investigators have used specific criteria to define new lesions, e.g. no lesion or less than 20% narrowing at first angiogram in combination with an increase of narrowing by at least 0.2 or 0.4 mm[7,12,], or the development of lesions causing >20% narrowing if there is an increase in narrowing of at least 15%[6]. These definitions make it possible to understand what the investigators actually mean. However, if these criteria are used, the term 'new lesions' is no longer appropriate. We feel that, with current techniques, it is more accurate to use a descriptive terminology, such as 'progression in normal or slightly abnormal segments' instead of the term 'new lesion'.

New occlusions and segments distal to occlusions

If a segment becomes occluded, it is obvious that the MOD is reduced to zero. To evaluate correctly the change in MSD in the case of a new occlusion is more complicated. Some investigators have assigned a value of zero to the MSD of the newly occluded segment[6]. This, however, may lead to serious overestimation of the significance of new occlusions, e.g. progression from subtotal narrowing to occlusion may cause an unrealistically large change of MSD. Other options, such as measuring the mean diameter of the portion of the arterial segment that is still open, are hardly meaningful. Therefore, it appears that there is only one possibility left; that is to exclude from the MSD analysis entirely segments which have become occluded during follow-up. New occlusions are then only accounted for by changes in MOD or they may be treated as a separate category.

Segments distal to occlusions (either at baseline or follow-up) cannot be adequately assessed, even in the presence of good collateral flow. This is clearly demonstrated by postoperative studies in which occluded portions of coronary arteries are supplied by bypass grafts; often the distal artery appears to be wider than anticipated preoperatively or lesions may become visible which could not be recognized before. There appears to be consensus that arterial segments distal to occlusions should not be included in analysis of progression although this is not specifically mentioned in several studies.

Segments influenced by percutaneous transluminal coronary angioplasty (PTCA) or coronary artery bypass surgery (CABG)

If it is the purpose of a study to assess the influence of non-mechanical interventions (drugs, diet, etc.) on progression and regression of coronary atherosclerosis, then segments or lesions modified by PTCA or CABG should be excluded from the primary analysis (they may, of course, be included in a separate analysis). If PTCA or other catheter intervention is performed, we suggest that the entire artery concerned should be excluded because, apart from the treated lesion, all portions have usually been subjected to the potential trauma of guide-wire manipulation. For patients who underwent CABG, we used, in REGRESS, the following algorithm which provided satisfactory results: if a particular segment in a coronary artery was grafted and no occlusions were present at baseline coronary arteriography, all segments in the same artery were considered to be influenced by the bypass graft; if occlusions were present, all segments which were filled directly by the native system were considered to be not influenced by the bypass graft and only the segments distal to the occlusion were considered to be influenced[11].

Relative versus absolute measurements and use of vasodilators

As explained above, measurements in absolute values are mandatory for some parameters (e.g. change in MSD) and to be preferred for other parameters (e.g. change in degree of narrowing) although we recognize that the extensive clinical experience gained with the relative measurements (percentage narrowing) represents a certain advantage. Absolute diameter measurements require calibration of the angiogram. A convenient way to do so is to use the catheter as a scaling device. The actual catheter size may be measured but using the manufacturer's specifications yields satisfactory results with some catheters[14].

An important aspect of study design concerns the administration of vasodilators before or during coronary arteriography. Recently, it has been shown that lowering of serum cholesterol may restore endothelial function and consequently reduce vasomotor tone[15]. If no endothelium-independent vasolidators are given, this can lead to differences in angiographic outcome between treatment groups which are not solely due to progression or regression. Unfortunately, in many studies[2,7,9,10], vasodilators were not or not consistently used and therefore the angiographic beneficial effect of lipid-lowering might be partly due to diminished vasomotor tone.

The angiographic data as continuous or categorical variables

Using the angiographic data as categorical variables, that is separating patients into progressors, regressors, patients showing no change and those showing a mixed reaction, has the advantage that it characterizes the reaction observed in patients in a clinically meaningful manner. The main problem related to this type of analysis is that such a division requires that threshold values to define pro- and regression be adopted (e.g. two times the standard deviation of the measurements) and thus smaller changes, even if they are numerous, are not included in the analysis. Therefore, if it is the main objective of the study to determine whether there is a difference between placebo and treatment groups, it is more appropriate to use the angiographic data as continuous variables. One should realize, however, that this may lead to difficult-to-interpret results in terms of individual clinical benefit. If, for instance, a patient shows progression of 1 mm of a certain lesion and a total of 10 segments are analysed, then the average change for such a patient will be 0.1 mm if the other segments remain the same. The treatment effect may be further 'diluted' if average values for groups of patients are determined. Using the angiographic data as continuous variables, it is also difficult to account for simultaneously occurring progression and regression, which may happen in an individual patient or with a group of patients. In this respect, a categorical approach has the advantage that it allows identification of 'mixed responders' although it does not provide an index of the net effect of both progression and regression in patients either. It would seem that the only way to describe such changes adequately is to characterize patients by two numbers reflecting total progression and total regression respectively.

Primary vs secondary endpoints and definition of subgroups

Most angiographic studies have used primary and secondary endpoints. There is some merit in this: looking at the angiographic changes from different standpoints may lead to a better understanding of the dynamics of progression and regression and the factors which may influence this process. However, investigators may be inclined to base their conclusions on secondary endpoints if the primary endpoints fail to demonstrate a significant treatment effect or, conversely, if a primary endpoint is positive, the secondary endpoints tend to be neglected if they are negative. Considering the large number of potential endpoints, this may easily lead to unjustified conclusions.

The same is true for subgroup analyses. For instance, in one study[1] the primary endpoint, namely average change of % stenosis, was not significantly different between placebo and treatment groups but a division of lesions causing respectively more or less than 50% narrowing showed a significant treatment effect in the first category. The authors considered this evidence of a beneficial effect of treatment; however, such results should be interpreted with great caution. This is demonstrated by another study which showed the opposite, that is an overall positive effect but practically no treatment effect in lesions causing more than 50% narrowing[7].

Shortcomings in reporting of analysis of coronary angiograms

The examples shown above were taken from reports in which it was stated how certain problems were dealt with. However, in a surprisingly large number of reports, the methods used to analyse the angiographic findings are insufficiently described. This adds considerably to the difficulty of comparing studies.

Conclusions and recommendations

Based upon theoretical considerations and experiences obtained in REGRESS[11], we come to the following conclusions and recommendations for angiographic intervention trials:

1. To describe adequately changes in the vessel wall, the primary endpoints should account for focal changes and global changes. Parameters like 'minimum obstruction diameter' and 'mean segment diameter' have proven merit.

2. Endothelium-independent vasodilators should be given before every catheterization. This should be repeated if necessary.

3. The term 'new lesion' should be avoided and, if a separate description is desirable, be replaced by 'progression in normal or slightly abnormal segments'.

4. In the primary analysis of progression in angiographic trials, segments influenced by bypass surgery or PTCA should be excluded (unless the study was designed to study such changes).

5. To demonstrate a treatment effect, using the angiographic data as continuous variables (preferably representing absolute values) is most appropriate.

6. Results relating to secondary endpoints and subgroup analyses should be interpreted with great caution.

References

1. Blankenhorn DH, Azen SP, Kramsch DM, et al. Coronary angiographic changes with lovastatin therapy. The Monitored Atherosclerosis Regression Study (MARS). The MARS Research Group. Ann Intern Med. 1993;119:969–76.
2. Brown G, Albers JJ, Fisher LD, et al. Regression of coronary artery disease as a result of intensive lipid-lowering therapy in men with high levels of apolipoprotein B. N Engl J Med. 1990;323:1289–98.
3. Haskell WL, Alderman EL, Fair JM, et al. Effects of intensive multiple risk factor reduction on coronary atherosclerosis and clinical cardiac events in men and women with coronary artery disease. The Stanford Coronary Risk Intervention Project (SCRIP). Circulation. 1994;89:975–90.

4. Kane JP, Malloy MJ, Ports TA, Phillips NR, Diehl JC, Havel RJ. Regression of coronary atherosclerosis during treatment of familial hypercholesterolemia with combined drug regimens. JAMA. 1990;264:3007–12.
5. Pitt B, Mancini GB, Ellis SG, Rosman HS, McGovern ME. Pravastatin limitation of atherosclerosis in the coronary arteries (PLAC I) [abstract]. J Am Coll Cardiol. 1994;23 Special issue:131A.
6. The MAAS Investigators. Effect of simvastatin on coronary atheroma: the Multicentre Anti-Atheroma Study (MAAS) [published erratum appears in Lancet. 1994;344:762]. Lancet. 1994;344:633–8.
7. Waters D, Higginson L, Gladstone P, et al. Effects of monotherapy with an HMG-CoA reductase inhibitor on the progression of coronary atherosclerosis as assessed by serial quantitative arteriography. The Canadian Coronary Atherosclerosis Intervention Trial. Circulation. 1994;89:959–68.
8. Sacks FM, Pasternak RC, Gibson CM, Rosner B, Stone PH. Effect on coronary atherosclerosis of decrease in plasma cholesterol concentrations in normocholesterolaemic patients. Harvard Atherosclerosis Reversibility Project (HARP) Group. Lancet. 1994;344:1182–6.
9. Schuler G, Hambrecht R, Schlierf G, et al. Regular physical exercise and low-fat diet. Effects on progression of coronary artery disease. Circulation. 1992;86:1–11.
10. Watts GF, Lewis B, Brunt JN, et al. Effects on coronary artery disease of lipid-lowering diet, or diet plus cholestyramine, in the St Thomas' Atherosclerosis Regression Study (STARS). Lancet. 1992;339:563–9.
11. Jukema JW, Bruschke AV, van Boven AJ, et al. Effects of lipid lowering by pravastatin on progression and regression of coronary artery disease in symptomatic men with normal to moderately elevated serum cholesterol levels. The Regression Growth Evaluation Statin Study (REGRESS). Circulation. 1995;91:2528–40.
12. Quinn TG, Alderman EL, McMillan A, Haskell W. Development of new coronary atherosclerotic lesions during a 4-year multifactor risk reduction program: the Stanford Coronary Risk Intervention Project (SCRIP). J Am Coll Cardiol. 1994;24:900–8.
13. Bruschke AV, Padmos I, Buis B, Van Benthem A. Arteriographic evaluation of small coronary arteries. J Am Coll Cardiol. 1990;15:784–9.
14. Reiber JH, Jukema W, van Boven A, van Houdt RM, Lie KI, Bruschke AV. Catheter sizes for quantitative coronary arteriography. Cathet Cardiovasc Diagn. 1994;33:153–5; discussion 156.
15. Gould KL, Martucci JP, Goldberg DI, et al. Short-term cholesterol lowering decreases size and severity of perfusion abnormalities by positron emission tomography after dipyridamole in patients with coronary artery disease. A potential noninvasive marker of healing coronary endothelium. Circulation. 1994;89:1530–8.

PART THREE

Angiographic lipid-lowering clinical trials

7. The Cholesterol Lowering Atherosclerosis Study (CLAS)

L. CASHIN-HEMPHILL

Summary

The Cholesterol Lowering Atherosclerosis Study (CLAS) was a landmark serial angiographic trial. It was the first randomized controlled prospective trial to conclusively demonstrate the angiographic benefit of lipid lowering therapy, first at two and subsequently more pronounced at four years. Recently, long-term clinical follow-up has been completed.

Study design/lipid response

The Cholesterol Lowering Atherosclerosis Study (CLAS)[1,2] at the University of Southern California was conducted between 1980 and 1987. Elective baseline angiography was followed by two-year angiography in 162 participants and four-year angiography in 103 participants. The treated group received niacin 4–12 g/day plus colestipol 30 g/day. The CLAS study population consisted of men between the ages of 40 and 59 who had had previous coronary artery bypass graft surgery. The entry cholesterol range was from 185 to 350 mg/dl (average 246 mg/dl). The changes in lipid levels during the trial were the greatest and were maintained for the longest period of any angiographic trial to date. The total cholesterol of the drug group dropped 27% to 178 mg/dl and that of the placebo group 4% to 233 mg/dl. The HDL-cholesterol of the drug group increased 37% to 60 mg/dl while the placebo group showed no change. The LDL-cholesterol fell 43% from 170 to 96 mg/dl in the drug-treated group and that of the placebo group dropped 4% to 160 mg/dl. Finally, the triglycerides of the drug group dropped 22% and the placebo group 6% throughout the four years.

Two- and four-year angiographic results

The baseline and follow-up angiograms were read by an independent panel of expert angiographers. The film pairs – baseline vs two years and baseline vs four years – were read side-by-side and the angiographers were blind, not only to the drug vs placebo status of the patient, but also to the temporal order of the films. Based on their overall assessment of change in both the native coronary arteries and the bypass grafts, the angiographers were asked to assign a global change score to each film pair: 0 – no demonstrable change; 1 – definitely discernible,

A.V.G. Bruschke et al. *(eds): Lipid-lowering therapy and progression of atherosclerosis, 81–106*
© 1996 *Kluwer Academic Publishers.*

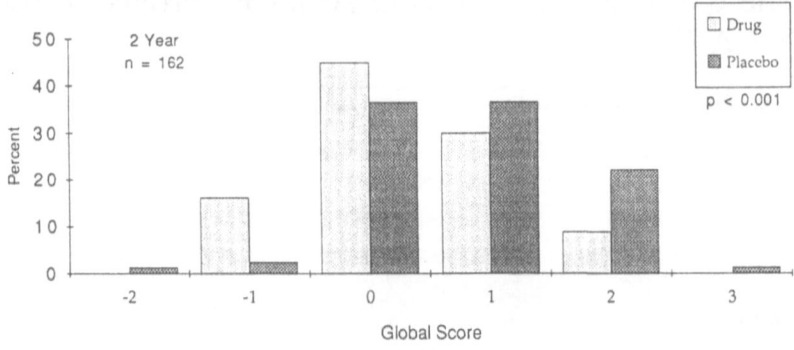

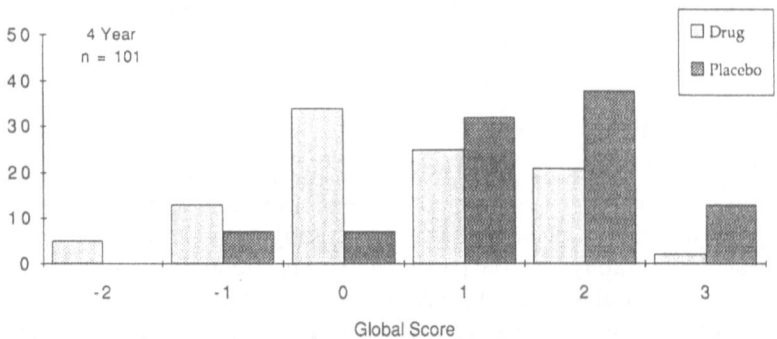

Figure 7.1.   Assessment of overall angiographic change at two and four years in the cholesterol lowering atherosclerosis study. (A positive global score = progression.)

2 – intermediate and 3 – extreme. They were also asked to designate a plus or a minus sign depending on whether they thought the right-hand film was worse or better than the left-hand film. After all the film pairs were read, the blinding to the temporal order of the angiograms was broken and global change scores, from –3 for extreme regression to +3 for extreme progression, were tallied. At two years, the distribution of global scores for the drug group shifted to the left – indicating stability or regression – compared with the placebo group (Figure 7.1). At four years, this gap widened: 13% of placebo patients showed extreme progression vs 2% of the drug-treated group. At the same time, 50% of drug patients remained stable or improved vs only 15% of placebo patients. The average global score at two years in the drug group was 0.4 and at four years 0.5. For the placebo group, the average global score was 0.8 at two years and increased to 1.4 at four years. This growing disparity in global score was based on an increasing difference in changes taking place in the native arteries and bypass grafts (Table 7.1). After two years, 10% of drug vs 22% of placebo patients developed new lesions in native arteries. By the end of four years, these numbers were 14 and

Table 7.1. Progression of lesions and development of new lesions at two and four years in the cholesterol lowering atherosclerosis study.

	CLAS I (2 years)			CLAS II (4 years)		
	Drug	Placebo	p	Drug	Placebo	p
Native vessels						
% Subjects with new lesions	10.0	22.0	(0.03)	14.3	40.4	(0.001)
% Subjects with progressing lesions	43.8	56.0	(>0.05)	44.6	74.5	0.001
Number of progressing lesions/subject	1.0	1.4	(0.03)	0.9	2.0	(0.0002)
Bypass grafts						
% Subjects with new lesions	18.0	30.0	(0.04)	16.0	38.3	(0.006)

Table 7.2. Treatment group comparisons of number of subjects with events, event rate, and % reduction in event rate.

	Drug group		Placebo group			
	Number of subjects	Event rate/100 y	Number of subjects	Event rate/100 y	% Reduction with drug vs placebo	p value*
All coronary events	22	4.37	34	7.60	42	0.03
MI and death	8	1.48	21	4.18	64	0.007
Coronary death	2	0.36	6	1.07	67	0.16
MI	7	1.29	19	3.78	66	0.008

*Mantel-Cox.

40, respectively. The percentage of patients with at least one lesion progressing in the native vessels was 44 in the drug-treatment group vs 56 in the placebo group at two years. At four years, the drug group showed no significant change while three quarters of placebo patients had at least one lesion progressing. The average number of progressing lesions per subject among placebo patients was slightly greater than the drug group in CLAS I but more than twice as many in CLAS II. In the bypass grafts, there was also a significant and widening difference in the percentage of subjects with new lesions, favouring the drug-treated group. QCA analysis of the full CLAS I cohort is confirmatory of those results. The mean per-subject change in % diameter stenosis in the drug-treated group was +0.35 (±5.47) vs +2.65 (±5.47) in the placebo group ($p < 0.01$; unpublished results).

Long-term follow-up

Recently, up to ten years of clinical follow-up has been completed on the CLAS population (median follow-up, seven years after second angiogram)[3]. Cardiovascular event data collected over this time period are: symptom related revascularization, non-fatal myocardial infarction and cardiac death. Treatment group comparisons of number of subjects with events, event rates and % reduction of events for drug vs placebo are presented in Table 7.2. The drug group had fewer subjects with myocardial infarction, cardiac death, combined

Table 7.3. Relative risks for all coronary events adjusted for treatment group and CLAS II continuation status.

	Relative risk (95% CI)	*p*
GCS		0.007*
Regression	1.0	—
No change	1.7 (0.5, 5.7)	0.40
Progression	2.3 (0.7, 7.8)	0.17
QCA change in % stenosis		<0.001*
<−2.4	1.0	—
−2.4−4.4	2.8 (1.1, 7.4)	0.03
≥4.4	5.2 (1.9, 13.9)	0.001
All lesions†	2.4 (1.5, 3.7)	<0.001
Native arteries	1.5 (1.1, 2.2)	0.02
Bypass grafts	1.6 (1.2, 2.1)	0.001

*Likelihood ratio test for trend; †relative risk per 10% change in % stenosis.

MI and cardiac death and all cardiac events including revascularization. The percentage reduction in event rate, which takes into account time to event, was 42% for all events, 64% for MI plus cardiac death, 67% for cardiac death alone, and 66% for MI alone. The relative risks for all coronary events by global change score and change in % stenosis by quantitative coronary angiography are presented in Table 7.3. It can be seen that both global change score and QCA are predictive of future cardiac events as well as QCA of native arteries vs bypass grafts.

Conclusion

In conclusion, short-term angiographic benefit of niacin/colestipol therapy has been demonstrated in CLAS both by human panel analysis and quantitative coronary angiography. This short-term benefit with both endpoints is predictive of long-term cardiovascular event reduction.

References

1. Blankenhorn DH, Nessim SA, Johnson RL, Sanmarco ME, Azen SP, Cashin-Hemphill L. Beneficial effects of combined colestipol−niacin therapy on coronary or atherosclerosis and coronary venous bypass grafts [published erratum appears in JAMA. 1988;259:2698]. JAMA. 1987;257:3233−40.
2. Cashin-Hemphill L, Mack WJ, Pogoda JM, Sanmarco ME, Azen SP, Blankenhorn DH. Beneficial effects of colestipol−niacin on coronary atherosclerosis. A 4-year follow-up. JAMA. 1990;264:3013−17.
3. Cashin-Hemphill L, Mack WJ, LaBree L, et al. Coronary progression predicts future cardiac events [abstract]. Circulation. 1993;88(4 Suppl):I363.

8. Clinical efficacy and safety of pravastatin treatment in symptomatic patients – the REGRESS trial

J. W. JUKEMA, A. J. VAN BOVEN, J. H. C. REIBER,
A. H. ZWINDERMAN, K. I. LIE and A. V. G. BRUSCHKE on behalf of
the REGRESS Study Group, Interuniversity Cardiology Institute, Utrecht,
The Netherlands

Summary

Intensive lowering of serum cholesterol may retard progression of coronary
atherosclerosis in selected groups of patients. However, in almost all studies,
patients with a (nearly) normal serum cholesterol level as well as patients who
were likely to undergo a cardiac revascularization procedure have been excluded
from the trials. Thus, few data are available about the potential benefit of serum
cholesterol reduction in the broad range of patients with coronary atherosclerosis
and normal to moderately elevated serum cholesterol levels, who undergo
various forms of treatment. The Regression Growth Evaluation Statin Study
(REGRESS) addresses this group of patients.

REGRESS is a double-blind placebo-controlled multicentre study to assess
the effect of two years' treatment with the HMG-CoA reductase inhibitor,
pravastatin, on progression and regression of coronary atherosclerosis in 885
male patients with a serum cholesterol between 4 and 8 mmol/L (155 and
310 mg/dl) using quantitative coronary arteriography. Clinical events were also
analysed and an extensive safety analysis was performed.

REGRESS showed that, in symptomatic men with significant coronary atherosclerosis and normal to moderately elevated serum cholesterol, undergoing
various forms of treatment, pravastatin slows progression of coronary
atherosclerosis and reduces the number of new clinical events. This can be
achieved in a relatively easy and well-tolerated manner. No serious side effects
were recorded during the pravastatin therapy, and the incidence of minor side
effects was less than 1%.

Introduction

Several studies have demonstrated that intensive lowering of serum total
cholesterol or low density lipoprotein (LDL) cholesterol may retard progression
of coronary atherosclerosis in selected groups of patients[1-13]. However, in most
studies, patients with a (nearly) normal serum cholesterol level as well as
patients who were likely to undergo a cardiac revascularization procedure were
excluded from the trials. Therefore, much less is known about the potential
benefit of serum cholesterol reduction in the broad range of patients with coronary

A.V.G. Bruschke et al. *(eds): Lipid-lowering therapy and progression of atherosclerosis, 85–106.*
© 1996 *Kluwer Academic Publishers.*

atherosclerosis who have normal to moderately elevated serum cholesterol levels and undergo various forms of primary treatment, including medical management, percutaneous transluminal coronary angioplasty (PTCA) or coronary artery bypass surgery (CABG). The Regression Growth Evaluation Statin Study (REGRESS) specifically addresses this large group of patients which represents the majority of patients seen in clinical practice. The effect of lipid reduction by the 3-hydroxy-3-methylglutaryl-coenzyme A (HMG-CoA) reductase inhibitor, pravastatin, was assessed in a randomized study design using quantitative coronary arteriography to determine the effect of two years of treatment on progression and regression of coronary atherosclerosis.

Since HMG-CoA reductase inhibitors have now been widely approved and marketed for therapeutic use for a growing number of indications, and safety features of a (secondary) prevention drug are of great importance for evaluating the (non-financial) cost – benefit ratio, an extensive safety analysis of pravastatin treatment within the REGRESS study was performed. The safety aspects together with the clinical and angiographic results of the REGRESS study will be discussed in this chapter.

Methods

Study design

REGRESS is a double-blind placebo-controlled multicentre study to assess the effect of two years' treatment with the HMG-CoA reductase inhibitor, pravastatin, on progression and regression of angiographically documented coronary atherosclerosis in male patients with a serum cholesterol between 4 and 8 mmol/L (155 – 310 mg/dl). The study was conducted under the auspices of the Interuniversity Cardiology Institute of the Netherlands (ICIN), Utrecht, the Netherlands. Eleven hospitals in the Netherlands participated in the study (seven university and four non-university hospitals). Each participating hospital appointed a centre co-ordinator who was responsible for patient recruitment, conduct of the study and data collection. The trial was approved by the ethics committees of each of the participating institutions. Written informed consent was obtained from each patient.

Following certification, according to the inclusion and exclusion criteria, the patients were divided into one of three groups according to the type of primary management elected at the participating centre. The groups were: a percutaneous transluminal coronary angioplasty (PTCA) group, a coronary artery bypass grafting (CABG) group and a medical management group. In each group patients were randomized to receive pravastatin, 40 mg once daily, or placebo.

Patients and physicians were blinded to the result of randomization throughout the study.

The complete enrolment procedure and quantitative coronary angiography methods are described in detail elsewhere[14].

Endpoints of the trial

The angiographic endpoints of this trial were defined before the study was unblinded. The primary endpoint of the trial was a comparison between the pravastatin and placebo groups for:

1. Change in average mean obstruction segment diameter (MSD) on a by-patient basis, and
2. Change in average minimum obstruction diameter (MOD) on a by-patient basis.

Because PTCA and CABG procedures may influence progression considerably, we excluded, in the primary analysis, lesions and segments modified or conceivably modified by PTCA or CABG[14].

Clinical events during the trial

The following clinical events were analysed, according to prespecified criteria[14]:

1. Myocardial infarction (fatal or non-fatal);
2. Coronary heart disease death (other than known fatal myocardial infarction);
3. Non-scheduled PTCA or CABG: PTCA and CABG not planned in the original group division of REGRESS (e.g. PTCA in the medical management group, CABG in the PTCA group, second PTCA in the PTCA group, etc.);
4. Stroke and transient ischaemic attack (TIA);
5. Death (all other).

Investigational plan safety monitoring

Adverse events

Clinical adverse events (AEs) were defined as illnesses, signs or symptoms which appeared or worsened during the course of the study. Investigators were instructed to document the occurrence of clinical AEs, both those volunteered by the subjects and those elicited by general questioning, at all scheduled visits. All investigators were required to report the nature, severity and action taken relating to any AEs and to express their opinion regarding the relationship between the AE and the study medication.

Serious adverse events (SAEs) were defined as those AEs that were fatal, immediately life-threatening, permanently disabling, cancer, associated with an overdose, or those that required overnight or prolonged hospitalization. In such cases, the investigator, in addition to filling out the AE page of the case record form (CRF), was to send immediately to the medical monitor a completed serious adverse event report (SAER). The SAERs were completed whenever an SAE occurred, regardless of its attribution to study therapy. The investigator was required to telephone immediately or rapifax any SAE that was not cited in the Investigator brochure, in addition to sending in a SAER and filling out the CRF.

Based on the investigator's attribution, AEs were classified as adverse drug experiences (ADEs) or concomitant events (CEs). Adverse drug experiences were defined as those events occurring during double-blind therapy that were regarded by the investigator as related, possibly related, or of undetermined relationship to the study medication. Concomitant events were defined as those AEs that the investigator considered unrelated to the study medication. Laboratory abnormalities could have been either ADEs or CEs, based upon the opinion of the investigator. Randomization group-scheduled PTCAs and CABGs were collected in the AE database and were included in the AE summary tables, but were not included in the evaluation of serious adverse events.

Adverse events that began or worsened after randomization were considered treatment emergent. Adverse events that began in the dietary lead-in phase and recurred after randomization were not considered treatment emergent, unless either or both of the following occurred afterward: the AE worsened or the investigator classified the AE as an ADE (an ADE is always considered of greater intensity than a CE). Recurrent or continuing treatment-emergent AEs were counted once only at the time of highest intensity, as indicated above.

Laboratory tests

The Lipid Reference Laboratory of the Central and Clinical Laboratory of AZR Hospital Dijkzigt, provided all lipoprotein values for high density lipoprotein cholesterol (HDL-C), total cholesterol (total-C), and triglycerides (TGs). The laboratory tests listed below were performed after an overnight fast of at least ten hours:

- Plasma lipoproteins: total cholesterol (total-C), high density lipoprotein cholesterol (HDL-C), triglycerides (TGs); low density lipoprotein cholesterol (LDL-C) was calculated with the formula: LDL-C (mmol/L) = total-C − [HDL-C + (0.45 × TG)].

- Haematology: haematocrit, haemoglobin, white blood cell (WBC) count, WBC differential, platelet estimate.

- Clinical chemistry: aspartate aminotransferase (AST), alanine amino-transferase (ALT), and creatine kinase (CK), blood urea nitrogen (BUN), creatinine, total protein, glucose, and, if indicated, tri-iodothyronine (T_3), thyroxine (T_4), and thyroid stimulating hormone (TSH).

- Urinalysis (UA): performed on a freshly voided morning specimen.

Investigators reviewed results of the laboratory tests and entered any clinically relevant laboratory abnormalities on the AE page of the CRF, indicating the relationship of the abnormal result to the test drugs. Any safety laboratory test with an abnormality that met the criteria for marked abnormalities (MA), as defined in Appendix A, and that could possibly be attributed to the test drug was repeated immediately. If the repeat value was abnormal, the test was repeated as appropriate (or at intervals not greater than every 2 weeks if the drug was discontinued) until the value returned to normal or the abnormality was judged due to other causes.

Other safety assessments

Other safety tests included a complete medical history, physical examinations, a chest X-ray, and 12-lead electrocardiograms (ECG) at specified intervals during the study.

Presentation of safety data

The extent of exposure to study medications, deaths, discontinuations from therapy due to AEs, treatment-emergent AEs, MAs occurring during double-blind therapy are provided in the Safety results section.

Medically important AEs and MAs that qualify for detailed description are presented in the relevant section discussing that body system or laboratory parameter and include:

1. Serious AEs or MAs as defined earlier;
2. Adverse events or MAs that were statistically significantly different in their rate of occurrence between treatment groups;
3. Adverse events or MAs that were potentially clinically significant but did not meet the criteria for serious adverse events listed above;
4. Adverse events or MAs for which there was significant precedent in animal models or that had been reported in association with compounds similar to the investigational drug.

Statistical analyses

Baseline characteristics of the different patient groups were compared and tested for balance with Pearson's Chi-square test, Student's t-test or one-way analysis of variance (ANOVA), where appropriate. The effects of treatment on the lipid levels were assessed with mixed model ANOVA, with random patients effects and fixed treatment and time effects. Kaplan–Meier curves were used to estimate time to first coronary event or death, and the treatment groups were compared using the log rank test and Cox regression model. Finally, the angiographic effect of treatment on MSD was assessed using analysis of covariance with baseline levels as covariates. The effect of treatment on MOD was analysed with non-parametric methods (Mann–Whitney test, rank ANOVA) because of the extremely skewed distribution of MOD. Therefore, we presented the median MOD and the median change of MOD to illustrate treatment effects. Differences between hospitals with respect to these effects were investigated using mixed model ANOVA. A p value of 0.05 or less was considered to be significant. The SPSS and BMDP (1L,2L,5V) statistical packages were used to perform the calculations.

With regard to the safety analyses, the AE data set included all randomized subjects and the events were counted up to and including 30 days after discontinuation of therapy. The clinical laboratory data set included all available data.

Clinical AEs were coded using the Bristol–Myers Squibb dictionary which is based on the International Classification of Disease (ICD-9) dictionary. Every code was mapped to a primary term on which all subsequent analyses and tabulations were based. Recurrent or continuing treatment-emergent AEs were counted only once, up to and including 30 days after discontinuing study treatment. The AE frequency rates were calculated by the number of subjects who experienced the AE as a proportion of the total number of subjects in that treatment group. Between-group comparisons of the AE frequency rates were assessed by Fisher's exact test.

The frequency of MAs of laboratory analyses was assessed for both treatment groups and statistically compared by Fisher's exact test.

Results

Study population, baseline characteristics and adverse events

Between December 1989 and December 1991, a total of 1068 patients was initially included and underwent a first coronary arteriography. Of these, 183 patients were not randomized for several reasons, mostly because of non-qualifying lipid measurements or non-qualifying coronary arteriograms. A total of 885 patients were randomized, that is 230 in the PTCA group, 282 in the CABG group and 373 in the medical management group. In some cases, after randomization by the referring physician, the primary treatment was changed from that initially decided upon (e.g. PTCA instead of CABG). In total, 107 patients had no pair of matching angiograms, 48 in the placebo group and 59 in the pravastatin group. The treatment groups were well balanced with respect to baseline characteristics and concomitant medication, especially antithrombotics[14].

Effect of treatment on serum lipid levels

Lipid levels in the placebo group did not change significantly during the study. In the pravastatin group, maximum lipid reduction was achieved within two months. Total cholesterol and LDL-cholesterol and triglycerides were lowered significantly, that is, total cholesterol dropped by 20%, LDL-cholesterol dropped by 29%, and triglycerides dropped by 7%. HDL-cholesterol increased significantly by 10% during the study period. Lipid values during the study are displayed in Figure 8.1.

Clinical events

The clinical events of the study patients, according to treatment allocation, are shown in Figure 8.2. Of the 152 clinical events, 140 (92%) were cardiac events,

8 (5%) were of cerebrovascular origin and 4 (3%) were non-cardiovascular events. In the placebo group, there were 12 and in the pravastatin group there were 7 non-fatal myocardial infarctions, a reduction of 42%. In the placebo group, 47 patients and, in the pravastatin group, 20 patients needed a non-scheduled PTCA (a reduction of 57%). The incidence of the other clinical events, including the non-cardiac events, did not differ between the two treatment groups. After two years of treatment, 89% (95% confidence interval (CI) 86–92%) of the patients in the pravastatin group and 81% (CI 77–85%) of the patients in the placebo group were without clinical events ($p = 0.002$).

Angiographic findings

Of the 885 patients enrolled in the trial, a second angiogram was obtained in 778 patients (88%). For the primary analysis, the angiographic data of 125 patients (56 patients in the placebo group and 69 patients in the pravastatin group) could not be used because all coronary segments of these patients were considered influenced by a performed PTCA or CABG (see Endpoints of the trial). There were no differences in baseline characteristics between the patients with and those without a second angiogram, except for a slightly greater age, a somewhat larger proportion of patients with multivessel disease and a higher New York Heart Association angina class, in the group without an (informative) second angiogram, which is to be expected. In total, 4209 coronary segments, with a mean of 6.6 (SD 3.0) per patient, containing 4340 stenoses, with a mean of 6.8 (SD 4.0) per patient, were measured quantitatively and included in the primary analysis.

Baseline MSD and MOD did not differ significantly between the treatment groups. Both groups showed net progression, having smaller MSDs and MODs at follow-up than at baseline. However, in the placebo group, mean MSD decreased 0.10 mm (from 2.82 to 2.72 mm), whereas, in the pravastatin group, mean MSD decreased 0.06 mm (from 2.80 to 2.73), $p = 0.019$. MOD behaved similarly: in the placebo group, the median MOD decrease was 0.09 mm (from 1.88 to 1.78 mm), whereas, in the pravastatin group, the median MOD decrease was 0.03 mm (from 1.85 to 1.81 mm), $p = 0.001$. The relative changes in MSD and MOD during the study are shown in Figure 8.3.

Relationship between baseline lipid levels, change in MOD and MSD and occurrence of clinical events

In Figure 4, the median change in MOD is given for patients (in quartiles) treated with placebo or pravastatin with respect to different levels of baseline LDL-cholesterol and triglycerides. In patients with a baseline LDL-cholesterol <3.8 mmol/L (147 mg/dl), the median change in MOD was −0.10 mm in the placebo group, and −0.03 mm in the pravastatin group. The effect of pravastatin could therefore be estimated as a reduction in progression of 0.07 mm in 2 years.

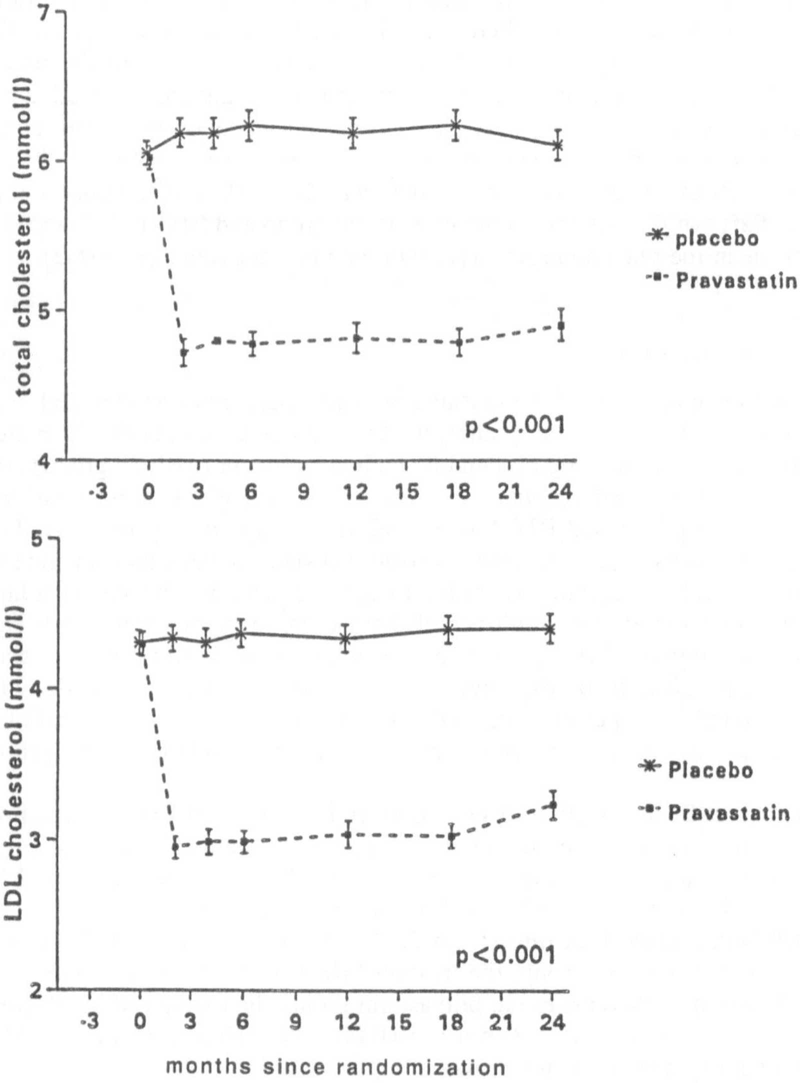

Figure 8.1. Changes in total cholesterol, LDL-cholesterol, high density lipoprotein (HDL) cholesterol and triglycerides during the study.

In patients with a baseline LDL-cholesterol between 3.8 and 4.3 mmol/L (147 and 166 mg/dl) the thus-defined pravastatin effect was 0.04 mm; in patients with a baseline LDL-cholesterol between 4.3 and 4.8 mmol/L (166 and 186 mg/dl) the effect was 0.06 mm; and, in patients with baseline LDL-cholesterol levels >4.8 mmol/L (186 mg/dl), it was 0.04 mm. The effect of pravastatin did not differ significantly between the four subgroups with regard to LDL-cholesterol levels ($p > 0.38$). For the other baseline lipid values (total cholesterol, HDL-cholesterol

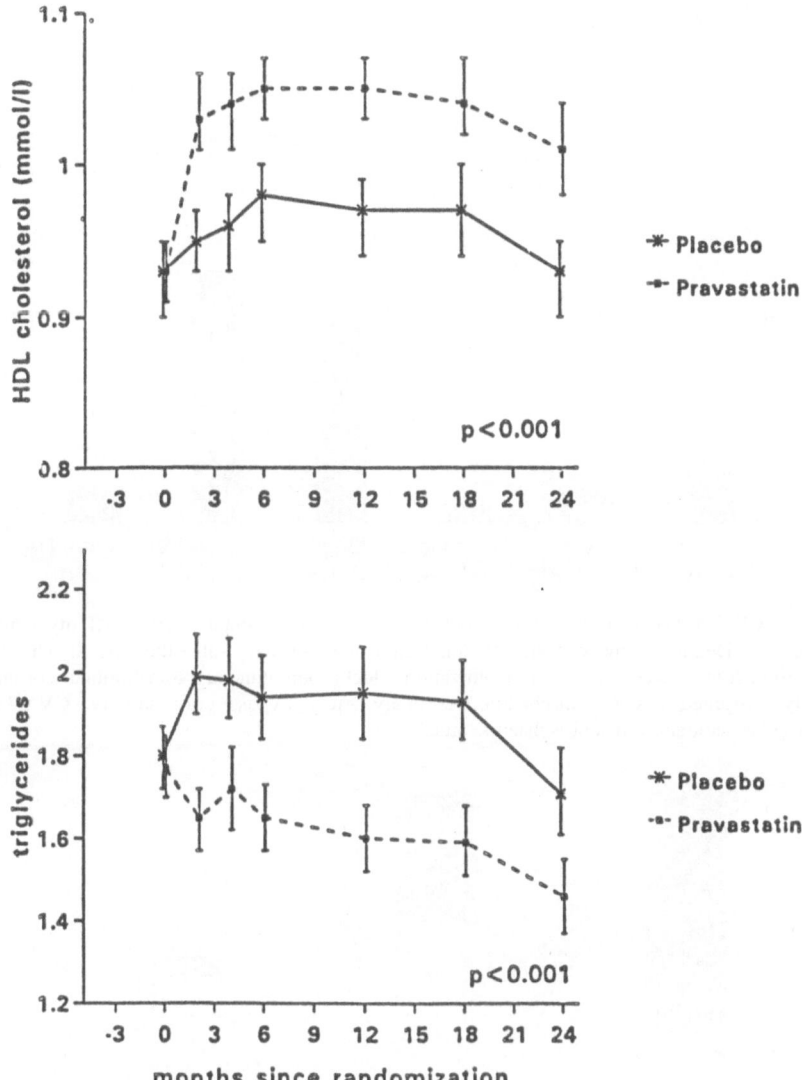

Figure 8.1.   continued

and triglycerides), essentially the same results were obtained. With respect to MSD, the pravastatin effect also did not differ between the subgroups with regard to lipid levels.

No interaction could be demonstrated between baseline lipid levels, baseline patient characteristics and the change in MOD−MSD or the occurrence of clinical events during the study.

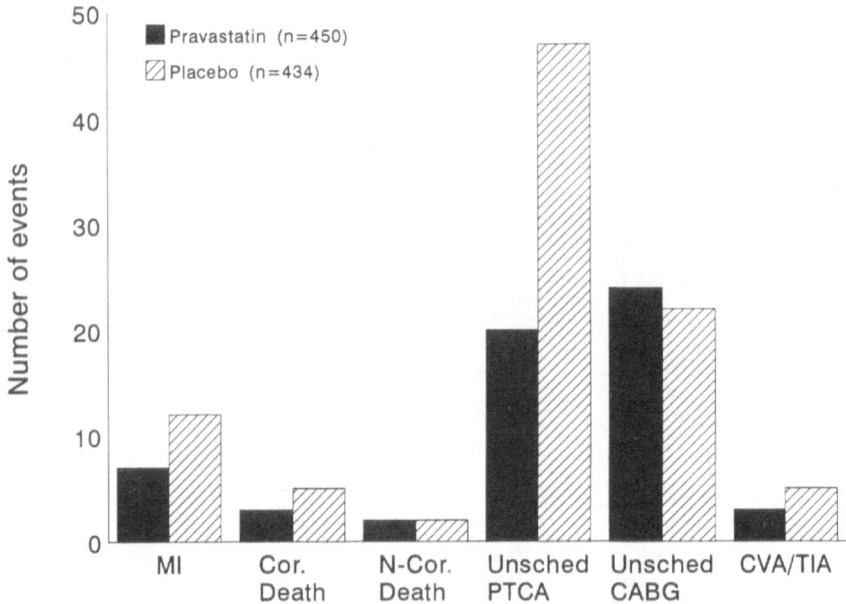

Figure 8.2. Clinical events of the study patients according to treatment allocation. MI, myocardial infarction; Cor. Death, coronary death; N-Cor. Death, non-coronary (all other) death; Unsched PTCA, unscheduled (according to randomization block) percutaneous transluminal coronary angioplasty; Unsched CABG, unscheduled coronary artery bypass graft surgery; CVA/TIA, cerebrovascular accident/transient ischaemic attack.

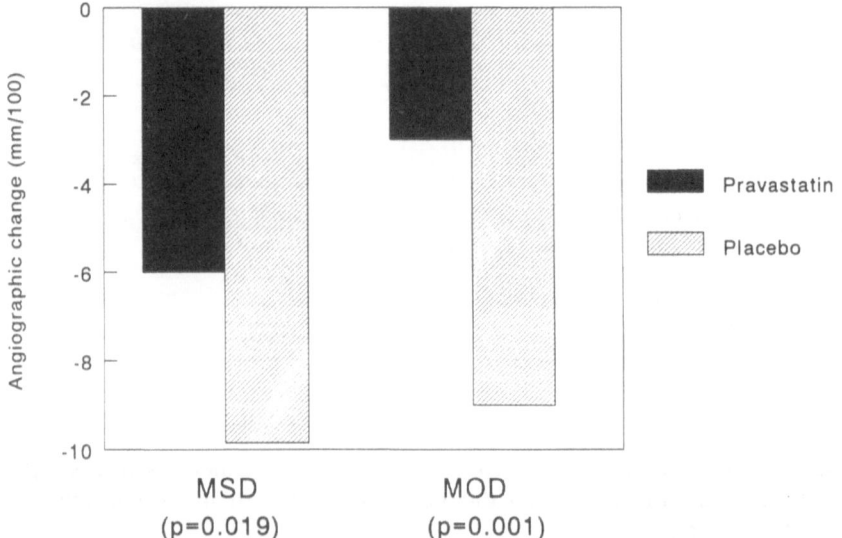

Figure 8.3. Change in mean segment diameter and median minimum obstruction diameter in mm/100 for the pravastatin vs the placebo group during the study. MSD, mean segment diameter; MOD, minimum obstruction diameter.

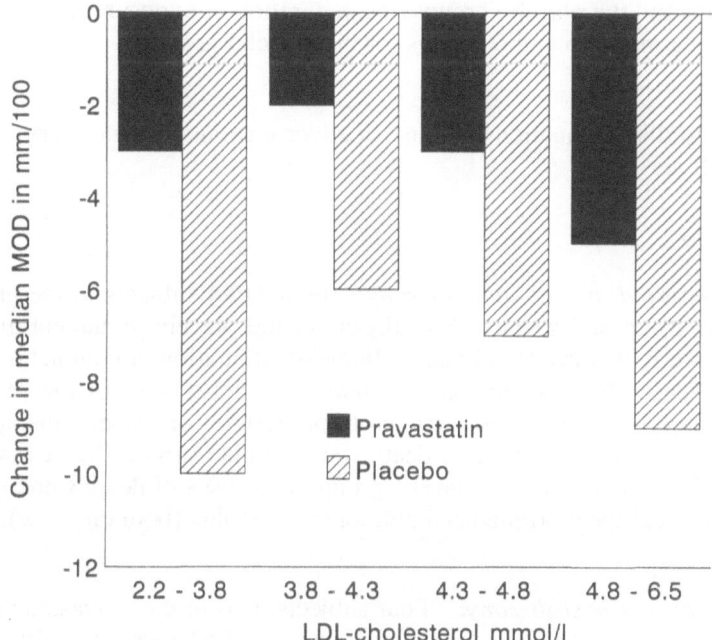

Figure 8.4. Change in median minimum obstruction diameter (MOD) in mm/100 related to baseline LDL-cholesterol level (patient quartiles) for the pravastatin vs the placebo group during the study.

Table 8.1. Deaths, discontinuations because of adverse events*, serious adverse events, and all adverse events reported by treatment group.

	Number (per cent) of subjects	
	Pravastatin group $n = 450$	Placebo group $n = 435$
Deaths†	4 (0.9)	7 (1.6)
Discontinuations	18 (4.0)	11 (2.5)
SAEs†	130 (28.9)	146 (33.6)
All AEs†	369 (82.0)	380 (87.4)

*Includes laboratory abnormalities.
†Occurred while on study therapy or ≤30 days after discontinuation of study therapy.

Safety results

Overall summary of safety results and extent of exposure

An overall summary of safety results, including deaths, discontinuations from study therapy because of adverse events (including laboratory abnormalities), serious adverse events, and all adverse events is shown in Table 8.1. Exposure to study medications for all 885 subjects randomized did not differ between the pravastatin and the placebo groups (mean duration of exposure was 687 days for the pravastatin group and 693 days for the placebo group).

Deaths and discontinuations because of adverse events or laboratory abnormalities

DEATHS

Deaths reported during study therapy: Four (1%) subjects in the pravastatin treatment group and seven (2%) subjects in the placebo treatment group died while on study therapy or ≤30 days after discontinuation or completion of study therapy. These eleven deaths are summarized below. None of the deaths were reported as related or possibly related to pravastatin or placebo therapy. In the pravastatin group, the causes of death were: cardiac origin (3 cases) and leptospirosis (1 case); and, in the placebo group, the causes of death were: cardiac (5 cases), cerebral haemorrhage and pulmonary embolus (both one case).

Deaths reported post-therapy: Four subjects, two in the pravastatin-treatment group and two in the placebo-treatment group, died more than 30 days after study therapy was discontinued.

In the pravastatin group, two patients died, of thyroid and lung cancer respectively, and, in the placebo group, two patients died of lung cancer.

DISCONTINUATIONS FROM STUDY THERAPY BECAUSE OF ADVERSE EVENTS OR LABORATORY ABNORMALITIES

Randomized subjects who stopped study therapy prematurely because of an AE or laboratory abnormality and did not restart were termed discontinued. Eighteen (4%) of the 450 pravastatin-treated subjects and 11 (3%) of the 435 placebo-treated subjects permanently discontinued study therapy because of AEs or laboratory abnormalities. In the pravastatin treatment group, five subjects were discontinued because of events reported as related or possibly related to study therapy. In the placebo treatment group, one subject was discontinued because of an event reported as possibly related to study therapy. None of the events was serious in nature. Another pravastatin-treated subject was discontinued 65 days after randomization because of conjunctivitis. Although the investigator reported the event as related to pravastatin on the CRF, he also stated that the condition could have been viral in origin. The remaining pravastatin-treated subject who discontinued because of an event reported as related to pravastatin had a complicated clinical course ('jaundice' with normal liver function tests, gastrointestinal discomfort and co-ordination disturbance in a 53-year-old man with a history of MI, hypertension, angina, intermittent claudication and multiple sclerosis). While the investigator did state that the subject's co-ordination

Table 8.2. Number (per cent) of subjects experiencing serious adverse events by treatment group and body system.

| Body system | Number (per cent) of subjects) | | | |
| | Pravastatin treatment group $n=450$ | | Placebo treatment group $n=435$ | |
	AEs	ADEs*	AEs	ADEs*
Cardiovascular	97 (21.6)	16 (3.6)	108 (24.8)	23 (5.3)
Dermatological	1 (0.2)	0	1 (0.2)	0
Endocrine/metabolic/electrolyte	1 (0.2)	0	1 (0.2)	0
Gastrointestinal	6 (1.3)	2 (0.4)	6 (1.4)	1 (0.2)
General	11 (2.4)	1 (0.2)	12 (2.8)	2 (0.4)
Haematopoietic	1 (0.2)	0	3 (0.7)	2 (0.4)
Immunology/sensitivity disorder	1 (0.2)	0	0	0
Musculoskeletal/connective	3 (0.7)	0	8 (1.8)	0
Nervous	3 (0.7)	2 (0.4)	6 (1.4)	3 (0.7)
Renal/genitourinary	4 (0.9)	2 (0.4)	8 (1.8)	1 (0.2)
Respiratory	12 (2.7)	3 (0.7)	9 (2.1)	0
Special senses	1 (0.2)	1 (0.2)	1 (0.2)	1 (0.2)

*AEs reported by investigators as related, possibly related or of unknown relationship to pravastatin or placebo.

problems were possibly related to the underlying disease, he still reported these events as related to pravastatin.

SERIOUS ADVERSE EVENTS

Twenty-nine per cent of pravastatin-treated subjects (130/450) and 34% of placebo-treated subjects (146/435) experienced SAEs during treatment or ≤ 30 days after discontinuation or completion of study therapy. Cardiac procedures (PTCA or CABG) scheduled by stratum as part of the protocol did not require an SAE report and therefore were not included in SAE analysis. Table 8.2 shows the frequency of SAEs for both treatment groups alphabetically by body system. Serious adverse events categorized in the cardiovascular body system were by far the most commonly reported in both treatment groups as expected because of the subjects' underlying coronary artery disease.

Clinical adverse events

Eighty-two per cent (369/450) of subjects in the pravastatin treatment group and 87% (380/435) of subjects in the placebo treatment group experienced AEs during the study. In 57% of subjects in the pravastatin treatment group and 63% of subjects in the placebo treatment group, those AEs were reported as ADEs, most of which were reported by the investigators as being of unknown relationship to the study drug.

Table 8.3.   Most common* adverse events by primary term.

| Adverse events | Number (per cent) of subjects) | | | |
| | Pravastatin treatment group $n=450$ | | Placebo treatment group $n=435$ | |
	AEs	ADEs†	AEs	ADEs†
Invasive cardiovascular procedure	173 (38.4)	34 (7.6)	195 (44.8)	45 (10.3)
Angina pectoris	94 (20.9)	50 (11.1)	114 (26.2)	58 (13.3)
Musculoskeletal pain	81 (18.0)	50 (11.1)	70 (16.1)	37 (8.5)
Fatigue	41 (9.1)	27 (6.0)	32 (7.4)	24 (5.5)
Chest pain**	38 (8.4)	11 (2.4)	32 (7.4)	11 (2.5)
Dizziness††	37 (8.2)	19 (4.2)	16 (3.7)	12 (2.8)
Subjective rhythm disturbance	33 (7.3)	15 (3.3)	26 (6.0)	10 (2.3)
Dyspnoea	30 (6.7)	12 (2.7)	18 (4.1)	9 (2.1)
Pain in abdomen	25 (5.6)	16 (3.6)	35 (8.0)	26 (6.0)
Dyspepsia/heartburn	22 (4.9)	16 (3.6)	25 (5.7)	20 (4.6)
Peripheral vascular disease (arterial)	22 (4.9)	9 (2.0)	20 (4.6)	11 (2.5)

*Ten most common events in the pravastatin treatment group (both dyspepsia/heartburn and peripheral vascular disease occurred in 22 subjects in the pravastatin treatment group); †AEs reported by investigators as related, possibly related or of unknown relationship to pravastatin or placebo; **Chest pain of non-cardiac, non-musculoskeletal or unknown origin; ††Statistically different between groups ($p \leq 0.05$) in frequency of AEs; ADEs were not tested.

FREQUENCY OF EVENTS BY BODY SYSTEM

Adverse events occurred with similar frequency in both treatment groups for all body systems with the exception of the respiratory system, which showed a statistically significant difference ($p \leq 0.05$) between the two treatment groups in overall totals (19% pravastatin vs 14% placebo). This was primarily due to more reports of dyspnoea, chronic obstructive pulmonary disease and sinus abnormalities in the pravastatin treatment group, although none of these individual AEs occurred at a statistically significantly higher frequency in the pravastatin versus the placebo group.

The rate at which investigators reported AEs to be ADEs (reported as related, possibly related, or of unknown relationship to study drug) was similar when comparing within-body systems by treatment group.

MOST COMMON EVENTS

Table 8.3 shows the most commonly reported events in decreasing order of frequency. Commonly reported AEs occurred with similar frequency in both treatment groups with the exception of dizziness, which occurred statistically more frequently in the pravastatin treatment group ($p \leq 0.05$). None of the pravastatin-treated subjects discontinued study medication due to this event, and no episodes of dizziness were reported as severe in intensity.

Clinical laboratory data evaluation

OVERVIEW OF LABORATORY RESULTS

In general, laboratory abnormalities occurring in subjects were asymptomatic. Only two subjects were discontinued from the study because of laboratory results. One subject in the pravastatin treatment group was discontinued from the study with moderate transient elevations of alanine aminotransferase (ALT) and γ-glutamyltransferase (GGT) after 61 days of therapy and did not fulfil the MA criteria. These findings were probably related to the CABG procedure which had been performed on the previous day. One placebo-treated subject was discontinued because of elevations of aspartate aminotransferase (AST) and ALT. These abnormalities subsequently resolved over several months and were not associated with a known aetiology.

MARKED ABNORMALITIES

Laboratory MAs occurred with relatively similar frequencies when comparing the pravastatin (8%) and placebo (11%) treatment groups. Marked abnormalities of hepatic transaminase (AST and ALT) and creatine kinase (CK) values are more fully discussed, as elevations of these analyses are of relevant interest with HMG-CoA reductase inhibitor therapy.

Hepatic transaminases: The MA criteria for AST and ALT are defined as greater than three times the upper limit of normal. Two pravastatin-treated subjects (0.5%) and two placebo-treated subjects (0.3%) each demonstrated one isolated AST value meeting MA criteria during active treatment. Measurements of AST returned to normal without discontinuation of therapy, and MAs did not recur. No MAs of AST were reported by the investigators as AEs. No MAs of ALT were reported in either treatment group.

As mentioned earlier, therapy was discontinued in one subject in the pravastatin treatment group with single elevations of ALT and GGT, but the values did not qualify as MAs.

Thus, MAs in hepatic transaminase levels were uncommon and limited to AST. The MAs occurred with similar frequency in both treatment groups and were not clinically significant.

CREATINE KINASE

Eleven subjects (2.4%) in the pravastatin treatment group and 15 subjects (3.5%) in the placebo treatment group had elevations of CK that met the MA criteria of four times pretreatment value. Two of the subjects in the pravastatin treatment group had MAs that were reported as AEs and judged by the investigator to be related to study therapy.

None of the MAs of CK occurring in either treatment group were associated with myopathic syndromes or caused discontinuation of study therapy.

REGRESS safety conclusions

Serious adverse events occurred with similar frequency in both treatment groups (pravastatin, 29%; placebo, 34%). The most common SAEs that occurred during this study were cardiovascular in nature as would be expected because of the subjects' coronary artery disease. There were no serious AEs clearly attributed to pravastatin therapy that were reported in this trial.

Overall AEs (both serious and non-serious AEs) occurred with similar frequency in the pravastatin (82%) and placebo (87%) groups. Adverse events reported in the respiratory system occurred at a statistically significantly higher rate in pravastatin-treated subjects (19%) versus placebo-treated subjects (14%; $p \leq 0.05$). This was largely because of more reports of dyspnoea, chronic obstructive pulmonary disease, and sinus abnormalities in the pravastatin treatment group, although none of these primary terms occurred at a statistically significantly higher frequency rate in the pravastatin vs the placebo treatment group. Of the most commonly occurring events in pravastatin-treated subjects, only dizziness occurred at a statistically significantly higher rate in pravastatin-treated subjects (8%) vs placebo-treated subjects (4%; $p \leq 0.05$). There were no reports of myositis or rhabdomyolysis in this study.

In general, laboratory abnormalities occurring in both treatment groups during this trial were asymptomatic. Only one pravastatin-treated subject was discontinued from the study because of transient elevations of ALT and GGT, which were probably unrelated to study therapy.

Discussion

Angiographic findings and clinical events

In this study, pravastatin had a significant beneficial effect on both a priori established endpoints, that is, mean segment diameter (MSD) and mean obstruction diameter (MOD). We elected to use two primary endpoints since they reflect different manifestations of progression (or regression) of coronary atherosclerosis and it is conceivable that a drug has a beneficial effect on only one of these aspects. Changes in MSD reflect mainly changes that affect a coronary artery or segment in a diffuse manner, whereas changes in MOD reflect mainly changes in degree of narrowing of atherosclerotic lesions and the development of new lesions.

Although cardiac events did not represent a primary endpoint, we included cardiac events in this report because of their clinical significance and because they may influence the outcome of the analysis of progression. The latter is particularly true for patients who needed PTCA or CABG during follow-up. It is highly probable that progression in these patients with usually increasing (or at least not improving) symptoms was more pronounced than it was in patients in whom the clinical condition did not call for mechanical intervention (the fact that perhaps plaque instability and not gradual progression is the underlying cause in some of these patients is of secondary importance in this context). However, progression leading to initially non-scheduled interventions is not immediately apparent in the analysis of progression because segments in which PTCA is performed and segments influenced by bypass grafts should be excluded from primary analysis of progression and regression. There are two options to deal with this problem. The first option is to analyse angiograms made before the intervention. This, however, was not feasible in our study because, in many instances, these angiograms were not made according to the standards required for QCA follow-up angiograms. Furthermore, the variable time interval between baseline angiogram and pre-intervention angiogram would have made a correct interpretation of the findings very difficult. Therefore, we chose the second option, that is, we analysed events separately for differences between the placebo and the pravastatin group. Apart from being of direct clinical importance, the markedly lower event rate in the pravastatin group corroborates the angiographic finding of reduced progression.

Safety and side effects

In general, HMG-CoA reductase inhibitors seem effective and well tolerated, according to safety studies and large clinical trials[15-17]. Although there may be differences in safety profile between the three main HMG-CoA reductase inhibitors (lovastatin, simvastatin and pravastatin) on theoretical grounds, almost no long-term large trials comparing their safety profiles directly have been published so far. The multicentre comparative trial of lovastatin and pravastatin – follow-up of only 18 weeks – showed similar safety profiles for both agents[18]. Therefore, in this overview, we describe safety features of the HMG-CoA class drugs in general, derived from important placebo-controlled studies unless explicitly stated. Thus far, a number of (possible) side effects of the administration of HMG-CoA reductase inhibitors, and lipid lowering in general, have been described or given extra attention because of results of animal studies. The side effects are:

1. Elevation of hepatic transaminases,
2. Creatine kinase elevations and myopathy,
3. Ocular lens opacities,
4. Central nervous system effects, and
5. Cancer and violent death.

Elevation of hepatic transaminases

Transaminase elevations have been reported in virtually all clinical trials of HMG-CoA reductase inhibitors. For instance, in the Expanded Clinical Evaluation of Lovastatin Study (EXCEL), monitoring 8425 patients treated with lovastatin or placebo, the percentage of patients with an elevation of trans-aminases three times the upper limit of normal increased dose-dependently from 0.1% on placebo and 20mg/day to 1.5% on 80mg/day[15]. In the Scandinavian Simvastatin Survival Study (4S), monitoring 4444 patients treated with simvastatin, 10–40mg/day, or placebo, the percentage of patients with an elevation of transaminases above three times the upper limit of normal was 1.5% for placebo and 2.2% for simvastatin[16]. In the Pravastatin Multinational Study (1062 patients, pravastatin 20–40mg/day or placebo), these figures were 0.2% for placebo and 1.1% for pravastatin[17], and, in REGRESS, 0.4% for placebo as well as for pravastatin.

Currently, it can be recommended that liver function tests be monitored every 6 weeks during the first few months of treatment and periodically thereafter, and to stop the drug if transaminases increase above three times the upper limit of normal.

Creatine kinase elevations and myopathy

Creatine kinase (CK) elevations can result from exercise or minor muscle trauma and are often not drug-related. In EXCEL, 29–35% of patients on lovastatin had CK elevations at some time during the study, but this was also present in 29% of patients on placebo[15]. Muscle symptoms developed in 7–9% of patients both on placebo and on lovastatin. Frank myopathy was observed in 5 of 6582 patients receiving active drug (0.08%), but no rhabdomyolysis developed. In 4S (simvastatin), an increase in CK to more than 10 times the upper limit of normal occurred in 1 patient (0.05%) in the placebo group and in 6 patients (0.3%) in the simvastatin group, respectively, but in none of the latter was this high level maintained in a repeat sample or accompanied by muscle pain or weakness[16]. A single case of rhabdomyolysis occurred in a woman taking simvastatin, 20mg/day; she recovered when treatment was stopped. In the Pravastatin Multinational Study, elevations of creatine kinase to values more than 4 times the upper limit of normal occurred in 8 (1.5%) and 14 (2.6%) patients in the placebo and pravastatin groups, respectively. The elevations were not associated with musculoskeletal symptoms and did not lead to discontinuation of double-blind treatment[17]. In REGRESS, 2.4% of the patients in the pravastatin group and 3.5% of the patients in the placebo group had CK elevations of more than four times pretreatment value. None of the increases in CK were associated with myopathic syndromes or caused discontinuation of study therapy.

Thus, it appears that it is not useful to monitor CK levels in order to detect the development of myopathy; patients should be instructed to contact their physician if muscle symptoms occur.

Lens opacities

Based on experimental work with extremely high doses of lovastatin in dogs, there has been concern that HMG-CoA reductase inhibitors may cause cataracts in humans. However, careful follow-up with slit-lamp examinations of a large number of patients on HMG-CoA reductase inhibitors for several years has not revealed an increased incidence of lens opacities and therefore regular ophthalmological examinations are no longer required[19,20].

Central nervous system effects

A small percentage of patients complain about central nervous system effects, such as headache and insomnia, during treatment with HMG-CoA reductase inhibitors[21,22]. A causal relationship between HMG-CoA reductase inhibitors and these adverse effects remains unclear because of the high prevalence of these symptoms in untreated patients. The EXCEL study of lovastatin showed no significant excess of headache (approximately 3% for the placebo as well as for the lovastatin groups). Central nervous system effects have been claimed to be a consequence of the lipophilic nature of lovastatin and simvastatin compared with the hydrophilic compound of pravastatin. A small placebo-controlled study in 12 healthy individuals performed in a sleep laboratory revealed significant influences on sleep in the group on lovastatin, which were not found in the group on pravastatin[23]. It was suggested that this is caused by lovastatin (in contrast to pravastatin) crossing the blood–brain barrier. Indeed, lovastatin could be detected in the cerebrospinal fluid of normal volunteers, whereas pravastatin could not[24]. However, additional well-controlled studies did not indicate any deleterious effect on sleep of the three different HMG-CoA reductase inhibitors[18,25].

The clinical relevance of these findings has not yet been established.

Cancer and violent death

Some trials raised concern over excess of violent death or increased risk from cancer due to lipid-lowering therapy[26,27]. In the 4S study, the number of cancer and violent deaths was 42 in the placebo group and 39 in the simvastatin group, during a median follow-up period of 5.4 years, whereas total mortality was reduced in the simvastatin group versus the placebo group by 42%. REGRESS showed no excess mortality from cancer or violent death in the pravastatin group.

In a careful meta-analysis, reviewing systematically published data on mortality from causes other than ischaemic heart disease, derived from the 10 largest cohort studies, two international studies, and 28 randomized trials, Law et al. concluded that there was no evidence that a low or reduced serum cholesterol concentration increased mortality from cancer or violent death[28]. However, we must bear in mind that the long-term safety of HMG-CoA reductase inhibitors is not completely known because we have no information available yet about side effects of HMG-CoA reductase inhibitors when taken for decades.

Clinical implications and conclusion

REGRESS has demonstrated that pravastatin monotherapy slows progression of coronary artery disease and reduces clinical events in symptomatic patients with normal to moderately elevated serum cholesterol, who undergo various forms of therapy, including PTCA and CABG. This can be achieved in a relatively easy and well-tolerated manner. There were no new safety issues identified with pravastatin therapy in this study. The favourable safety profile of pravastatin that has been previously observed in other trials in this subject population is confirmed here.

The retardation of progression and reduction of cardiac events which could be achieved by cholesterol reduction in a wide range of patients with normal to moderately elevated serum cholesterol levels raises the question whether cholesterol lowering should be an integral part in the management of patients with coronary atherosclerosis, almost regardless of initial serum cholesterol level. The present study and recently reported other studies at least justify serious consideration of this option. However, for several reasons, administration of lipid-lowering drugs on such a large scale may not be achievable and therefore future studies should be directed towards identifying patients who will benefit most.

Acknowledgement

The REGRESS study was sponsored by Bristol–Myers Squibb Company, Princeton, New Jersey.

References

1. Brensike JF, Levy RI, Kelsey SF, et al. Effects of therapy with cholestyramine on progression of coronary arteriosclerosis: results of the NHLBI Type II Coronary Intervention Study. Circulation. 1984;69:313–24.
2. Arntzenius AC, Kromhout D, Barth JD, et al. Diet, lipoproteins, and the progression of coronary atherosclerosis. The Leiden Intervention Trial. N Engl J Med. 1985;312:805–11.
3. Blankenhorn DH, Nessim SA, Johnson RL, Sanmarco ME, Azen SP, Cashin-Hemphill L. Beneficial effects of combined colestipol–niacin therapy on coronary atherosclerosis and coronary venous bypass grafts [published erratum appears in JAMA. 1988;259:2698]. JAMA. 1987;257:3233–40.
4. Buchwald H, Varco RL, Matts JP, et al. Effect of partial ileal bypass surgery on mortality and morbidity from coronary heart disease in patients with hypercholesterolemia. Report of the Program on the Surgical Control of the Hyperlipidemias (POSCH). N Engl J Med. 1990; 323:946–55.
5. Brown G, Albers JJ, Fisher LD, et al. Regression of coronary artery disease as a result of intensive lipid-lowering therapy in men with high levels of apolipoprotein B. N Engl J Med. 1990;323:1289–98.
6. Kane JP, Malloy MJ, Ports TA, Phillips NR, Diehl JC, Havel RJ. Regression of coronary atherosclerosis during treatment of familial hypercholesterolemia with combined drug regimens. JAMA. 1990;264:3007–12.
7. Schuler G, Hambrecht R, Schlierf G, et al. Regular physical exercise and low-fat diet. Effects on progression of coronary artery disease. Circulation. 1992;86:1–11.

8. Watts GF, Lewis B, Brunt JN, et al. Effects on coronary artery disease of lipid-lowering diet, or diet plus cholestyramine, in the St Thomas' Atherosclerosis Regression Study (STARS). Lancet. 1992;339:563–9.

9. Blankenhorn DH, Azen SP, Kramsch DM, et al. Coronary angiographic changes with lovastatin therapy. The Monitored Atherosclerosis Regression Study (MARS). The MARS Research Group. Ann Intern Med. 1993;119:969–76.

10. Waters D, Higginson L, Gladstone P, et al. Effects of monotherapy with an HMG-CoA reductase inhibitor on the progression of coronary atherosclerosis as assessed by serial quantitative arteriography. The Canadian Coronary Atherosclerosis Intervention Trial. Circulation. 1994;89:959–68.

11. The MAAS Investigators. Effect of simvastatin on coronary atheroma: the Multicentre Anti-Atheroma Study (MAAS) [published erratum appears in Lancet. 1994;344:762]. Lancet. 1994;344:633–8.

12. Pitt B, Ellis SG, Mancini GB, Rosman HS, McGovern ME. Design and recruitment in the United States of a multicenter quantitative angiographic trial of pravastatin to limit atherosclerosis in the coronary arteries (PLAC I). Am J Cardiol. 1993;72:31–5.

13. Haskell WL, Alderman EL, Fair JM, et al. Effects of intensive multiple risk factor reduction on coronary atherosclerosis and clinical cardiac events in men and women with coronary artery disease. The Stanford Coronary Risk Intervention Project (SCRIP). Circulation. 1994;89:975–90.

14. Jukema JW, Bruschke AV, van Boven AJ, et al. Effects of lipid lowering by pravastatin on progression and regression of coronary artery disease in symptomatic men with normal to moderately elevated serum cholesterol levels. The Regression Growth Evaluation Statin Study (REGRESS). Circulation. 1995;91:2528–40.

15. Bradford RH, Shear CL, Chremos AN, et al. Expanded Clinical Evaluation of Lovastatin (EXCEL) study results. I. Efficacy in modifying plasma lipoproteins and adverse event profile in 8245 patients with moderate hypercholesterolemia. Arch Intern Med. 1991;151:43–9.

16. The Scandinavian Simvastatin Survival Study Group. Randomised trial of cholesterol lowering in 4444 patients with coronary heart disease: the Scandinavian Simvastatin Survival Study (4S). Lancet. 1994;344:1383–9.

17. The Pravastatin Multinational Study Group for Cardiac Risk Patients. Effects of pravastatin in patients with serum total cholesterol levels from 5.2 to 7.8 mmol/liter (200 to 300 mg/dl) plus two additional atherosclerotic risk factors. The Pravastatin Multinational Study Group for Cardiac Risk Patients. Am J Cardiol. 1993;72:1031–7.

18. The Lovastatin Pravastatin Study Group. A multicenter comparative trial of lovastatin and pravastatin in the treatment of hypercholesterolemia. The Lovastatin Pravastatin Study Group. Am J Cardiol. 1993;71:810–5.

19. Boccuzzi SJ, Bocanegra TS, Walker JF, Shapiro DR, Keegan ME. Long-term safety and efficacy profile of simvastatin. Am J Cardiol. 1991;68:1127–31.

20. Laties AM, Shear CL, Lippa EA, et al. Expanded clinical evaluation of lovastatin (EXCEL) study results. II. Assessment of the human lens after 48 weeks of treatment with lovastatin. Am J Cardiol. 1991;67:447–53.

21. Dujovne CA, Chremos AN, Pool JL, et al. Expanded clinical evaluation of lovastatin (EXCEL) study results: IV. Additional perspectives on the tolerability of lovastatin. Am J Med. 1991;91(1B):25S–30S.

22. Hunninghake DB, Knopp RH, Schonfeld G, et al. Efficacy and safety of pravastatin in patients with primary hypercholesterolemia. I. A dose–response study. Atherosclerosis. 1990;85:81–9.

23. Vgontzas AN, Kales A, Bixler EO, Manfredi RL, Tyson KL. Effects of lovastatin and pravastatin on sleep efficiency and sleep stages. Clin Pharmacol Ther. 1991;50:730–7.

24. Botti RE, Triscari J, Pan HY, Zayat J. Concentrations of pravastatin and lovastatin in cerebrospinal fluid in healthy subjects. Clin Neuropharmacol. 1991;14:256–61.

25. Eckernas SA, Roos BE, Kvidal P, et al. The effects of simvastatin and pravastatin on objective and subjective measures of nocturnal sleep: a comparison of two structurally different HMG CoA reductase inhibitors in patients with primary moderate hypercholesterolaemia. Br J Clin Pharmacol. 1993;35:284–9.

26. Law MR, Thompson SG. Low serum cholesterol and the risk of cancer: an analysis of the published prospective studies. Cancer Causes Control. 1991;2:253–61.
27. Wysowski DK, Gross TP. Deaths due to accidents and violence in two recent trials of cholesterol-lowering drugs. Arch Intern Med. 1990;150:2169–72.
28. Law MR, Thompson SG, Wald NJ. Assessing possible hazards of reducing serum cholesterol. BMJ. 1994;308:373–9.

9. Familial Atherosclerosis Treatment Study

V. M. G. MAHER

Summary

The Familial Atherosclerosis Treatment Study (FATS) was a randomized double-blind placebo-controlled trial that investigated the effects on coronary artery disease of two intensive lipid-lowering strategies compared with a more conventional approach in a group of men at high risk of future cardiac events. It demonstrated that, with intensive lipid-lowering treatment, it is possible to halt the progression and induce regression of coronary atherosclerosis in a selected population of men. It was the first angiographic regression study to demonstrate a significant benefit of lipid-lowering treatment in reducing cardiovascular events. Subsequent analyses from FATS have highlighted that, while angiographic change is maximal in the more severe baseline stenoses, the major clinical benefits are thought to relate to stabilization of moderate stenoses.

The concept that rupture of moderately stenosing lipid-rich plaques underlies most cardiovascular events has initiated intense research to identify these plaques and the individuals likely to have them. Recent evidence from FATS has highlighted that only individuals with previous cardiac symptoms developed events during the study, previously asymptomatic individuals being spared. Thus individuals with previous angina or myocardial infarction should be considered more likely to have these vulnerable plaques. Another interesting observation in FATS is that the benefits of lipid-lowering are not only confined to those with very high LDL-cholesterol (LDLc) levels. In fact, the individuals in FATS whose qualifying LDLc levels at baseline were in the lower half of the LDLc distribution were more likely to have other derangements of lipoprotein metabolism, have an increased risk of clinical events but were likely to respond better to lipid-lowering strategies. This has brought up the idea that certain building blocks used in plaque development may generate more vulnerable yet more treatable lesions. Further analyses of FATS are ongoing and long-term follow-up of the FATS patients will hopefully uncover more answers to the difficult questions posed by coronary atherosclerosis.

A.V.G. Bruschke et al. *(eds): Lipid-lowering therapy and progression of atherosclerosis, 107–113.*
© 1996 *Kluwer Academic Publishers.*

Study design

Patients

One hundred and forty-six men, 62 years old or younger, with coronary artery disease (CAD), who had a positive family history of coronary heart disease (CHD) and apolipoprotein B-100 levels > 125 mg/dl, were involved.

Randomization

Following enrolment, all patients received an American Heart Association Step 1 diet and were randomized according to age, smoking history and three lipoprotein phenotypic patterns to receive either niacin 4 g/day plus colestipol 30 g/day, or to lovastatin 40 mg/day plus colestipol 30 g/day, or to a conventional strategy which included placebos for lovastatin and colestipol, except for those patients whose baseline low-density lipoprotein cholesterol (LDLc) levels exceeded the 90th population percentile, who received colestipol 30 g/day.

Clinic visits and laboratory tests

Patients visited the Northwest Lipid Research Clinic monthly for 1 year and every other month for the rest of the 2.5-year study. Plasma lipoproteins were measured at baseline and quarterly thereafter. The haematocrit, renal function and liver function tests were performed at baseline and every 6 months throughout the study.

Arteriography

All patients underwent coronary angiography at baseline which was repeated after 2.5 years in 120 patients who completed the study protocol. At the baseline catheterization, five views of the left coronary system and two of the right were obtained. These views gave at least one clear look at each coronary segment and formed four pairs of views suitable for biplane quantitative analysis. The use of nitrates and other vasoactive drugs, and the sequence of arteriographic projections, X-ray field, and catheter size were recorded; these conditions were duplicated as exactly as possible in the follow-up study 2.5 years later.

Arteriographic analysis

Change in the severity of coronary disease was assessed both visually and quantitatively by two trained observers blinded to the patient's identity, treatment group and film sequence. Films were viewed simultaneously side-by-side at five-fold magnification in a dual overhead-projector system, from which a detailed coronary map was drawn locating all lesions causing stenoses of at least 20%.

Visual assessment

By direct visual comparison and using the aid of a 'paper caliper' technique, lesions were classified as 'unchanged', 'definitely changed' or 'possibly changed'.

Quantitative assessment

All lesions so classified were traced, digitized and processed by methods developed and validated in our laboratory. The minimum lumen diameter and the diameter of the nearest normal segment were measured in millimeters with the catheter used as a scaling device. The two principle measures of disease were the minimum diameter (DM) and the percent stenosis (%Sprox) of the nine proximal coronary segments. Disease change between the two time points was expressed as Δ%Sprox.

Results

The randomization worked very well with the niacin–colestipol, lovastatin–colestipol and conventionally treated groups having almost equal numbers of patients of similar age and body mass index, who had hypertension, smoked, had previous myocardial infarctions, and who had similar baseline disease severity and lipoprotein levels. The mean LDLc at baseline was 4.9 mmol/L (189 mg/dl) (88th percentile for 50-year-old American men). It fell by 7% in the conventionally treated patients, by 46% in the lovastatin–colestipol-treated patients and by 32% in the niacin–colestipol-treated patients. The apolipoprotein B-100 level fell comparably with the LDLc level. The mean HDLc level was 0.98 mmol/L (38 mg/dl) at baseline, rose 5% in the conventionally treated patients, 15% in the lovastatin–colestipol-treated patients and 43% in the niacin–colestipol-treated patients.

Disease change

The average stenosis of the worst lesion in the nine proximal arterial segments was 34%. Over 2.5 years, this value increased on average by 2.1% stenosis in the conventionally treated patients. By contrast, it decreased by 0.7% with lovastatin and colestipol and by 0.9% with niacin plus colestipol ($p < 0.003$). The minimum lumen diameter for the nine proximal segments averaged 1.9 mm for all patients. It decreased by 0.05 mm with conventional treatment but increased by 0.012 mm in the lovastatin and colestipol group and by 0.035 mm in the niacin and colestipol group ($p < 0.01$).

Progression and regression

Using a > 10% change in diameter stenosis as indicating true change since 10.2% is 3 SD of the repeat-measurement variance, patients were classified as 'progressors' if a lesion in any segment progressed by 10% or more without regression in any segment. Patients were considered 'regressors' if a proximal lesion regressed by 10% or more without any lesion progressing. Progression occurred in 46% of patients treated conventionally, in 21% of those treated with lovastatin–colestipol and in 25% of the niacin–colestipol-treated patients. Regression occurred in 11% of conventionally treated patients, in 32% of patients treated with lovastatin–colestipol and in 39% of the niacin–colestipol group.

Clinical events

Death, myocardial infarction or ischaemia requiring revascularization occurred in 15 of the 146 enrolled patients. Events occurred in 10 out of 52 patients originally assigned to conventional treatment compared with only 3 out of 46 patients assigned to lovastatin–colestipol and 2 out of 48 patients originally assigned to niacin–colestipol ($p=0.01$).

Correlates of disease change

The average percent change in the worst lesions of the nine proximal coronary artery segments correlated significantly with the % change in apoB, LDLc, HDLc, systolic blood pressure, body weight, Lp(a) levels and therapy code (placebo = 1, colestipol = 2, lovastatin–colestipol = 3, niacin–colestipol = 4). In a multivariate analysis, only the % change in apoB (or LDLc), HDLc and systolic blood pressure were significant correlates. Interestingly, the therapy code failed to compete in the multivariate analysis against the risk variables, suggesting that the benefit of therapy is through their action on these risk variables.

Lessons from FATS

Initial observations

In this select population of men at high risk of a future cardiac event, a conventional approach to treatment of hyperlipidaemia resulted in a high incidence of disease progression and clinical events over a very short time period[1]. In contrast, by radically altering serum lipoprotein levels, it was possible to arrest disease progression, induce disease regression and reduce cardiovascular events by 73%. It was also observed as appreciated in other studies that lesions >50% stenosed at baseline were more likely to change as a result of lipid-lowering therapy than less severe lesions. A key observation was that the lesions responsible for the majority of the cardiovascular events in the study were moderate 30–70% stenoses at baseline.

Subsequent observations from subgroup analyses

Since its original publication in 1990, many new and important observations have emerged from FATS. The earliest of these was a more detailed study of the impact of baseline lesion severity on disease change as a result of lipid-lowering therapy[2]. Categorizing the baseline lesions according to stenosis severity into mild (10–40% stenoses), moderate (40–70% stenoses) and severe (70–98% stenoses), it was observed that intensive lipid-lowering therapy decreases, by about four-fold, the likelihood of definitive lesion progression among mild and moderate lesions but does not appear to reduce the chance of progression of the small number of severe lesions studied. It was also observed that the lesions most likely to regress were the more severe stenoses with less marked changes occurring in the milder stenoses in response to lipid-lowering therapy. Thus, more severe stenoses undergo the greatest change with lipid-lowering therapy. Another lesion-related observation was that only 12% of all intensively treated lesions regressed and that the total amount of regression averaged 1–2%. However these modest angiographic disease changes were associated with a 70–80% reduction in cardiovascular events. This paradox of minimal angiographic change and marked event reduction has also been observed in other studies. To understand this phenomenon, one needs to appreciate how plaques change from stable quiescent lesions into the unstable culprit lesions which precipitate clinical events.

Pathological studies have demonstrated that plaque rupture is an important underlying feature precipitating cardiovascular events. These plaques usually have a large lipid-rich core and a thin foam-cell-laden smooth-muscle-cell-deficient fibrous cap. Angiographic studies, particularly FATS, have highlighted that the angiographic lesions responsible for clinical events are often only mildly stenosed. Thus, many clinical events arise from rupture of these mildly stenosed lipid-rich lesions. From animal studies, it has been observed that portions of the lipid component of similar-typed lesions can regress with intense lipid-lowering treatment. One possible explanation, therefore, for the angiographic change versus clinical event reduction paradox is that lipid-lowering strategies deplete the lipid component of the small number of these lipid-rich vulnerable plaques. While this is not angiographically spectacular, it renders these lesions more stable and less likely to rupture.

It is quite understandable, therefore, that identifying individuals with these vulnerable plaques has become a major goal in treating coronary artery disease. While no definitive stenosis characteristics on coronary angiography pin-point high-risk plaques, serial coronary angiograms over a 2–3-year time interval has helped to identify disease progressors who are more likely to experience clinical events[3,4] and, by inference, are more likely to have a number of these lipid-rich plaques. This could be taken one step further by assuming that coronary angiograms are 'normal' at birth and that any stenoses on angiograms in adult life indicate that these patients are progressors. Therefore, one should not hesitate to administer lipid-lowering treatment to all patients with documented CAD. Although this is helpful for individuals with angiographic documentation of their disease, it is not a practical way to screen a large population. Other strategies to identify at-risk patients are therefore necessary.

Recently in FATS[5], it was observed that patients who were asymptomatic at

Table 9.1. Influence of baseline cardiac symptoms on the angiographic and clinical outcome in FATS.

	Conventional treatment		Intensive treatment	
	Symptomatic	Asymptomatic	Symptomatic	Asymptomatic
Progressors	48%	38%	24%**	19%*
Regressors	15%	0%	36%**	31%*
Clinical events	10 of 38	0 of 14	5 of 76**	0 of 18

Clinical events = death, myocardial infarction, unstable ischaemia requiring bypass or angioplasty. * = $p < 0.05$ asymptomatic patients: conventional vs intensive treatment; ** = $p < 0.01$ symptomatic patients: conventional vs intensive treatment. Progressors = ≥10% stenosis progression without any significant regression; regressors = ≥10% stenosis regression without any significant progression.

entry into the study ($n = 29$) had less-marked baseline disease than previously symptomatic patients ($n = 91$). Interestingly, the asymptomatic patients had a reduction in disease progression and increase in disease regression as a result of lipid-lowering therapy similar to that of patients who were symptomatic at entry (Table 9.1). One key difference between these groups was that clinical events only occurred in patients who were previously symptomatic. These data would suggest that a history of angina or myocardial infarction is an important predictor of future events and that all such patients should be considered as having lipid-rich vulnerable plaques and likely to benefit from lipid-lowering strategies. It was also noted that ischaemia on baseline exercise tolerance tests was associated with a greater proximal disease progression among asymptomatic patients. This subgroup of asymptomatic patients may also be considered at a greater risk of future events and thus may also be a reasonable indication to treat such patients with lipid-lowering therapy.

Are lipid profiles helpful in deciding which patients are more likely to incur clinical events? In FATS, it was observed that the benefits of lipid-lowering therapy are not confined to those with very high LDLc levels[6]. Of the 120 patients completing the 30-month protocol, 60 had a baseline LDLc <90th percentile (mean LDLc 152 mg/dl) and 60 had LDLc levels >90th percentile (mean LDLc 221 mg/dl). Thirty-one patients had levels <160 mg/dl (mean LDLc = 134 mg/dl) and 89 had >160 mg/dl (mean LDLc = 205 mg/dl). Patients with LDLc <90th percentile had an angiographic benefit from therapy similar to that of patients with LDLc levels >90th percentile at baseline (Table 9.2). The same was true for patients whose baseline LDLc levels were above or below 160 mg/dl. Interestingly, the majority of clinical events in FATS occurred in patients with LDLc levels <90th percentile or <160 mg/dl. These patients had significantly higher triglyceride levels and significantly lower HDLc levels than the patients with high LDLc levels. One possible explanation for the difference is that modestly raised LDLc levels in the presence of high triglyceride and low HDLc levels form a type of atherosclerotic plaque that is much more prone to rupture and cause clinical events. This lipid profile may therefore help to identify high-risk patients in the population. If this were the case, its recognition would

Table 9.2. Influence of baseline LDLc levels on angiographic and clinical outcome in FATS.

LDLc level	n	LDLc	HDLc	TG	% Δ diameter stenosis		Clinical events	
					Intensive	Conventional	Intensive	Conventional
<90th	60	152	35***	261***	−1.50	2.3**	2 of 42	8 of 29**
≥90th	60	221	41	159	−0.20	1.9*	3 of 52	2 of 23
<160mg/dl	31	134	33†	302†	−4.2	3.3†	2 of 20	6 of 15*
≥160mg/dl	89	205	40	178	0.2	1.6	3 of 74	4 of 37

Baseline lipids: *** = $p<0.001$ for <90th vs ≥90th, † = $p<0.005$ for <160 vs ≥160mg/dl. Disease change and clinical events: * = $p<0.05$, ** = $p<0.01$, † = $p<0.0005$ for intensive vs conventional treatment. LDLc = low-density lipoprotein cholesterol, HDLc = high-density lipoprotein cholesterol, TG = triglycerides. Values are means. Clinical event numbers were based on an intention-to-treat analysis (146 men).

be very important as the presence of this lipid profile was also associated with the greatest reduction in clinical events from lipid-lowering therapy in FATS. These observations unearth the concept that differences in the building blocks used for plaque development may be critical to how vulnerable plaques become and how well they stabilize with lipid-lowering strategies.

Many new aspects of FATS are currently being investigated to add even more hypothesis-generating information to uncover ways to control coronary atherosclerosis. Despite the valuable lessons learned from FATS, certain limitations of this study must be considered. The population involved in FATS were selected to include only men under 62 years of age who had apolipoprotein B-100 levels in excess of 125 mg/dl and had a positive family history for CHD. Therefore, a large portion of patients with coronary artery disease were excluded and thus the findings of this study cannot be extrapolated to the broad population of patients with CAD. FATS follow-up angiographic and clinical studies are ongoing which will hopefully help answer more questions related to this select population of men and generate hypotheses to apply to other at-risk populations of patients.

References

1. Brown BG, Albers JJ, Fisher LD, et al. Regression of coronary artery disease as a result of intensive lipid-lowering therapy in men with high levels of apolipoprotein B. N Engl J Med. 1990;323:1289–98.
2. Brown BG, Zhao X-Q, Sacco DE, Albers JJ. Lipid lowering and plaque regression. New insights into prevention of plaque disruption and clinical events in coronary disease. Circulation. 1993;87:1781–91.
3. Buchwald H, Matts JP, Fitch LL, et al. Change in sequential coronary arteriograms and subsequent coronary events. JAMA. 1992;268:1429–33.
4. Waters D, Craven TE, Lesperance J. Prognostic significance of progression of coronary atherosclerosis. Circulation. 1993;87:1067–76.
5. Zhao X-Q, Brown BG, Hillger L, et al. Effects of intensive lipid-lowering therapy on the coronary arteries of asymptomatic subjects with elevated apolipoprotein B. Circulation. 1993;88:2744–53.
6. Stewart BF, Brown BG, Zhao Z-Q, et al. Benefits of lipid-lowering therapy in men with elevated apolipoprotein B are not confined to those with very high low-density lipoprotein cholesterol. J Am Coll Cardiol. 1994;23:899–906.

10. Pravastatin Limitation of Atherosclerosis in the Coronary Arteries (PLAC 1): A Summary

G. B. J. MANCINI

Abstract

PLAC 1 is a double-blind randomized placebo-controlled trial assessing the efficacy of monotherapy with an HMG-CoA reductase inhibitor (pravastatin) in altering the atherosclerotic process. This trial was an angiographic trial undertaken in the United States and was completed in early 1994. Despite the fact that angiographic endpoints were the prime focus during the planning and execution of the trial, significant impact was seen in the area of clinical events, particularly fatal and non-fatal myocardial infarctions. The latter were significantly reduced in the treated patients. These results were paralleled by a significant slowing of progression in the treated patients. Importantly, the angiographic effects were predominant in prevention of new lesion formation and in slowing the progression of mild/moderate lesions with less than 50% diameter stenosis at baseline. Current concepts suggest that the latter two categories of lesions are the most important in linking angiographic outcomes with clinical events. PLAC 1 is the first trial to show concomitantly statistically significant effects in clinical endpoints and angiographic endpoints in the category of new and/or mild stenoses. These results are compatible with the concept of plaque stabilization.

Methods

Pravastatin Limitation of Atherosclerosis in the Coronary Arteries (PLAC 1) is a multicentre prospective randomized placebo-controlled trial of the effect of lipid-lowering therapy on the progression and regression of coronary disease[1]. The major goals were to evaluate the effects of pravastatin on angiographic parameters of progression and regression and to evaluate these in the context of only moderate increases of low density lipoprotein (LDL) cholesterol.

The study was initiated in early 1988 and randomization ended after a 30-month recruitment period. All follow-up angiography was completed in 1993 and the angiographic analyses were completed in late 1993. Clinical endpoints were first published in the spring of 1994[2] and the angiographic endpoints were presented at the 1994 meeting of the American College of Cardiology.

During patient screening, angiography was to include at least two relatively orthogonal views of all coronary segments, central placement of the catheter, use of catheters of 6 French or greater in size, administration of nitroglycerin and

A.V.G. Bruschke et al. (eds): Lipid-lowering therapy and progression of atherosclerosis, 115–118.

detailed documentation of the sequence of injections during the procedure, including the angles of view. Quantitative angiography was used during the screening phase to ensure that these procedural factors were adhered to and that the presence of at least one stenosis of ≥50% could be documented.

Patients qualified for randomization if, after diet stabilization, their LDL-cholesterol concentrations were ≥130 and <190 mg/dl and triglycerides were ≤350 mg/dl. Pravastatin (40 mg) or placebo was administered once daily at bedtime.

During a 30-month recruitment period, 44 145 patients were screened, 1114 were enrolled and 706 were excluded prior to randomization. Thus, 408 patients were randomized. The most frequent reason for excluding patients during the screening and dietary lead-in phases was a low serum cholesterol level. That is, a large proportion of the patients identified largely through cardiac catheterization for established coronary disease had cholesterol concentrations considered to be normal or only modestly increased. There were 54 patients in the enrolled cohort that were excluded because of a technically inadequate angiogram.

The study design included a certification procedure undertaken by the Core Angiography Laboratory. This certification occurred early in the screening phase and was not limited to those patients that were suitable for enrolment in every other respect. There are 895 angiograms screened at baseline. Approximately 10% of these were rejected. The top three reasons for rejection were excessive streaming of contrast material, excessively poor image quality (reflected by an inordinate need to edit automatically determined edges) and the absence of a qualifying stenosis ≥50%. This overall rejection rate of 10% was a result of continuous feedback from the Core Angiographic Laboratory to the investigative sites about the reasons for film rejection. Early in the study, up to 29% of films in any given month were rejected whereas, in the intermediate and terminal stages of recruitment, the rejection rate was minimal.

Pravastatin or placebo was administered as two 20-mg tablets at bedtime and the dosage remained fixed for the duration of the study unless safety considerations dictated a reduction. The assignment was balanced within strata defined by clinical characteristics such as myocardial infarction, percutaneous transluminal coronary angioplasty and stable or unstable angina. This stratification also was undertaken based on LDL-cholesterol concentration ranges of 130–169 and 170–189 mg/dl.

In anticipation of increases in cholesterol beyond the 190 mg/dl range, a provision for treating patients who, during the study, had three consecutive levels above this threshold was incorporated. This included an initial change from a Step 1 to a Step 2 diet. If, after a month, this did not bring the LDL below 190 mg/dl, then cholestyramine resin was added in a titrated fashion up to 6 packets per day. If this was not successful, then 5–10 mg of open-label pravastatin was provided. A patient from the other treatment group, matched by age, sex and upper tertile of LDL-cholesterol concentration, was selected to undergo the more aggressive Step 2 dietary intervention or to receive pravastatin placebo. This was done to preserve the blinding during the study.

Results

Long-term lipid results included 18% and 26% reductions in serum total cholesterol and LDL-cholesterol, respectively, and an 8% increase in high density lipoprotein cholesterol. The predefined clinical endpoints (occurring after 90 days of treatment to ensure lipid lowering and out of deference to the lack of expected angiographic changes within this time period) showed unexpectedly positive results. In the pravastatin group, only 5 myocardial infarctions were noted whereas there were 17 in the placebo group (logrank $p = 0.005$). For the combined endpoints of non-fatal infarction plus death and non-fatal infarction plus coronary artery disease death, there were 8 and 7 in the privastatin group vs 19 and 18 in the placebo group, respectively (logrank $p = 0.017$ and 0.014, respectively).

The rate of progression of angiographic atherosclerosis was diminished by approximately 50% based on diameter stenosis, mean diameter, and minimum diameter measurements. Importantly, these effects were limited to those segments with baseline stenoses $\leq 50\%$. In addition, there were fewer patients in the privastatin group demonstrating new lesion formation than in the placebo group. The clinical endpoint results appear to be concordant, therefore, with dominant effects on new lesion formation and progression of modest lesions which are the substrate of most clinical events. This finding is in keeping with the concept of plaque stabilization which complements the overall demonstration of morphological improvement in the angiograms through lipid lowering.

Discussion

The PLAC 1 angiographic results are in keeping with another recently completed trial, the Canadian Coronary Atherosclerosis Intervention Trial[3]. The major difference is that the latter trial did not show a significant reduction in clinical events. Despite this, data continue to accumulate from all such trials that outcome, not just angiography, is improved by aggressive lipid lowering as can now be most easily achieved with the statin class of drugs.

All of the recent regression trials can be viewed as secondary prevention trials. Law and co-workers[4] have recently undertaken an extensive meta-analysis of lipid-lowering trials and focused their conclusions in males and in the context of an intervention amounting to approximately a 10% fall in total cholesterol. The expected reduction in coronary heart disease predicted by that study is compatible with the results shown in PLAC 1 when the larger magnitude of cholesterol reduction in PLAC 1 is taken into account. That is, a reduction of events in the PLAC 1 study of approximately 50% was seen in the context of a total cholesterol reduction of approximately 20%. This is compatible with the Law study showing a reduction of coronary heart disease events in middle-aged males of about 25%, with only a 10% net fall in total cholesterol. The PLAC 1 study will also add further weight to the positive meta-analyses of angiographic trials that are appearing in the literature[5-7].

References

1. Pitt B, Ellis SG, Mancini GB, Rosman HS, McGovern ME. Design and recruitment in the United States of a multicenter quantitative angiographic trial of pravastatin to limit atherosclerosis in the coronary arteries (PLAC I). Am J Cardiol. 1993;72:31–5.
2. Pitt B, Mancini GB, Ellis SG, Rosman HS, McGovern ME. Pravastatin limitation of atherosclerosis in the coronary arteries (PLAC I) [abstract]. J Am Coll Cardiol. 1994;23 Special Issue:131A.
3. Waters D, Higginson L, Gladstone P, et al. Effects of monotherapy with an HMG-CoA reductase inhibitor on the progression of coronary atherosclerosis as assessed by serial quantitative arteriography. The Canadian Coronary Atherosclerosis Intervention Trial. Circulation. 1994;89:959–68.
4. Law MR, Wald NJ, Thompson SG. By how much and how quickly does reduction in serum cholesterol concentration lower risk of ischaemic heart disease? BMJ. 1994;308:367–72.
5. Rossouw JE, Lewis B, Rifkind BM. The value of lowering cholesterol after myocardial infarction [Review]. N Engl J Med. 1990;323:1112–9.
6. Superko HR, Krauss RM. Coronary artery disease regression. Convincing evidence for the benefit of aggressive lipoprotein management [Review]. Circulation. 1994;90:1056–69.
7. Vos J, de Feyter PJ, Simoons ML, Tijssen JG, Deckers JW. Retardation and arrest of progression or regression of coronary artery disease: a review. [Review]. Prog Cardiovasc Dis. 1993;35:435–54.

11. The Multicenter Anti-Atheroma Study (MAAS)

THE MAAS INVESTIGATORS

Summary

The Multicentre Anti-Atheroma Study (MAAS) is a randomized double-blind clinical trial of 381 patients with mild coronary artery disease and moderate hyper-cholesterolaemia assigned to simvastatin (20 mg daily) or placebo treatment for 4 years.

Quantitative coronary arteriography was performed at baseline, 2 years and 4 years, and 167 placebo patients (89%) and 178 simvastatin patients (92%) had matched angiograms for analysis. The two primary outcome measures were:

1. The difference in change over 4 years in the mean lumen diameter of all coronary segments (a measure of diffuse atherosclerosis), treatment effect 0.06 mm in favour of simvastatin (95% CI 0.02–0.10), and
2. The difference in change over 4 years in the minimum lumen diameter of all lesions (a measure of focal atherosclerosis), treatment effect 0.08 mm in favour of simvastatin (95% CI 0.03–0.14). The treatment effect was similar in diseased and non-diseased segments.

On a per-patient basis, progression occurred less often in the simvastatin group, 23% vs 32% of the patients, and regression was more frequent, 18% vs 12% of the patients. Significantly, more new lesions and new total occlusions developed in the placebo group, 25% vs 14% and 11% vs 5%, respectively. There was no difference in clinical outcome.

In conclusion, monotherapy with 20 mg simvastatin daily during a 4-year period results in a significant stable amelioration of the lipid profile, which is associated with retardation of progression of diffuse and focal coronary atherosclerosis.

Introduction

The Multicenter Anti-Atheroma Study (MAAS), involving 11 centres in Europe, was conducted to study whether reducing lipoproteins with 20 mg simvastatin daily over a period of 4 years could reduce, relative to placebo, the progression of focal and diffuse coronary atherosclerosis in mildly symptomatic patients with moderate hypercholesterolaemia and mild angiographic coronary artery disease.

The MAAS comprises three serial coronary angiograms (baseline, 2 years and

A.V.G. Bruschke et al. *(eds): Lipid-lowering therapy and progression of atherosclerosis, 119–130.*
© 1996 *Kluwer Academic Publishers.*

4 years) and investigates the treatment effect of simvastatin over time in diseased and non-diseased coronary segments. The main results have recently been reported[1].

Patients and methods

The design, baseline characteristics, randomization and conduct of the MAAS trial have been published previously[2].

The inclusion criteria were:

1. Age 30–67 years.
2. At least two coronary artery segments visibly involved with atherosclerosis, but not totally occluded and neither requiring angioplasty or bypass surgery nor previously 'undergone' percutaneous transluminal coronary angioplasty (PTCA).
3. At least five segments in the qualifying angiogram suitable for quantitative analysis in at least two projections each.
4. Mean of two successive total serum cholesterol determinations 5.5–8.0 mmol/L.
5. Mean of two successive fasting serum triglyceride determinations less than 4.0 mmol/L.
6. Informed consent obtained.

The exclusion criteria were:

1. Myocardial infarction (MI) or unstable angina within six weeks before the qualifying angiogram
2. Previous coronary artery bypass surgery (CABG).
3. Angioplasty or major surgery within three months before the qualifying angiogram.
4. 'Qualifying angiography' more than 60 days prior to enrolment.
5. Clinical congestive heart failure or an ejection fraction less than 30%.
6. Diastolic blood pressure > 100 mmHg despite treatment.
7. Serum creatinine > 150 μmol/L.
8. Fasting blood sugar > 6.7 mmol/L, fasting venous plasma glucose > 7.8 mmol/L or diabetes requiring therapy other than diet.
9. Secondary hypercholesterolaemia due to hypothyroidism, nephrotic syndrome or other causes.
10. Abnormal liver function tests.
11. Recent history of hepatitis, biliary obstruction or cholelithiasis.
12. Partial ileal bypass.
13. Gross obesity: i.e. > 1.5 times the ideal weight.
14. Use of lipid-lowering drugs, oestrogens or steroids within six weeks of randomization.
15. Alcohol or drug abuse; psychosocial, physical, or mental condition which makes completion of the trial unlikely.

Lipoprotein measurements

Prior to blood sampling, the patient must have been fasting for 12 hours and been in a sitting position for 15 minutes. All lipid measurements: total cholesterol, HDL, triglycerides, apo-lipoprotein A-1 and B were performed in a central Lipid Reference Laboratory (LRL) in Rotterdam which is standardized in the programme of the Center for Disease Control, Atlanta, USA[3-7]. LDL was calculated using the Friedewald formula[8]. Lipoprotein(a) (Lp(a)) was analysed yearly by the Lipid Laboratory at Hammersmith Hospital, London with enzyme-linked immunosorbent assay (Tint Elize, Biopool, Umer, Sweden).

Coronary angiography and quantitative analysis

Coronary angiography was performed according to standards required for quantitative analysis[9]. Five minutes prior to angiography, 5 mg isosorbide dinitrate was given sublingually to induce standardized vasodilation.

All films were sent to the Angiographic Reference Laboratory for analysis. Two members of the Angiographic Committee reassessed the film and selected all possible coronary segments (RCA: 3 segments; LCX: 3–4 segments; LAD: 3 segments; left main: 1 segment) which appeared suitable for quantitative analysis. This required adequate filling with contrast medium, acceptable film contrast, suitable anatomy (no overlap or foreshortening). A qualifying angiogram was accepted only if at least 5 coronary segments were analysable (preferably in two orthogonal views). If this criterion was not met, patients were excluded retroactively. All available segments in views matched to the qualifying angiogram were analysed at follow-up. Quantitative analysis of coronary artery segments was carried out by the computer-assisted cardiovascular angiography analysis system (CAAS)[10].

Two primary efficacy parameters were adopted[9,11]:

1. A measure of **diffuse** coronary atherosclerosis: the per-patient average of mean lumen diameters (mm) of all coronary segments, angiographically non-diseased (diameter stenosis <20%) and diseased (diameter stenosis ≥20%).
2. A measure of **focal** coronary atherosclerosis: the per-patient average of minimum lumen diameters (mm) of all angiographically diseased segments (diameter stenosis ≥20%).

Furthermore, the per-patient average of the percentage diameter stenosis of all angiographically diseased segments (diameter stenosis ≥20%) is reported.

Progression of any segment was defined as either total occlusion of a previously patent segment or an increase of ≥15% diameter stenosis at follow-up of a lesion of ≥20% diameter stenosis present at baseline, or the development of a new lesion. A **new lesion** was defined as a segment with a diameter stenosis ≥20% at follow-up which had a diameter stenosis <20% at baseline, provided there was ≥15% diameter stenosis increase between baseline and follow-up.

Regression of any segment was defined as the appearance of patency of a previously occluded segment, or a decrease of ≥15% diameter stenosis at follow-up of a lesion existing at baseline and still present at follow-up, or the disappearance of a lesion (defined as a decrease of ≥15% diameter stenosis in a segment with a diameter stenosis ≥20% at baseline which has a diameter stenosis <20% at follow-up).

From this classification of segments, the following four categories of patients were defined:

– **Progressor** (at least one segment progressed and none regressed),
– **Mixed responder** (at least one segment regressed and also at least one segment progressed),
– **Stable** (no segments regressed or progressed) and
– **Regressor** (at least one segment regressed and none progressed).

Statistical methods

Continuous variables are presented as means and standard deviations; categorical variables as total number and percentages. Treatment effects were defined as the differences between the treatment groups in change between baseline and follow-up and are reported as point estimates with 95% confidence intervals. For comparisons between treatment groups unpaired *t*-tests were performed, comparisons within groups were evaluated with paired *t*-tests. For categorical outcome measures, rate ratios and 95% confidence intervals are reported and Chi-square tests were performed. For all hypothesis tests a two-sided p value <0.05 was considered significant.

Results

From March 1988 to November 1989, a total of 404 patients were randomized to receive simvastatin, 20 mg daily, or placebo treatment. Twenty-three patients have been excluded from this report because of ineligibility.

In 381 patients, an approved baseline angiogram was available, 345 had a final angiogram (272 four years, 73 two years), and 272 had baseline as well as a 2- and 4-year angiogram. In the 345 patients with a final angiogram, 5262 projections were analysed of 2679 coronary segments of which 1323 were angiographically diseased.

For the 381 patients (193 simvastatin, 188 placebo), the baseline characteristics are shown in Table 11.1. The treatment groups were well balanced.

The effects of simvastatin on serum lipids are shown in Table 11.2 and Figure 11.1.

The effects of simvastatin on the angiographic findings are shown in Table 11.3. There were 36 randomized patients (21 placebo, 15 simvastatin) without a final angiogram, which leaves 167 placebo and 178 simvastatin patients for analysis of primary outcomes.

Compared with placebo, the simvastatin group had less progression: treatment

Table 11.1. Baseline characteristics for all patients included in the study.

	Placebo ($n=188$)	Simvastatin ($n=193$)
Mean age (years)	54.9 (±7.1)	55.6 (±7.3)
Male	165 (88%)	171 (89%)
Current smoker	38 (20%)	53 (27%)
Obese (body mass index ≥30 kg/m²)	18 (10%)	15 (8%)
Systolic blood pressure (mmHg)	132 (±16)	132 (±17)
Diastolic blood pressure (mmHg)	80 (±8)	80 (±8)
Current angina		
None	57 (30%)	65 (34%)
Grade 1 or 2	116 (62%)	117 (61%)
Grade 3 or 4	15 (8%)	11 (5%)
Vessel disease*		
None	78 (42%)	77 (40%)
One	68 (36%)	72 (37%)
Two	30 (16%)	34 (18%)
Three	12 (6%)	10 (5%)
Previous myocardial infarction	101 (54%)	106 (55%)
Previous PTCA	83 (44%)	94 (49%)

*Visual assessment – a vessel was considered diseased when there was a stenosis of >50%.

effect on diffuse disease 0.06 mm and on focal disease 0.08 mm. Combining these two primary endpoints into a single test statistic produced a significant difference between simvastatin and placebo, $p=0.006$.

The changes between baseline and final angiogram in mean and minimum lumen diameter for segments with different degrees of stenosis at baseline are shown in Figures 11.2 and 11.3. Both angiographically non-diseased segments (diameter stenosis <20%) and mild to moderately diseased segments (diameter stenosis 20–50%) showed similar progression of disease and treatment effects, whereas the progression of disease and treatment effect were larger in severely diseased segments (diameter stenosis ≥50%).

There were 129 placebo and 143 simvastatin patients who had matched angiograms at baseline, 2 years and 4 years. In Figures 11.4 and 11.5, the mean changes at 2 years and 4 years compared with baseline are depicted. All measures of diffuse disease and focal disease showed rather similar time patterns which were consistent with a gradual and significant progression in patients on placebo and no significant overall change in patients on simvastatin.

Figure 11.6 shows a classification of patients on simvastatin and placebo according to angiographic improvement/worsening on their final angiogram compared with baseline. The simvastatin group had a smaller proportion of patients with progression and a higher proportion of patients with regression compared with placebo with an overall trend of $p=0.02$. Significantly fewer

124   The MAAS Investigators

Table 11.2. Serum lipid levels before and during treatment for all patients included in the study.

	Placebo			Simvastatin			Treatment effect*
	n	Baseline[1]	During[2]	n	Baseline[1]	During[2]	Difference (95% CI)
Total cholesterol (mmol/L)	184	6.43 (±0.82)	6.45 (±0.77)	189	6.35 (±0.73)	4.94 (±0.75)	−1.42 (−1.55, −1.29)
LDL-cholesterol (mmol/L)	184	4.47 (±0.77)	4.50 (±0.70)	189	4.38 (±0.69)	3.02 (±0.68)	−1.39 (−1.49, −1.25)
HDL-cholesterol (mmol/L)	184	1.11 (±0.27)	1.08 (±0.25)	189	1.10 (±0.30)	1.18 (±0.30)	0.10 (0.07, 0.13)
Triglycerides (mmol/L)	184	1.84 (±0.85)	1.92 (±0.93)	189	1.92 (±0.95)	1.68 (±0.79)	−0.33 (−0.45, −0.20)

n=Number of patients; CI=confidence interval; standard deviations in brackets. [1]Each patient's baseline values are the mean of two prerandomization measurements; [2]each patient's value during treatment is the mean of all available measurements during 4 years follow-up; *all treatment effects are significant ($p<0.001$).

Table 11.3. Changes per patient and treatment effects in quantitative coronary angiographic measurements during 4 years treatment.

	Placebo			Simvastatin			Treatment effect (95% CI)
	n	Baseline	Change	n	Baseline	Change	
Diffuse coronary atherosclerosis							
Mean lumen diameter (mm)	167	2.82 (±0.41)	−0.08 (±0.26)	178	2.84 (±0.38)	−0.02 (±0.23)	0.06 (0.02, 0.10)
Focal coronary atherosclerosis							
Minimum lumen diameter (mm)	166	1.91 (±0.39)	−0.13 (±0.27)	175	1.93 (±0.38)	−0.04 (±0.25)	0.08 (0.03, 0.14)

n=Number of patients; CI=confidence interval; standard deviations in brackets.

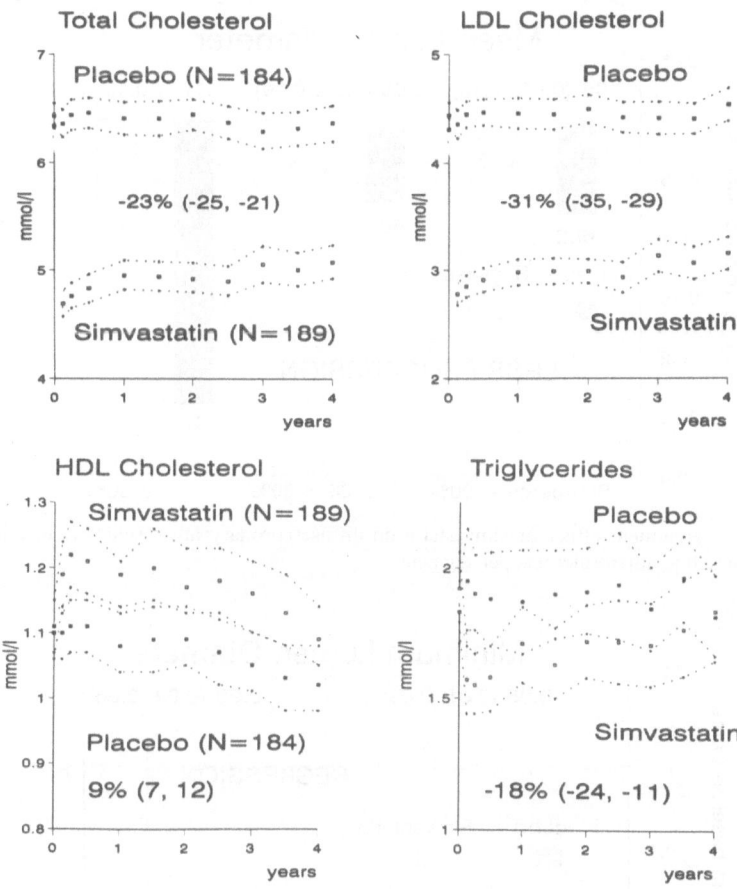

Figure 11.1. Effects of simvastatin on total cholesterol, LDL-cholesterol, HDL-cholesterol and triglycerides.

patients with new lesions, 28 versus 48, and fewer total occlusions, 8 vs 18, developed in the simvastatin group.

The occurrence of clinical events during 4 years follow-up is reported in Table 11.4. The differences between the groups are not statistically significant.

Discussion

In this multicentre study, monotherapy with simvastatin, 20 mg daily, reduced total cholesterol and LDL by one third and triglycerides by one fifth and increased HDL by one tenth. In the placebo group, no changes in lipids or in bodyweight occurred in spite of diet counselling at the beginning of the study.

Quantitative coronary angiography after 2 and 4 years showed a gradual progression of both diffuse and focal disease in the placebo group, whereas, in the simvastatin group, no progression of diffuse disease and only a small

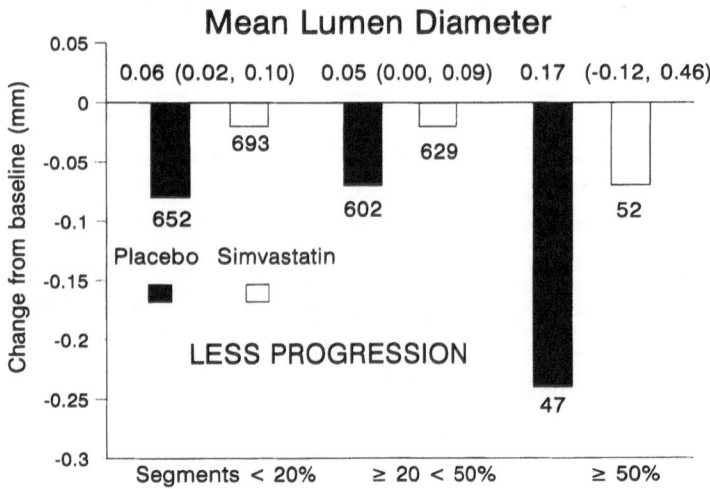

Figure 11.2. Treatment effect of simvastatin on diffuse coronary atherosclerosis in relation to severity of baseline atherosclerosis per segment.

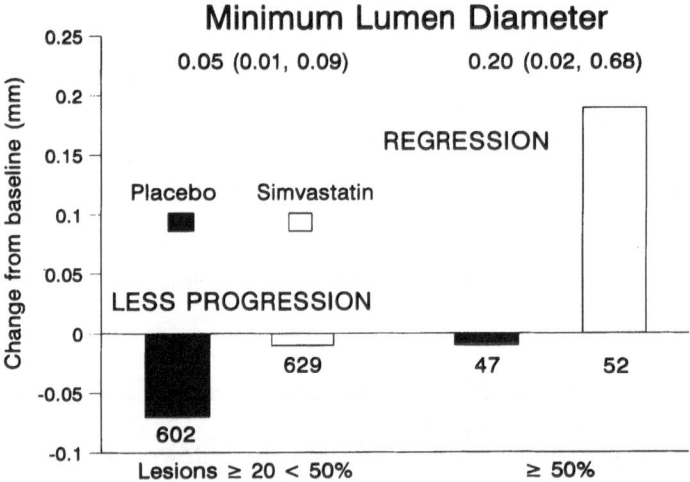

Figure 11.3. Treatment effect of simvastatin on focal coronary atherosclerosis in relation to severity of baseline lesions.

progression of focal disease occurred. The lipid changes in the simvastatin group were associated with a retardation of both diffuse and focal coronary athero-sclerosis in diseased and non-diseased coronary segments. The changes found in MAAS, 0.06 mm on diffuse disease and 0.08 mm on focal disease, are of almost the same magnitude as in other trials[12-18] using quantitative coronary angiography. At first sight, these observed angiographic changes appear to be

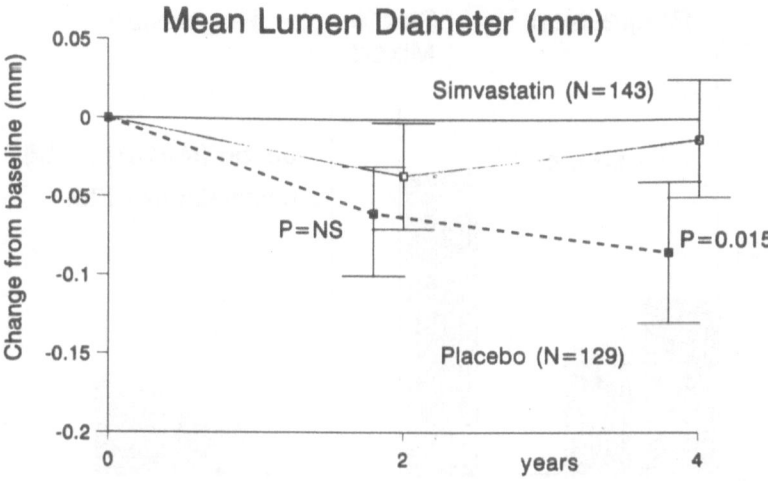

Figure 11.4. Treatment effect of simvastatin on diffuse coronary atherosclerosis at 2 and 4 years follow-up.

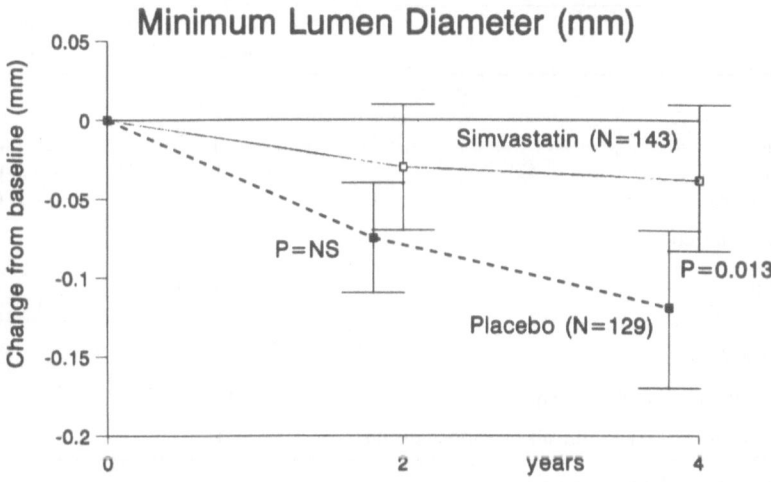

Figure 11.5. Treatment effect of simvastatin on focal coronary atherosclerosis at 2 and 4 years follow-up.

clinically insignificant, but, if these changes could be maintained over years, taking into account that coronary atherosclerosis progresses over decades, a substantial favourable effect on the lumen size might develop. Also, these relatively small angiographic changes have been shown to portend future beneficial effects on the occurrence of clinical events. Two serial quantitative angiographic studies[19,20], where patients were categorized into progressors and

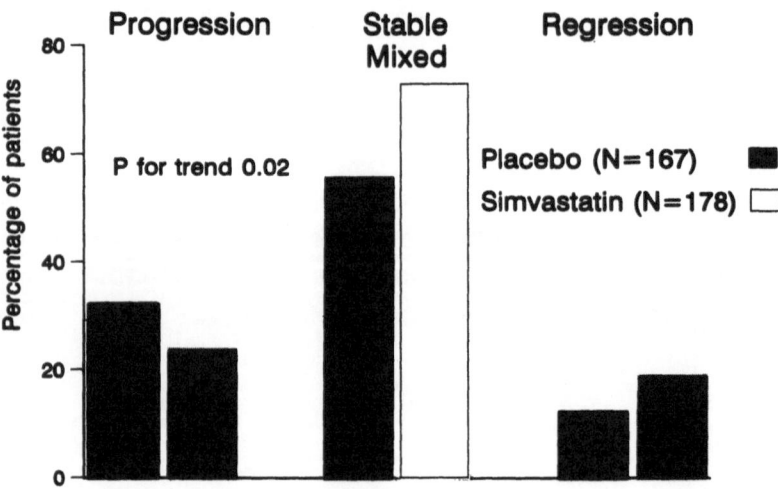

Figure 11.6.   Treatment effect of simvastatin on progression/regression per patient.

Table 11.4.   Clinical events during 4 years follow-up.

	Placebo (n = 188)	Simvastatin (n = 193)
Death		
Total	11	4
Cardiac	4	4
Sudden	1	0
Other causes	6	0
Myocardial infarction		
Total	7	11
Fatal MI	2	1
Non-fatal MI	5	10
CABG or PTCA	34	23
Hospitalization for unstable angina	18	15
Patients with at least one of the above cardiac events	51	40

All figures indicate number of patients.

non-progressors, indicated that the minimal angiographic progression was associated with a higher incidence of clinical events in progressors than non-progressors.

The MAAS trial is the first large quantitative angiographic trial to examine the effect of lipid lowering on both angiographically non-diseased segments and diseased segments. The findings show that the magnitude of progression and of the treatment effect in the non-diseased segments was similar to that of the mild and moderately diseased segments, indicating that both angiographically diseased and non-diseased segments benefit from lipid lowering. However, the treatment effect was largest in the severely diseased segments. There was a significant increase in minimum lumen diameter, and thus regression of focal disease, in lesions with a diameter stenosis ≥50%. This is in agreement with the MARS[13], the STARS[17] and the FATS[15] trials where the treatment effect was also more pronounced in the severe lesions, but opposed to the findings in the CCAIT[12] where the greatest benefit was found in the mild lesions.

The number of patients in our trial showing progression was reduced by 29% and the number of patients showing regression was increased by 55%. These figures resemble the results of the MARS[13] trial, 29% and 88%, and of the CCAIT[12], 34% and 47%, for progression and regression, respectively. Furthermore, the number of patients with new lesions and progression to total occlusion were significantly reduced in the simvastatin group. The prevention of the occurrence of angiographically new lesions, also found in the CCAIT trial[12], may be particularly important since lesions which tend to rupture are often non-severe lipid-rich lesions.

In this trial, there was no significant difference in the incidence of clinical events between the placebo and simvastatin groups. The sample size and duration of MAAS do not permit firm conclusions regarding the impact of simvastatin on the risk of cardiovascular events. The large POSCH[20] study with a follow-up of almost ten years, assessing the effects of ileal bypass surgery, showed a significant decrease of 35% in cardiac death and non-fatal myocardial infarction. This clinical benefit was preceded by a retardation of coronary atherosclerosis already present after 3 years.

The results of the MAAS trial and other angiographic trials indicate that lowering of atherogenic lipoproteins is associated with retardation of the atherosclerotic process and that this angiographic benefit accumulates over time. The need for longer follow-up is illustrated by the results of primary prevention trials that showed significant reductions in total coronary events only after about 5–6 years of treatment[21].

These observations all support the lipid hypothesis that amelioration of the lipid profile beneficially influences the course of coronary atherosclerosis which should result in an improved long-term clinical outcome. Serial angiographic studies show that the atherosclerotic process can be retarded by a relatively short-term intervention (2–4 years).

References

1. MAAS Investigators. Effect of simvastatin on coronary atheroma: The Multicenter Anti-Atheroma Study (MAAS) [Published erratum appears in Lancet. 1994;344:762]. Lancet. 1994; 344:633–8.
2. Dumont JM and the MAAS Research Group. Effect of cholesterol reduction by simvastatin on progression of coronary atherosclerosis: design, baseline characteristics, and progress of the Multicenter Anti-Atheroma Study (MAAS). Controlled Clin Trials. 1993;14:209–28.
3. Myers GL, Cooper GR, Winn CL, Smith LSJ. The centers for disease control. National Heart, Lung and Blood Institute lipid standardization program. Clin Lab Med. 1989;9:105–35.

4. Boerma GJM, Jansen AP, Jansen RTP, Leijnse B, van Strik R. Minimizing interlaboratory variation in routine assay of serum cholesterol through the use of serum calibrators. Clin Chem. 1986;32:943–7.
5. Kattermann R, Jaworek D, Möller G, et al. Multicenter study of a new enzymatic method of cholesterol determination. J Clin Chem Clin Biochem. 1984;22:245–51.
6. Warnick GR, Nguyen P, Albers JJ. Comparison of improved precipitation methods for quantitation of the high density lipoprotein cholesterol. Clin Chem. 1985;31:217–24.
7. Bucolo G, David H. Quantitative determination of serum triglycerides by use of enzymes. Clin Chem. 1973;19:475–82.
8. Friedewald WT, Levy RI, Fredrickson DS. Estimation of plasma low-density lipoprotein cholesterol without the use of the preparative ultracentrifuge. Clin Chem. 1972;18:499–502.
9. de Feyter PJ, Serruys PW, Davies MJ, et al. Quantitative coronary angiography to measure progression and regression of coronary atherosclerosis: value, limitations, and implications for clinical trials. Circulation. 1991;84:412–23.
10. Reiber JHC, Kooijman JC, Slager JC, et al. Computer assisted analysis of the severity of obstructions from coronary cineangiograms. A methodological Review. Automedica. 1984;5:219–38.
11. Pocock SJ, Geller NS, Tsiatis AA. The analysis of multiple endpoints in clinical trials. Biometrics. 1987;43:487–98.
12. Waters D, Higginson L, Gladstone P, et al. Effect of monotherapy with an HMG CoA reductase inhibitor upon the progression of coronary atherosclerosis as assessed by serial quantitative arteriography: the Canadian Coronary Atherosclerosis Intervention Trial (CCAIT). Circulation. 1994;89:959–68.
13. Blankenhorn DH, Azen SP, Kramsch DM, et al. Coronary angiographic changes with Lovastatin therapy – MARS. Ann Intern Med. 1993;119:969–76.
14. Ornish D, Brown SE, Scherwitz LW, et al. Can lifestyle changes reverse coronary heart disease? Lancet. 1990;336:129–33.
15. Brown G, Albers JJ, Fisher LD, et al. Regression of coronary artery disease as a result of intensive lipid-lowering therapy in men with high levels of apolipoprotein-B. N Engl J Med. 1990;323:1289–98.
16. Kane JP, Malloy MJ, Ports TA, et al. Regression of coronary atherosclerosis during treatment of familial hypercholesterolemia with combined drug regimens. JAMA. 190;264:3007–12.
17. Watts GF, Lewis B, Brunt JNH, et al. Effects on coronary artery disease of lipid-lowering diet, or diet plus cholestyramine, in the St Thomas Atherosclerosis Regression Study (STARS). Lancet. 1992;339:563–9.
18. Haskell WL, Alderman EL, Fair JM, et al. Effects of intensive multiple risk factor reduction on coronary atherosclerosis and clinical cardiac events in men and women with coronary artery disease. The Stanford Coronary Risk Intervention Project (SCRIP). Circulation. 1994;89:975–90.
19. Waters D, Craven TE, Lespérance J. Prognostic significance of progression of coronary atherosclerosis. Circulation. 1993;87:1067–75.
20. Buchwald H, Matts JP, Fitch LL, et al. for the Program on the Surgical Control of the Hyperlipidemias (POSCH) Group. Changes in sequential coronary arteriograms and subsequent coronary events. JAMA. 1992;268:1429–33.
21. Holme I. Relation of coronary heart disease incidence and total mortality to plasma cholesterol reduction in randomized trials: use of meta-analysis. Br Heart J. 1993;69(1 Suppl):S42–7.

12. Lessons from the Monitored Atherosclerosis Regression Study (MARS) and beyond: atherosclerosis progression/regression responses to therapy depend on lesion size and composition

D. M. KRAMSCH

Summary

MARS and other angiographic trials revealed that aggressive LDL-cholesterol reduction regressed only advanced fibrous–fatty plaques while younger cell proliferative lesions progressed further. We, therefore, tested the antioxidant/antiproliferant Ca^{2+}-antagonist amlodipine in cynomolgus monkeys on atherogenic diet. Amlodipine did not lower elevated LDL-cholesterol but suppressed the rises in circulating oxidized LDL, insulin and triglycerides, resulting in significant atherosclerosis suppression and suggesting amlodipine as an effective adjunct to lipid-lowering therapy.

Introduction

Atherosclerotic vascular disease remains the leading cause of death and morbidity in industrialized nations[1,2] in spite of the fact that many risk factors associated with coronary and other atherosclerotic vascular disease, such as hypercholesterolaemia, hypertension, diabetes mellitus, central obesity and smoking have been identified and substantial progress has been made in risk-factor prevention programmes. Hypercholesterolaemia, especially elevations of low density lipoprotein cholesterol (LDL-C), has been thought to be the chief cause of atherosclerotic disease[3]. Consequently, efforts have principally focused on decreasing plasma LDL-C as a means of preventing, arresting or reversing the atherosclerotic disease process. As a substantial number of pertinent trials have already been completed, it is warranted to take stock as well as to assess how far lipid-lowering therapy has brought us and where we go from here.

Limitations of lipid-lowering therapy for atherosclerotic arterial disease

The Cholesterol Lowering Atherosclerosis Study (CLAS) was the first trial to shed a realistic light on what can be expected to be achieved by maximal reduction of LDL-C to levels below 100 mg/dl (2.59 mm/L)[3,4]. CLAS was a randomized placebo-controlled angiographic trial in which the treatment regimens consisted of placebo or a combination of high-dose niacin (mean 4.3 g/day) and colestipol (mean 29 g/day) with substantial dietary saturated fat restrictions in both groups. Similar maximal LDL-C reductions were achieved in

A.V.G. Bruschke et al. *(eds): Lipid-lowering therapy and progression of atherosclerosis, 131–141.*
© 1996 *Kluwer Academic Publishers.*

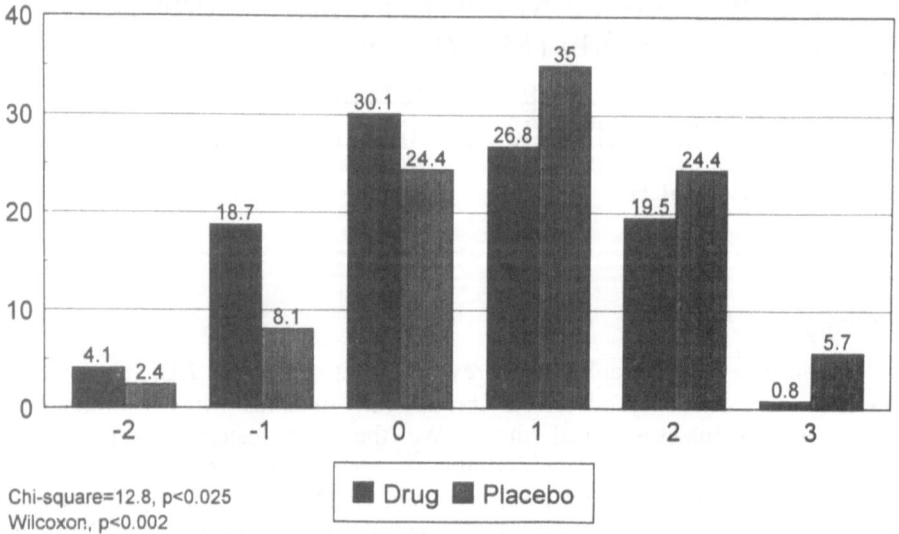

Figure 12.1. Global change score of coronary arteries in MARS comparing angiograms at baseline and after two years as estimated by a panel of expert angiographers. 0 = no change; 1 = small change; 2 = intermediate change; 3 = large change; − = regression. In the drug-treated group, only a total of 52.9% of the patients did not progress (0) or showed small (−1) or intermediate (−2) regression of lesions. On the other hand, 47.1% of the drug-treated patients did reveal atherosclerosis progression in spite of maximal lowering of LDL-cholesterol to 86 mg/dl.

our recently completed Monitored Atherosclerosis Regression Study (MARS) in which patients received lovastatin (80 mg/dl) and a slightly more relaxed low-fat diet[5]. Other recent angiographic trials, such as the Familial Atherosclerosis Treatment Study (FATS)[6] and the Program on Surgical Control of Hyperlipidemias (POSCH)[7] achieved similar drastic reductions of LDL-C.

In spite of these aggressive reductions in LDL-C levels, arrest of atherosclerosis progression – determined either by panel reading of angiograms or quantitative coronary angiography (QCA) – occurred only in about 50–60% of patients while, in about 40–50% of the patients, atherosclerosis further progressed, as shown for example by the results of MARS (Figure 12.1). This notion was reinforced when other parameters in native vessels and bypass grafts were analysed after 2 years of treatment at the end of CLAS I[3] and after 4 years of treatment at the end of CLAS II[4]. Compared with placebo, maximal drug treatment for four years resulted in reducing, by about one half, the number of subjects with angiographically new lesions in native coronary arteries and bypass grafts, but it did not abolish the occurrence of substantial new lesion formation in the other half.

The reasons for these phenomena appear to be that other factors which cannot be influenced by LDL-C reduction alone operate independently to promote atherogenesis. Among the likely candidates for these independent atherogenic

Table 12.1. Significant risk factors (+) for coronary lesion progression measured by quantitative computer angiography in the MARS study.

	Placebo group ($n = 106$)		Lovastatin group ($n = 114$)	
	<50% stenosis	≥50% stenosis	<50% stenosis	≥50% stenosis
Univariate analysis				
ΔTC/HDL-C	+	+	NS	NS
ΔLDL-C/HDL-C	NS	+	NS	NS
OT triglycerides	NS	NS	+	NS
ΔAPO-CIII-HP	NS	NS	+	NS
Multivariate analysis				
ΔTC/HDL-C	+	+	NS	NS
OT LDL-C/HDL-C	NS	NS	NS	+
OT APO-CIII-HP	NS	NS	+	NS

+ = significant relative risk (95% CI); NS = not significant; TC/HDL-C = total cholesterol/high density lipoprotein-cholesterol; APO-CIII-HP = apolipoprotein CIII heparin precipitate (marker for triglyceride-rich lipoprotein; VLDL); LDL-C = low density lipoprotein-cholesterol; Δ = absolute change from baseline; OT = on trial value.

factors are oxidized LDL, triglyceride-rich lipoproteins and unopposed smooth muscle cell proliferation[8]. The CLAS study has demonstrated for the first time that coronary atherosclerosis further progresses when triglyceride-rich lipoproteins are not reduced simultaneously with maximal LDL-C lowering[9]. The MARS trial[10] confirmed these CLAS findings, revealing that for lesions of <50% stenosis at baseline, triglyceride-rich lipoproteins are one of the driving forces of lesion progression, once LDL-C has been removed aggressively (Table 12.1).

A small but significant lesion regression was demonstrated by maximal LDL-C reduction in the following percentages of subjects: 16.2% in CLAS I[3], 17.9% in CLAS II[4], 23% in MARS[5], and 33% in FATS[6] compared with much smaller percentages of subjects showing regression in the placebo groups of these trials. A startling result of MARS[5] was the clear-cut difference in the response to maximal LDL-lowering to 86 mg/dl (2.2 mm/L) between angiographic lesions of ≥50% stenosis and those <50% stenosis at baseline (Figure 12.2). Significant arrest of lesion progression and regression was demonstrated only in the larger fibrous–fatty plaques of ≥50% stenosis, whereas the lesions of <50% stenosis did not stop progressing with maximal lowering of LDL-C alone. Five other angiographic trials[6,11–14] also showed a greater impact of LDL-C lowering on the more advanced larger (older) lesions than on the younger smaller intermediate lesions. The reason for this benefit may be that most of the advanced plaques of >50% stenosis contain lipid-rich necrotic cores which are often large (Figure 12.3a and b) and which apparently can be reduced by aggressive LDL-C lowering, resulting in a small reduction of lesion size up to a point. As most of these advanced older lesions are also severely fibrotic, it appears that any further reduction in lesion size is limited by the failure to remove these collagenous fibrous masses by our current treatment regimens as evidenced by the minimal additional plaque reversal after the extension of CLAS

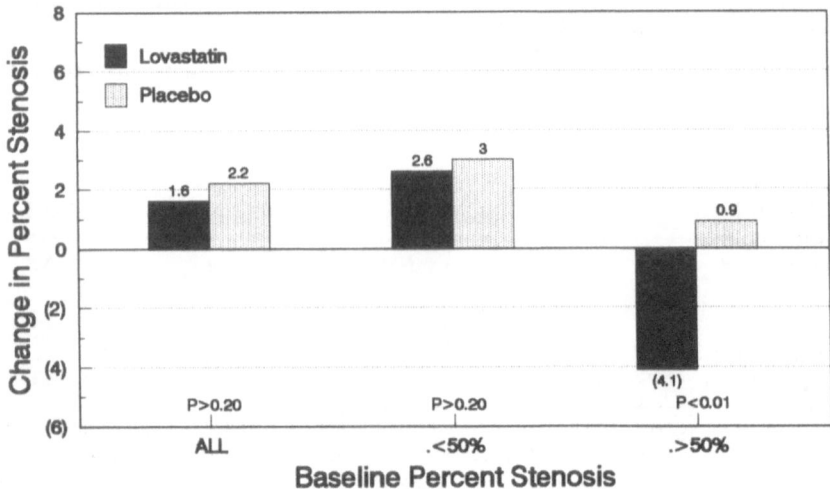

Figure 12.2. Quantitative computer analysis of MARS angiogram comparing change in lesions of <50% stenosis at baseline to those of ≥50% stenosis. Regression was achieved only in the larger fibrous–fatty lesions of ≥50% stenosis whereas lesions of <50% stenosis further progressed in spite of maximal lovastatin treatment with no statistical difference from placebo treatment.

I[3] for two years to CLAS II[4] (16.2% vs 17.9%, see above). The extension of FATS for two and one half more years also showed only minimal added lesion regression in spite of continued maximal LDL-C lowering by even triple lipid-lowering therapy[15].

It is of considerable interest that the younger intermediate lesions of <50% (angiographic) stenosis failed to stop progressing in MARS and five other trials with lipid-lowering regimens. These smaller lesions are presumed to be most dangerous because of their instability resulting from a younger and thinner fibrous cap, easily prone to rupture, covering a necrotic core[16]. This lesion type should have benefited most by maximal LDL-C reduction instead of continuing to grow. This apparent paradox is resolved if one takes into account the known differences in the composition of these intermediate lesions. The International Atherosclerosis Project[17] revealed that, up to age 54, only 20% of these smaller coronary lesions contain necrotic cores which could be reduced by lipid lowering and that, even after age 55, the incidence of necrotic cores in these lesions only rises to slightly more than 50%. Similarly, the study of Pathological Determinants in Youth (Robert W. Wissler, personal communication) showed necrotic cores only in 26% of intermediate lesions of the left-anterior descending coronary artery in subjects up to 35 years of age. In other words, while some of these intermediate lesions indeed contain such dangerous necrotic cores with thin fibrous caps and can be stabilized by lipid lowering (reducing clinical events), this is not the predominant type to be found in angiographically smaller lesions. The vast majority of these smaller lesions are of fibro-smooth muscle cell (SMC)-proliferative nature (Figure 12.3c) and appear to be prone to further

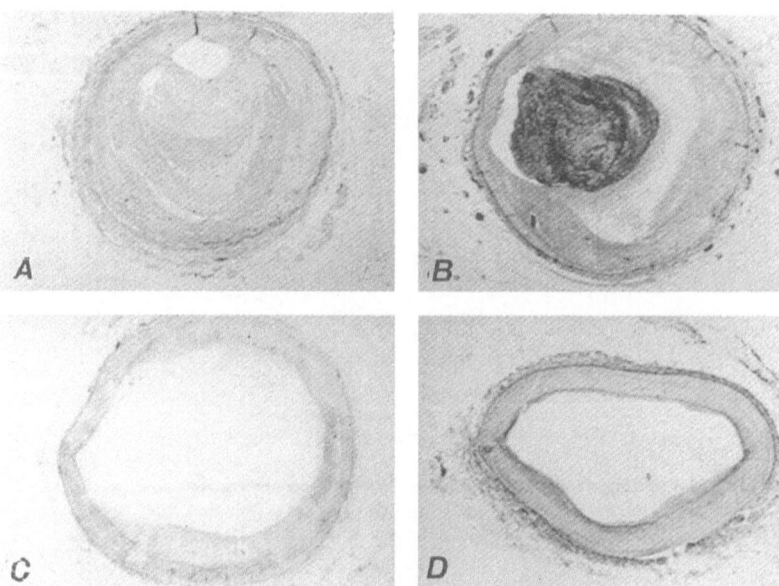

Figure 12.3.   Cross-sections through lesions of coronary artery. The top two lesions (a,b) are large fibrous–fatty (dark grey=collagen) plaques of >50% stenosis anatomically as well as angiographically. Both contain large lipid-rich necrotic cores (light-coloured areas) which can apparently be shrunk by lowering of LDL-cholesterol (LDL-C) resulting in lesion stabilization. At bottom right (d) is a fatty streak lesion which does not intrude much into the arterial lumen and which also can be reduced by lowering of LDL-C. In contrast, the intermediate lesions of angiographically <50% stenosis, as seen on the bottom left (c) and which constitute the still-progressing lesions in MARS, did not show a group response to maximal lowering of LDL-C. These lesions contain much less collagen (grey), consist predominantly of proliferating smooth muscle cells, and less than one-half of these younger lesions contain lipid-rich necrotic areas that can be shrunk by lipid lowering.

growth, once started, which apparently cannot be arrested by reduction of plasma LDL-C alone.

In contrast to these intermediate SMC-proliferative lesions, the earliest lesions of atherosclerosis, the macrophage derived foam cell lesions or fatty streaks (Figure 12.3d), which cannot be visualized by angiography but impose as intima-media thickening by ultrasound imaging, can be reduced in size by lipid lowering, at least as demonstrated with carotid artery ultrasonography[18,19]. There is recent evidence that oxidized LDL may also be particularly involved in the progression of early carotid artery atherosclerosis as the rate of progression correlated with a titre of autoantibodies against oxidized LDL[20].

The multifactorial genesis of atherosclerosis and some common pathways

It is clear from the above considerations that a variety of atherogenic mechanisms must be explored for their potential yield in treatment modalities for this multi-

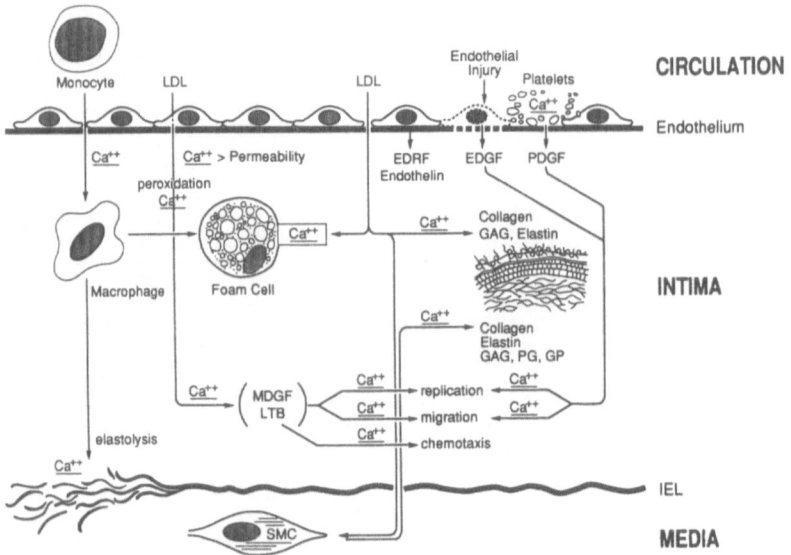

Figure 12.4. Schematic representation of current concepts of atherogenesis: Ca^{2+} = ionic calcium as second messenger in atherogenic processes; EDRF = endothelium-derived relaxing factor; EDGF = endothelium-derived growth factor; PDGF = platelet-derived growth factor; MGDF = macrophage-derived growth factor; GAG = glycosaminoglycans; PG = proteoglycans; GP = glycoprotein; IEL = internal elastic lamina; LDL = low density lipoprotein; LTB = leukotriene B; SMC = smooth muscle cell.

factorial disease; treatment modalities that go beyond lowering of conventional lipids. According to the current concepts of atherogenesis[21,22] depicted in Figure 12.4, the main processes leading to plaque formation include:

1. Increased permeability of the endothelium to macromolecules such as LDL, a process which is enhanced by endothelial cell constriction and subsequent opening of endothelial junctions in response to vasoconstrictive agents (e.g. catecholamines);
2. Blood cells such as monocyte/macrophages (Mφs) and lymphocytes also enter the intimal space readily, and platelets adhere to areas of functional endothelial injury or denudation;
3. Platelets secrete platelet-derived growth factors, the altered endothelium releases endothelial growth factor, macrophages release macrophage growth factor and many other growth factors, presumably including insulin and angiotensin II, come into play in the arterial intima during atherogenesis which all have in common that they recruit smooth muscle cells (SMC) from the media to migrate to the intima where they proliferate by mitosis;
4. These proliferated SMCs, along with Mφs, internalize lipids and oxidatively modified lipoproteins either by LDL receptors (SMCs) or scavenger receptors (Mφs); but more importantly these migrated SMCs synthesize and

secrete into the extracellular intimal space excessive amounts of collagen, elastin, glycosaminoglycans and other connective tissue elements – in other words, cause the formation of the significant human lesion which produces the clinical symptoms – the fibrous plaque.

In fact, one of the newer hypotheses of atherogenesis, building on concepts developed by earlier researchers, including ourselves[21], holds that the intimal connective tissue accumulation and alteration comes first and that this accumulated connective tissue traps LDL by tight binding[23,24]. Then, the longer LDL is kept resident in the arterial wall, the more it can become oxidized and attract Mφs which take it up and become foam cells in the process. It has been demonstrated by several researchers that glycated collagen[25] and glycosamino-glycans[26], both increased in diabetes mellitus, as well as collagen type I[27] and elastin[28], both increased in hypertension and atherosclerosis, all avidly bind LDL and cholesterol. We, therefore, can conceive that, at least in hypertension and in diabetes mellitus, the connective tissue accumulation and changes precede the lipid changes, including lipoprotein peroxidation, in the arterial wall. This may explain why large advanced plaques can be made to regress through lipid lowering only up to a point by removing intracellular lipids and extracellular lipids (e.g. from lipid-rich necrotic cores), leaving an irreducible rest: the amassed connective tissue. As the hallmarks of hypertension and diabetes mellitus are especially large depositions of altered intimal connective tissue in the arterial intima and throughout the thickened intima, it is understandable that halting and/or reversal of lesion progression in both conditions appears to be extremely difficult. This may account, at least in part, for the negative outcome of the Multicenter Isradipine Diuretic Atherosclerosis Study (MIDAS)[29] which employed a non-antioxidant dihydropyridine (isradipine) as an antiathero-sclerosis agent in patients with hypertension.

Another impasse is imposed by the apparent inability of maximal lipid lowering to arrest further progression and growth of the more SMC-proliferative (coronary) lesions of <50% angiographic stenosis[5,6,11-14]. As depicted in Figure 12.4, most processes of atherogenesis and particularly the proliferation and migration of SMCs and the secretion of connective tissue by these cells requires calcium ions (Ca^{2+}) as second messengers. It is not surprising then that Ca^{2+}-channel blockers, particularly the dihydropyridines, have been shown to suppress in (non-hypertensive) animal models the development and progression of atherosclerotic lesions, especially the SMC-proliferative component as well as the excessive secretion of connective tissue by these SMCs[30-32]. Consistent with these animal data are data obtained in non-hypertensive patients with coronary artery disease, indicating that the calcium channel blockers, nifedipine[33,34] and nicardipine[35] have an inhibiting effect on the formation of angiographically new (anatomically intermediate) lesions in coronary arteries, i.e. on precisely the SMC-proliferative phase of atherosclerosis that cannot be influenced by lipid-lowering agents[5]. It is noteworthy in this context that there is growing evidence from animal work that antioxidant therapy also can reduce the rate of progression

Table 12.2.   Antioxidant effect according to RO· and ROO· test.

	Antioxidant effect*	
	RO·	ROO·
Lacidipine	3.9×10^{-3}	3.4×10^{-3}
Amlodipine	1.0×10^{-3}	4.0×10^{-3}
Nicardipine	5.7×10^{-3}	Inactive
Verapamil	0.3×10^{-3}	Inactive
Probucol	0.7×10^{-3}	0.5×10^{-1}
Trolox	2.1×10^{-1}	1.8

*Reported values are the ratios between rate constants for reactions with alkoxyl and hydroperoxyl radicals of different compounds and crocin. The hydroperoxyl radicals are most predominantly involved in the peroxidation of lipids and lipoproteins.

of atherosclerosis[36–39]. Additionally, data from prospective human studies support a negative correlation between intake of antioxidants and coronary heart disease[40,41].

The role of amlodipine in atherosclerosis suppression

It is, therefore, of considerable interest that some of the new generation of Ca^{2+}-antagonists, the highly lipophilic dihydropyridine agents, amlodipine, nisoldipine and lacidipine[42,43] possess, in addition to their Ca^{2+}-antagonistic suppressive effect on SMC-proliferation and connective tissue accumulation, antioxidant properties not found in the older Ca^{2+}-antagonists, such as nifedipine, nicardipine, isradipine, verapamil and diltiazem, to name a few. These new-generation compounds have been shown to have marked inhibitory properties on oxygen free radicals involved in lipid peroxidation[42,43] (Table 12.2) as well as a pronounced stabilizing effect on cell membrane lipid bilayers[44].

We tested the antiatherosclerosis capacity of one of these antioxidant Ca^{2+}-antagonists, amlodipine, in non-human primates (cynomolgus monkeys) on a high-butter atherogenic diet at a dose of 2 mg amlodipine/kg body weight per day. At that dose, plasma amlodipine levels in the primates rose to (but did not exceed) therapeutic levels aimed for in humans, without affecting blood pressure or heart rate in the normotensive primates: C_{max} (6 h post-dosing) = 35 ng/dl; C_{min} (24 h post-dosing) = 12 ng/dl). We demonstrated that the drug normalized elevated plasma levels of in-vivo generated[45] circulating oxidized LDL (LDL^-) without reducing elevated total LDL-C levels[46]; it also normalized elevated serum insulin and triglyceride concentrations, effectively removing another independent atherogenic factor: triglyceride-rich lipoproteins[9]. This antioxidant Ca^{2+}-antagonist revealed a highly significant suppressive effect on atherosclerosis progression. It restored absent endothelial relaxing factor release by preventing LDL oxidation[47] and, while all 10 untreated monkeys on the atherogenic diet showed grade IV/IV atherosclerosis of aorta and coronary arteries, atherosclerosis was absent in systemic and coronary vessels in five of the 11 atherogenic-diet monkeys treated with amlodipine, mild (grade I and II) in 3, and more severe (grade III and IV) only in 2 of the treated animals[46-48]. The degree of protection from atherosclerosis correlated directly and highly significantly ($p < 0.0004$) with the circulating blood amlodipine levels.

We concluded that amlodipine, by the added (or synergistic) effects of blocking calcium movement into cells and of preventing LDL-oxidation, inhibited SMC proliferation and Mϕ infiltration; furthermore, it protected the endothelium and restored endothelium function, and prevented the rises in circulating insulin and triglyceride levels. These mechanisms appeared to act in concert to effect a remarkable suppression of the development and progression of atherosclerosis without reducing elevated plasma total cholesterol and LDL-C. The data indicate that amlodipine lends itself as an effective adjunct to lipid lowering or to monotherapy in atherosclerotic vascular disease.

References

1. Castelli WP. Epidemiology of coronary heart disease: the Framingham study. Am J Med. 1984;76:4–12.
2. American Heart Association. Heart and stroke facts: 1989–1990. Dallas, Tex.: American Heart Association; 1990.
3. Blankenhorn DH, Nessim SA, Johnson RL, Sanmarco ME, Azen SP, Cashin-Hemphill L. Beneficial effects of combined colestipol–niacin therapy on coronary atherosclerosis and coronary venous bypass grafts [published erratum appears in JAMA. 1988;259:2698]. JAMA. 1987;257:3233–40.
4. Cashin-Hemphill L, Mack WJ, Pogoda JM, Sanmarco ME, Azen SP, Blankenhorn DH. Beneficial effects of colestipol–niacin on coronary atherosclerosis. A 4-year follow-up. JAMA. 1990;264:3013–17.
5. Blankenhorn DH, Azen SP, Kramsch DM, et al. Coronary angiographic changes with lovastatin therapy. The Monitored Atherosclerosis Regression Study (MARS). The MARS Research Group. Ann Intern Med. 1993;119:969–76.
6. Brown G, Albers JJ, Fisher LD, et al. Regression of coronary artery disease as a result of intensive lipid-lowering therapy in men with high levels of apolipoprotein B. N Engl J Med. 1990;323:1289–98.
7. Buchwald H, Varco RL, Matts JP, et al. Effect of partial ileal bypass surgery on mortality and morbidity from coronary heart disease in patients with hypercholesterolemia. Report of the Program on the Surgical Control of the Hyperlipidemias (POSCH). N Engl J Med. 1990; 323:946–55.
8. Kramsch DM, Blankenhorn DH. Regression of atherosclerosis: which components regress and what influences their reversal [Review]. Wien Klin Wochenschr. 1992;104:2–9.
9. Blankenhorn DH, Alaupovic P, Wickham E, Chin HP, Azen SP. Prediction of angiographic change in native human coronary arteries and aortocoronary bypass grafts. Lipid and nonlipid factors. Circulation. 1990;81(2):470–6.
10. Hodis HN, Mack WJ, Azen SP, et al. Triglyceride- and cholesterol-rich lipoproteins have a differential effect on mild/moderate and severe lesion progression as assessed by quantitative coronary angiography in a controlled trial of lovastatin. Circulation. 1994;90:42–9.
11. Brensike JF, Levy RI, Kelsey SF, et al. Effects of therapy with cholestyramine on progression of coronary atherosclerosis: results of the NHLBI Type II Coronary Intervention Study. Circulation. 1984;69:313–24.
12. Arntzenius AC, Kromhout D, Barth JD, et al. Diet, lipoproteins, and the progression of coronary atherosclerosis. The Leiden Intervention Trial. N Engl J Med. 1985;312:805–11.

13. Ornish D, Brown SE, Scherwitz LW, et al. Can lifestyle changes reverse coronary heart disease? The Lifestyle Heart Trial. Lancet. 1990;336:129–33.
14. Watts GF, Lewis B, Brunt JN, et al. Effects on coronary artery disease of lipid-lowering diet, or diet plus cholestyramine, in the St Thomas' Atherosclerosis Regression Study (STARS). Lancet. 1992;339:563–9.
15. Stewart BF, Brown BG, Zhao XQ, et al. Coronary atherosclerosis regression is less pronounced during a second course of comparably effective lipid-lowering therapy [abstract]. Circulation. 1993;8(4 Suppl);I363.
16. Brown BG, Zhao XQ, Sacco DE, Albers JJ. Lipid lowering and plaque regression. New insights into prevention of plaque disruption and clinical events in coronary disease [Review]. Circulation. 1993;87(6):1781–91.
17. Tracy RE, Kissling GE. Age and fibroplasia as preconditions for atheronecrosis in human coronary arteries. Arch Pathol Lab Med. 1987;111:957–63.
18. Blankenhorn DH, Selzer RH, Crawford DW, et al. Beneficial effects of colestipol–niacin therapy on the common carotid artery. Two- and four-year reduction of intima-media thickness measured by ultrasound. Circulation. 1993;88:20–8.
19. Mack WJ, Selzer RH, Hodis HN. One-year reduction and longitudinal analysis of carotid intima-media thickness associated with colestipol/niacin therapy. Stroke. 1993;24:1779–83.
20. Salonen JT, Yla-Herttuala S, Yamamoto R, et al. Autoantibody against oxidised LDL and progression of carotid atherosclerosis. Lancet. 1992;339:883–7.
21. Kramsch DM. Calcium antagonists and atherosclerosis. Adv Exp Med Biol. 1985;183:323–48.
22. Ross R. The pathogenesis of atherosclerosis — an update [Review]. N Engl J Med. 1986; 314:488–500.
23. Carew TE, Pittman RC, Marchand ER, Steinberg D. Measurement in vivo of irreversible degradation of low density lipoprotein in the rabbit aorta. Predominance of intimal degradation. Arteriosclerosis. 1984;4:214–24.
24. Haberland ME, Fong D, Cheng L. Malondialdehyde-altered protein occurs in atheroma of Watanabe heritable hyperlipidemic rabbits. Science. 1988;241:215–18.
25. Cerami A, Vlassara H, Brownlee M. Protein glycosylation and the pathogenesis of atherosclerosis [Review]. Metabolism. 1985;34(12 Suppl 1):37–42.
26. Yla-Herttuala S, Solakivi T, Hirvonen J, et al. Glycosaminoglycans and apolipoproteins B and A-I in human aortas. Chemical and immunological analysis of lesion-free aortas from children and adults. Arteriosclerosis. 1987;7:333–40.
27. Hoover GA, McCormick S, Kalant N. Interaction of native and cell-modified low density lipoprotein with collagen gel. Arteriosclerosis. 1988;8(5):525–34.
28. Kramsch DM, Franzblau C, Hollander W. The protein and lipid composition of arterial elastin and its relationship to lipid accumulation in the atherosclerotic plaque. J Clin Invest. 1971; 50:1666–77.
29. Grimm RH Jr. Results of measurement of carotid intimal-medial thickness by ultrasound: the primary end point [abstract]. In: Abstracts of the satellite symposium Midas, a pivotal study in hypertension, of the 15th scientific meeting of the International Society of Hypertension, Melbourne, Australia, March 20, 1994. London: AVMD International Ltd.; 1994:18.
30. Weinstein DB, Heider JG. Antiatherogenic properties of calcium antagonists [Review]. Am J Cardiol. 1987;59(3):163B–72B.
31. Weinstein DB, Heider JG. Antiatherogenic properties of calcium antagonists. State of the art. Am J Med. 1989;86:27–32.
32. Henry PD, Bentley KI. Suppression of atherogenesis in cholesterol-fed rabbits treated with nifedipine. J Clin Invest. 1981;68:1366–9.
33. Loaldi A, Polese A, Montorsi P. Comparison of nifedipine, propranolol and isosorbide dinitrate on angiographic progression and regression of coronary arterial narrowings in angina pectoris. Am J Cardiol. 1989;64:433–9.
34. Lichtlen PR, Hugenholtz PG, Rafflenbeul W, Hecker H, Jost S, Deckers JW. Retardation of angiographic progression of coronary artery disease by nifedipine. Results of the International Nifedipine Trial on Antiatherosclerotic Therapy (INTACT). INTACT Group Investigators. Lancet. 1990;335:1109–13.

35. Waters D, Lesperance J, Francetich M, et al. A controlled clinical trial to assess the effect of a calcium channel blocker on the progression of coronary atherosclerosis. Circulation. 1990; 82:1940–53.
36. Carew TE, Schwenke DC, Steinberg D. Antiatherogenic effect of probucol unrelated to its hypocholesterolemic effect: evidence that antioxidants in vivo can selectively inhibit low density lipoprotein degradation in macrophage-rich fatty streaks and slow the progression of atherosclerosis in the Watanabe heritable hyperlipidemic rabbit. Proc Natl Acad Sci USA. 1987;84:7725–9.
37. Kita T, Nagano Y, Yokode M, et al. Probucol prevents the progression of atherosclerosis in Watanabe heritable hyperlipidemic rabbit, an animal model for familial hypercholesterolemia. Proc Natl Acad Sci USA. 1987;84:5928–31.
38. Bjorkhem I, Henriksson-Freyschuss A, Breuer O, Diczfalusy U, Berglund L, Henriksson P. The antioxidant butylated hydroxytoluene protects against atherosclerosis. Arterioscler Thromb. 1991;11:15–22.
39. Sparrow CP, Doebber TW, Olszewski J, et al. Low density lipoprotein is protected from oxidation and the progression of atherosclerosis is slowed in cholesterol-fed rabbits by the antioxidant N,N'-diphenyl-phenylenediamine. J Clin Invest. 1992;89:1885–91.
40. Manson JE, Gaziano JM, Jonas MA, Hennekens CH. Antioxidants and cardiovascular disease: a review [Review]. J Am Coll Nutr. 1993;12:426–32.
41. Stampfer MJ, Hennekens CH, Manson JE, Colditz GA, Rosner B, Willett WC. Vitamin E consumption and the risk of coronary disease in women. N Engl J Med. 1993;328(20):1444–9.
42. Janero DR, Burghardt B. Antiperoxidant effects of dihydropyridine calcium antagonists. Biochem Pharmacol. 1989;38:4344–8.
43. Herbaczynska-Cedro K, Gordon-Majszak W. Nisoldipine inhibits lipid peroxidation induced by coronary occlusion in pig myocardium. Cardiovasc Res. 1990;24:683–7.
44. Mason RP, Campbell SF, Wang SD, Herbette LG. Comparison of location and binding for the positively charged 1,4-dihydropyridine calcium channel antagonist amlodipine with uncharged drugs of this class in cardiac membranes. Mol Pharmacol. 1989;36:634–40.
45. Hodis HN, Kramsch DM, Avogaro P, et al. Biochemical and cytotoxic characteristics of an in vivo circulating oxidized low density lipoprotein (LDL−). J Lipid Res. 1994;35:669–77.
46. Kramsch DM, Sharma RC, Hodis HN, Hwang J, Lai M. Amlodipine prevents in vivo LDL-oxidation, preserves vitamin E, inhibits hyperinsulinemia and suppresses plaque growth [abstract]. J Am Coll Cardiol. 1994;23 Special Issue:437A.
47. Kramsch DM, Lium CR, Sharma RC, et al. Restoration of endothelial function in monkeys with atherogenic LDL levels through prevention of in vivo LDL oxidation and membrane lipid bilayer stabilization by amlodipine [abstract]. J Am Coll Cardiol. 1994;23 Special Issue:162A.
48. Sharma RC, Kramsch DM, Liu CR, Mack WJ. Non-invasive ultrasound demonstration of atherosclerosis progression and its suppression by the antioxidant calcium channel blocker amlodipine [abstract]. J Am Coll Cardiol. 1994;23 Special Issue:373A.

13. The St Thomas' Atherosclerosis Regression Study and an appraisal of its potential limitations

G. F. WATTS

Summary

The principal findings and potential limitations of the St Thomas' Atherosclerosis Regression Study (STARS) are presented. STARS was a randomized endpoint blinded study of the effects of lipid-lowering therapy on angiographic coronary artery disease (CAD) in male patients with hypercholesterolaemia. Both a fat-modified diet and diet-plus cholestyramine favourably influenced the course of CAD over 3 years. As discussed in this paper, the study did, however, have some limitations in respect of its sample size, use of angiography and generalizability of the findings.

Introduction

Developments in coronary angiography and quantitative methods for analysing angiograms have allowed the use of (so-called) 'regression trials' to more rigorously test the lipid hypothesis of atherosclerosis. By contrast to other lifestyle inter-vention trials[1-3], the St Thomas' Atherosclerosis Regression Study (STARS) used diet as a unifactorial mode of intervention[4].

Patients and Methods

Ninety men who had undergone coronary angiography for symptomatic angina were randomized to one of three groups: diet, diet+cholestyramine resin at an average dose of 14g per day, or usual care. Unlike other lifestyle intervention studies, mild to moderate hypercholesterolaemia (cholesterol 6.1 – 10 mmol/L) was an entry criterion. The interval between coronary angiograms averaged 39 months. Quantitative coronary angiography provided the primary endpoints[4].

The diet was designed to be readily complied with[5]. It included all usual food groups and permitted habitual use of alcohol to continue. Although weight loss was intended in overweight subjects, the mean weight did not differ significantly between the groups at the end of the study, nor did cigarette use or blood pressure. The diet comprised 27% energy from fat with a moderate increase of P:S ratio to 0.8 – 1.0, and intake of soluble fibre was increased; cholesterol intake was moderate, 100 mg per 1000 kcal per day. The diet was therefore broadly equivalent to the AHA phase 1 diet[6].

A.V.G. Bruschke et al. (eds): Lipid-lowering therapy and progression of atherosclerosis, 143–150.
© 1996 Kluwer Academic Publishers.

Table 13.1. Changes in angiographic endpoints by patient in the three treatment groups in STARS[4]. Mean (SEM) shown.

Changes observed	Usual care	Diet	Diet + resin	p value by ANOVA
MAWS (mm)	−0.201 (0.062)	0.003 (0.087)†	0.013 (0.051)**	0.012
MinAWS (mm)	−0.232 (0.068)	0.030 (0.086)*	0.117 (0.051)**	0.003
%DS	5.8 (1.8)	−1.1 (3.7)	−1.9 (1.1)***	0.077
EII (%)	2.0 (0.7)	0.0 (1.1)	−0.8 (0.5)***	0.066

MAWS = mean absolute width of segments; MinAWS = minimum absolute width of segments; %DS = percentage diameter stenosis; EII = edge-irregularity index.
*$p<0.05$; **$p<0.01$; ***$p<0.001$; †$p<0.06$, vs usual-care group.

Results

While plasma lipid levels in the usual-care group remained unchanged, the diet group showed mean reductions of 14.2% in serum cholesterol, 16.2% in LDL-cholesterol and 20% in triglycerides; HDL-cholesterol was unchanged. The reduction in serum cholesterol was consistent with that predicted by the Keys equation. In the diet + resin group, serum cholesterol fell 25.3% and LDL-cholesterol by 35.7%, while triglyceride and HDL-cholesterol did not change significantly.

Angiographic outcomes were analysed on both a per-patient and per-segment basis. The latter permitted measurements on 489 pairs of coronary artery segments, and allowed separate analyses of treatment effects on segments that showed mild, intermediate or severe disease. Seventy-four patients completed this study. Analysed by patient, the data showed a favourable global treatment effect with reduced incidence of progressive coronary narrowing (usual care 46%, diet 15%, diet + resin 12%; $p<0.02$), and an increased incidence of regression of disease (usual care 4%, diet 38%, diet + resin 33%; $p<0.01$); see Table 13.1. This was paralleled by the separate analyses of up to 10 proximal artery segments per patient, which showed that the progressive narrowing (revealed by all 4 angiographic endpoints) in the usual-care group was arrested or partly reversed with diet (see Table 13.2). The greater cholesterol lowering achieved with diet + resin was associated with more markedly favourable regression effects with widening of the lumen and reduction of irregularity of its diameter. It is probable that the greater benefit in the diet + resin group than in the diet-alone group in segmental analysis, but not in analysis by patient, reflects the greater number of measure-ments in the former.

STARS was unique in employing as one of the endpoints the mean absolute width of coronary segments, in addition to the more generally used measurement of percentage diameter stenosis. This allowed separate assessment of the effects of lipid lowering on segments that were minimally diseased at baseline, as well as more severely affected ones. As seen in Table 13.2, all degrees of baseline disease were favourably influenced by lipid lowering. As in trials with lipid-lowering drugs[7], the greatest benefit was shown in the most severely stenotic regions. However, segments containing 15–50% baseline stenosis (the most

Table 13.2. Angiographic changes by segments in STARS[4]. Mean (SEM) shown.

Changes observed	Usual care	Diet	Diet + resin	p value by ANOVA
All segments (n = 489)	(n = 157)	(n = 169)	(n = 163)	
MAWS (mm)	−0.131 (0.118)	0.011 (0.018)****	0.076 (0.074)***	0.002
MinAWS (mm)	−0.161 (0.111)	0.034 (0.116)***	0.086 (0.084)****	<0.0001
%DS	5.6 (3.6)	−0.5 (4.0)**	−1.5 (2.7)****	<0.0001
EII (%)	1.9 (1.3)	0.0 (1.4)†	−0.6 (0.9)****	0.001
<15% baseline stenosis (n = 208)	(n = 73)	(n = 72)	(n = 63)	
MAWS (mm)	−0.130 (0.142)	0.062 (0.082)*	0.055 (0.086)†	0.055
MinAWS (mm)	−0.198 (0.134)	0.011 (0.099)†	0.020 (0.090)*	0.044
%DS	8.8 (4.3)	4.4 (1.9)*	2.5 (1.5)*	0.035
EII (%)	2.8 (1.7)	0.8 (0.6)†	0.5 (0.6)*	0.033
15–50% baseline stenosis (n = 243)	(n = 75)	(n = 84)	(n = 84)	
MAWS (mm)	−0.099 (0.082)*	−0.085 (0.125)	0.094 (0.062)**	0.016
MinAWS (mm)	−0.122 (0.086)	0.012 (0.121)	0.105 (0.075)***	0.014
%DS	2.3 (2.5)	−1.2 (4.1)	−1.2 (2.4)	0.269
EII (%)	1.0 (0.9)	0.5 (1.5)	−0.3 (0.8)*	0.033
>50% baseline stenosis (n = 38)	(n = 9)	(n = 13)	(n = 16)	
MAWS (mm)	−0.406 (0.161)	0.345 (0.207)†	0.066 (0.084)	0.098
MinAWS (mm)	−0.187 (0.084)	0.423 (0.157)*	0.249 (0.098)*	0.075
%DS	7.4 (3.9)	−23.3 (7.9)*	−18.4 (4.7)**	0.050
EII (%)	2.0 (0.7)	−7.6 (2.9)*	−6.7 (1.6)†	0.078

MAWS = mean absolute width of segments; MinAWS = minimum absolute width of segments; %DS = percentage diameter stenosis; EII = edge-irregularity index.
*$p < 0.05$; **$p < 0.01$; ***$p < 0.001$; ****$p < 0.0001$; †$p < 0.06$, vs usual-care group.

frequent precursors of acute, full-thickness myocardial infarction) also showed improve-ment or retarded progression in both treatment groups, but most markedly in the diet + resin group.

Progression (change in mean segmental diameter) was directly related to the mean plasma concentration of LDL-cholesterol during the trial ($r = 0.40, p < 0.001$), the most significant association being attributed to the LDL_3 subfraction[8]. Regression or little change was the rule in patients who maintained a mean LDL-cholesterol of <3.5 mmol/L, and especially <3.0 mmol/L. Corresponding with the angiographic effects, the number of clinical cardiovascular events was significantly decreased in both intervention groups (see Table 13.3). Anginal symptoms were not significantly changed among the controls, whereas both intervention groups showed significant improvements ($p < 0.01$) in the severity of angina and Canadian Heart Association functional scores. Change in frequency of angina was significantly correlated with global changes in mean absolute width and minimum width of coronary segments.

Table 13.3. Cardiovascular events in STARS.

	Usual care	Diet	Diet + resin
Deaths (%)	10.7	3.7	0
Myocardial infarction (%)	7.1	3.7	4
Coronary surgery (%)	10.7	3.7	0
Angioplasty (%)	3.6	0	0
Stroke (%)	3.6	0	0
Total events (%)	35.7	11.1*	4**

*$p<0.05$; **$p<0.01$, vs usual-care group.

STARS also examined associations between the intake of nutrients (assessed by dietary history) and change in coronary luminal dimensions in the usual care and diet groups[9]. Significant inverse associations were seen between change in minimum absolute width of segments (i.e. progression of coronary artery disease) and intakes of energy, total fat, saturated fat, monounsaturated fat and cholesterol; but no associations were found with intakes of polyunsaturated fat, carbohydrate, fibre, alcohol or P : S ratio. In multiple regression analysis, intake of saturated fat ($p=0.03$) and the in-trial plasma LDL-cholesterol ($p=0.006$) were both independently associated with change in minimum absolute width of segments, after adjusting for other risk factors including treatment-group assignment. In more than one half of patients with regression of coronary artery disease, the daily intake of total fat and saturated fat was less than 61 g (27% energy) and 21 g (9% energy), respectively. These findings, which were compatible with an analysis of the placebo group in the CLAS trial[10], suggest that reduction in the intake of fat (in particular saturated fat) should be the primary goal for the nutritional management of coronary artery disease. Moreover, they demonstrate that diet may influence coronary atherosclerosis by mechanisms other than lipoprotein transport and these may include coagulation factors, platelet function, and oxidation of lipoproteins. From the results of correlational analyses, the therapeutic targets for stabilization/regression of CAD in at-risk patients were calculated to be a plasma LDL-cholesterol <3.5 mmol/L and a total fat intake <60 g/day (<30% energy), with total saturates <20 g/day (<10% energy).

Potential limitations of STARS

While the results achieved in STARS were impressive and in accordance with other sources of information[11-13], the study did have potential limitations with respect to its design, measurements, data analysis and clinical implications.

Trial design

The potential shortcomings of the trial design include the sample population studied and the randomization procedure[14]. STARS recruited a highly selected group of male patients with mild hypercholesterolaemia who underwent coronary angiography, but who did not have severe enough CAD to warrant surgical intervention. The patients were Caucasians, were highly motivated and came from the higher socioeconomic bracket. The relatively small number of patients undergoing angiography and the unwillingness of some to undergo a second angiogram accounted for the lower than expected accrual rate during recruitment in 1984–86. While the power calculation required that 60 patients be randomized per-treatment group, only half this number was achieved. The initial sample size was based on a previous angiographic trial of femoral atherosclerosis of relatively short duration[15,16]. Femoral atherosclerosis has, however, now been shown to regress at a lower rate than coronary atherosclerosis following lipid-lowering therapy[17]. Moreover, recent estimates employing quantitative coronary angiography and three-frame averaging suggest that, for 90% power and 10% relative difference in luminal dimensions between interventions, our trial sample size was statistically valid[18]. Nevertheless, a greater sample size would have reduced the confidence intervals of the trial endpoints. The randomization protocol in STARS required that all patients undergo a trial of tolerance to cholestyramine prior to formal randomization. Since a few patients were intolerant of this agent, this could have introduced bias[14]. Also, randomization did not employ a stratification procedure, but, in the final analysis group, characteristics were similar among the three treatments. Randomization of patients to a placebo group was ethically justified at the inception of the trial in 1984, since, at that time, treatment of mild-to-moderate hypercholesterolaemia in patients with CAD was not considered orthodox[19] and full informed consent was obtained. Since treatments of a very different nature were being compared[14], double-blinding was not a feasible technique in STARS. The trial did, however, employ blinded evaluation of outcome variables.

Angiography

The use of quantitative coronary angiography allows a more rigorous test of the lipid hypothesis of atherosclerosis in regression trials than in conventional clinical trials[20]. However, this technique does not directly examine atherosclerotic changes since it only assesses arterial luminal dimensions[21]. While these have been shown to be predictive of clinical events in other sequential studies[22], it would have been appropriate to include a non-invasive estimate of arterial wall contour, such as B-mode ultrasound of the carotid vessels, in the STARS protocol[23]. Use of percentage diameter stenosis is a particularly poor estimate of atherosclerosis, since it may be similar in arterial segments with different amounts of atherosclerosis. Although this has been the conventional angiographic outcome in many regression trials, STARS selected the change in mean absolute width of coronary segments as its primary endpoint. One major difficulty encountered was achieving good matching of coronary segments in paired angiograms sufficient to make reliable inferences about changes in luminal width. By contrast to the CLAS trials[24], STARS did not select patients to have the first angiogram and it is likely that technical factors associated with this confounded the matching procedure of all eligible segments. However, by contrast to other trials[7], STARS did not examine lesions alone and an average of 6 pairs of segments were analysed per patient.

Biochemical measurements

Besides the angiographic shortcomings, certain useful biochemical measurements were overlooked in STARS, some of which were unavoidable. At the commencement of the study, the lipid laboratory had not established assays for serum apolipoproteins and lipoprotein(a), so that information on potential changes in these variables during the trial was not available for the majority of patients. Moreover, no biochemical tests of compliance with diet and with abstention from smoking were employed[16]. Measurements of erythrocyte and/or adipose tissue fatty acid composition and plasma or urine nicotine levels would have been appropriate[25]. Monitoring of possible confounders of the experimental hypotheses should always be included in trial protocols. One potentially important shortcoming is that, although we assayed plasma vitamin E levels, we did not include other measurements of free radical activity[26]. The importance of oxidized LDL in atherosclerosis has, however, only been recognized recently[27]. The assessment of haemorrheological factors confounding the association between changes in lipoproteins and angiographic progression of CAD was only partially undertaken in STARS[28,29].

Data analysis

The methods of data analysis in STARS also requires mention. Angiographic data in regression trials can be expressed on either a per-patient or per-lesion (segment) basis[18]. The former averages the difference in available pairs of luminal measurements per patient and is equivalent to the global change score; it has clinical meaning but may lack statistical power. The latter pools segments from patients and treats them as independent variables; it is statistically powerful, but may be confounded by co-correlation of change within patients. STARS employed both approaches and, as anticipated, showed that the endpoint differences between diet and diet + resin were most significant with the lesional analysis[4]. The validity of lesional analysis was supported by the very low intraclass correlation for within-patient change. Because of differences in the number of segments available per patient, appropriate adjustments were also employed in the patient-based approach. Adjustments for differences in angiographic disease at baseline were not made, because of lack of significant statistical evidence for a correlation of baseline disease with the primary outcome variable. As in all other angiographic regression trials, intention-to-treat analysis was not possible[7,14], since patients who withdrew after randomization did not evidently undergo angiography. Intention-to-treat analysis was, however, carried out for clinical endpoints. Although these results were concordant with the angiographic changes, it must be conceded that STARS was not designed to test clinical events and that this post hoc analysis only achieved statistical significance after pooling all cardiovascular outcomes.

Clinical implications

As suggested earlier, the highly selected patients studied in STARS may limit the generalizability of the findings. This potential shortcoming applies to all regression trials since they have employed patients with specific recruitment characteristics. In broad terms, the clinical implications of STARS are restricted to the domain of the secondary prevention of CAD, inferences concerning primary prevention and other vascular beds being only by extension. It remains to be established also whether the conclusions also apply to women, to diabetics and to patients of different ethnic groups. From the therapeutic viewpoint, it is unlikely that a similar degree of compliance with diet or with resin therapy could be achieved at present in 'ordinary' clinical practice. STARS demonstrated the full potential of lipid-lowering therapy using highly motivated patients and therapists. The dietary regimen employed was, however, demonstrated to be highly effective in lowering plasma cholesterol in both an institutionalized and outpatient setting[5,30]. Design and testing of methods for increasing motivation among physicians and cardiologists and ensuring patient compliance with diet and, if required, drug therapy should be a priority for future clinical research[31,32].

Acknowledgement

I am grateful to Professor Barry Lewis for reviewing the manuscript.

References

1. Arntzenius AC, Kromhout D, Barth JD, et al. Diet, lipoproteins and the progression of coronary atherosclerosis. N Engl J Med. 1985;312:805–11.
2. Ornish D, Brown SE, Scherwitz LW, et al. Can lifestyle changes reverse coronary heart disease? The Lifestyle Heart Trial. Lancet. 1990;336:129–33.
3. Schuler G, Hambrecht R, Schlierf G, et al. Regular physical exercise and low-fat diet. Effects on progression of coronary artery disease. Circulation. 1992;86:1–11.
4. Watts GF, Lewis B, Brunt JNH, et al. Effects on coronary artery disease of lipid-lowering diet, or diet plus cholestyramine, in the St Thomas' Atherosclerosis Regression Study (STARS). Lancet. 1992;339:536–69.
5. Choudhury S, Jackson P, Katan MB, et al. A multifactorial diet in the management of hyperlipidaemia. Atherosclerosis. 1984;50:93–103.
6. Gotto AM Jr, Bierman EL, Connor WE, et al. Recommendations for the treatment of hyper-lipidemia in adults. A joint statement of the Nutrition Committee and the Council on Atherosclerosis. Circulation. 1984;69:1065A–90A.
7. Watts GF. Lipid-lowering therapy and regression of atherosclerosis. Endocrinol Metab. 1994;1: 71–87.
8. Watts GF, Mandalia S, Brunt JNH, et al. Independent associations between plasma lipoprotein subfraction levels and the course of coronary artery disease in the St Thomas' Atherosclerosis Regression Study (STARS). Metabolism. 1993;42:1461–7.

9. Watts GF, Jackson P, Brunt JNH, et al. Nutrient intake and progression of coronary artery disease. Am J Cardiol. 1994;73:328–32.
10. Blankenhorn DH, Johnson RL, Mack WJ, et al. The influence of diet on the appearance of new lesions in human coronary arteries. JAMA. 1990;263:1646–52.
11. Neaton JD, Wentworth D. Serum cholesterol, blood pressure, cigarette smoking, and death from coronary heart disease. Overall findings by age for 316,099 men. Arch Intern Med. 1992;152:56–64.
12. Blankenhorn DM, Kramsch DM. Reversal of atherosis and sclerosis. Circulation. 1989;79:1–7.
13. Holme I. An analysis of randomized trials evaluating the effect of cholesterol reduction on total mortality and coronary heart disease incidence. Circulation. 1990;82:1916–24.
14. Pocock SJ. Clinical trials: a practical approach. Chichester: John Wiley & Sons; 1983.
15. Duffield RGM, Lewis B, Miller NE, et al. Treatment of hyperlipidaemia retards progression of symptomatic femoral atherosclerosis: a randomized controlled trial. Lancet. 1983;2:639–42.
16. Azen S, Blankenhorn DH, Nessim S. Planning and evaluation of studies on atherosclerosis in controlled clinical trials. In: Malinow MR, Blaton VH, editors. Regression of atherosclerotic lesions: experimental studies and observations in humans. New York: Plenum; 1984:263–75.
17. Olsson A. Regression of femoral atherosclerosis. Circulation. 1991;83:698–700.
18. Gibson CM, Sandor T, Stone PH, et al. Quantitative angiographic and statistical methods to assess serial changes in coronary luminal diameter and implications for regression trials. Am J Cardiol. 1992;69:1286–90.
19. Oliver MF. Serum cholesterol – the knave of hearts and the joker. Lancet. 1981;2:1090–5.
20. Blankenhorn DM, Hodis HN. Arterial imaging and atherosclerosis reversal. Arterioscler Thromb. 1994;14:177–92.
21. Brown BG, Bolson EL, Dodge HT. Arteriographic assessment of coronary atherosclerosis: review of current methods, their limitations, and clinical applications. Arteriosclerosis. 1982;2:2–15.
22. Waters D, Craven TE, Esperance J. Prognostic significance of progression of coronary atherosclerosis. Circulation. 1993;87:1067–75.
23. Salonen JT, Salonen R. Ultrasound B-mode imaging in observational studies of atherosclerosis progression. Circulation. 1993;87(Suppl):II56–65.
24. Blankenhorn DH, Nessim SA, Johnson RL, et al. Beneficial effects of combined colestipol–niacin therapy on coronary atherosclerosis and coronary venous bypass grafts. JAMA. 1987;257:3233–40.
25. Katan MB, Birgelen AV, Deslypere JP, et al. Biological markers of dietary intake, with emphasis on fatty acids. Ann Nutr Metab. 1991;35:249–52.
26. Chait A. Methods for assessing lipid and lipoprotein oxidation. Curr Opin Lipidol. 1992;3:389–94.
27. Witztum JL. Role of oxidized low density lipoprotein in atherogenesis. Br Heart J. 1993;69(Suppl):12–8.
28. Hamsten A. Coagulation factors and hyperlipidaemia. Curr Opin Lipidol. 1991;2:266–71.
29. Watts GF, Mandalia S, Brunt JNH, et al. Metabolic determinants of the course of coronary artery disease in men. Clin Chem. 1995;40:2240–6.
30. Lewis B, Hammett F, Katan MB, et al. Towards an improved lipid-lowering diet: additive effects of changes in nutrient intake. Lancet. 1982;2:1310–13.
31. Mulcahy D, Kehely A, Fox K, et al. Risk reduction in patients with coronary artery disease: lipids and lost opportunities. Br J Cardiol. 1994;1:161–5.
32. Cohen MV, Byrne MJ, Levine B, et al. Low rate of treatment of hypercholesterolaemia by cardiologists in patients with suspected and proven coronary artery disease. Circulation. 1992;83:1294–304.

14. Effects of the lipid intervention in the Stanford Coronary Risk Intervention Project

E. L. ALDERMAN, A. McMILLAN and W. HASKELL

Summary

The Stanford Coronary Risk Intervention Project (SCRIP) randomized 300 subjects between intensive, multiple risk intervention and usual care. The change from entry to four-year follow-up angiograms in minimum lumen diameter of diseased segments in 245 subjects was analysed in relation to hypolipidaemic medication and lipid-related risk factors. Greater disease progression was associated with non-use of hypolipidaemic drugs and higher blood glucose and insulin levels.

Introduction

The SCRIP trial hypothesized that an intensive multifactor risk intervention would favourably alter the rate of lumen narrowing in men and women with coronary artery disease. Patients were randomized to a risk-reduction intervention or the usual care of their personal physicians. Risk-reduction subjects were provided with individualized programmes, involving a low-fat and low-cholesterol diet, exercise, weight loss, smoking cessation and medications to favourably alter lipid profiles. The dietary, exercise and blood pressure interventions led to significant reduction in fat and cholesterol intake, lowering of blood pressure, improved exercise capacity and reduced weight in the risk-reduction subjects compared with usual-care subjects. Lipid-lowering drugs were taken at any time during the four-year study by 93.3% of risk-reduction subjects vs 30.7% of usual-care subjects and similarly led to significant beneficial alterations in blood lipid profiles of risk reduction compared with usual-care subjects.

The main study results have previously been reported[1] and demonstrate that the rate of progression of the minimum lumen diameter within diseased coronary segments is 47% less in the risk-reduction group compared with the usual-care group. Multivariate analysis of the factors that contributed to the four-year reduction in the rate of change in the minimum diameter of disease segments yielded a best-fit two-variable model based on change in max METS and change in Framingham risk score (incorporates blood pressure, LDL-C, HDL-C and weight).

It is the purpose of this report to analyse the lipid responses to the drugs used

A.V.G. Bruschke et al. (eds): Lipid-lowering therapy and progression of atherosclerosis, 151–165.
© 1996 Kluwer Academic Publishers.

in SCRIP and to evaluate angiographic outcomes in relation to individual drugs and in relation to the altered lipid profiles. Both usual-care and risk-reduction subjects received lipid-altering drugs and lifestyle interventions to modify risk factors. For risk-reduction subjects, the success of these interventions depended on the individualized risk intervention programme. The management of usual-care subjects depended on the recommendations of their personal physicians. The analyses that follow include all SCRIP subjects (usual-care and risk-reduction, except as specified) in a single group, assessing the effects of lipid-lowering drugs and resultant changes in lipid-related measurements on four-year angiographic outcome.

Methods

Study population

The SCRIP study and design has previously been described[1]. In brief, SCRIP was a four-year randomized multiple-risk-factor intervention trial in men and women with coronary artery disease with the goal of altering the rate of coronary artery lumen narrowing. Three-hundred men and women (men: $n=259$; women: $n=41$), mean age 56 ± 7.4 years, with angiographically defined coronary athero-sclerosis were randomly assigned to the usual care of their own physician ($n=155$) or an individualized multifactor risk-reduction programme ($n=145$). Computer-assisted quantitative coronary arteriography, performed at baseline and four years later, provided the primary outcome measurement. The protocol and progress were reviewed prior to the study initiation and annually thereafter by the Stanford University Panel on Human Subjects in Medical Research, by committees on the use of human subjects at each of the participating hospitals and by the external Safety and Data Monitoring Committee appointed by the National Heart, Lung, and Blood Institute.

SCRIP risk-reduction programme

Patients assigned to risk reduction were provided with individualized programmes involving a low-fat and cholesterol diet, exercise, weight loss, smoking cessation and medications to favourably alter lipoprotein profiles. All risk-reduction subjects were instructed by a dietician in a low-fat, low-cholesterol and high-carbohydrate diet with a goal of <20% of energy intake from fat, <6% from saturated fat, and <75 mg of cholesterol per day. A physical activity programme was recommended, consisting of an increase in daily activities, such as walking, climbing stairs and household chores, and a specific endurance exercise training programme. A staff psychologist developed an individualized stop-smoking programme for smokers in the risk-reduction group. A major goal was to decrease low-density lipoprotein cholesterol (LDL-C) to <2.84 mmol/L (110 mg/dl), to decrease triglyceride concentrations below 1.13 mmol/L (100 mg/dl), and increase high-density lipoprotein cholesterol (HDL-C) concentrations above 1.42 mmol/L

(55 mg/dL). If the SCRIP staff concluded it unlikely that a risk-reduction subject would meet the maximum LDL-C goals within the first year without drug therapy, a cholesterol-lowering drug regimen was added.

A drug sequence similar to that now recommended by the National Cholesterol Education Program (NCEP) was followed, starting with a bile acid binding resin (colestipol) and, depending on subject response, adding or substituting other drugs including niacin, gemfibrozil, lovastatin (available only during last half of the study), and probucol. SCRIP differed from the NCEP ATP-1 approach to LDL-C reduction by setting an LDL-C target at 2.84 mmol/L (110 mg/dl) instead of 3.36 mmol/L (130 mg/dl), by using more aggressive guidelines for fat and cholesterol intake and by use of triple drug therapy when necessary. All lipid medications were provided to the risk-reduction subjects free of charge.

The risk-reduction subjects were provided verbal and written goals and instructions for their individualized risk-reduction plan. To track their progress, contact was maintained with the SCRIP staff using telephone and mail. Risk-reduction subjects returned every 2 or 3 months to the clinic to evaluate progress and provide additional assistance. During these visits, lipids, body weight and blood pressure were measured; diet, exercise and smoking programme assistance provided; and hypolipidaemic drugs evaluated and revised as needed.

Risk-factor evaluations

All subjects had their clinical status and risk factors evaluated at baseline prior to randomization and annually for four years. Blood pressure, cigarette usage, treadmill testing, dietary intake and physical activity were closely monitored using objective tools for data collection, details of which have been previously reported[1].

At baseline and annually, fasting plasma lipids and lipoproteins were measured during two clinic visits. The two values were averaged for each subject to represent the subject at baseline and for each year in the study. Plasma concentrations of total cholesterol (T-C), triglycerides (TG), LDL-C and HDL-C were directly measured. Plasma glucose concentration was measured using the glucose oxidase method[2] and insulin concentration by radioimmunoassay[3].

SCRIP angiographic acquisition protocol

Baseline coronary arteriograms were obtained in a uniform manner at baseline and follow-up with the requirement that nitroglycerin be administered prior to coronary injections. Coronary catheters with metallic cylindrical markers near their distal end provided a sharp calibration edge for quantitation, which reduces measurement variation when using computer-assisted measurement techniques[4].

Subjects were eligible for the study if at least one major coronary artery showed a segment with visually apparent disease that was unaffected by revascularization procedures. Neither a qualifying segment nor any vessel proximal to it could contain a lesion ≥70% in diameter reduction, nor could the vessel have been grafted or instrumented by a prior revascularization procedure. Visually normal segments were quantitated at enrolment; however, these segments were not included in the primary analysis of the SCRIP hypothesis.

All consenting subjects had protocol-mandated follow-up arteriograms obtained four years following the baseline arteriogram. Use of marker catheters, prior nitroglycerin administration and replication of projection angles were performed as at the baseline study. If a subsequent four-year arteriogram was not obtainable, the results of earlier clinically indicated angiograms were included as long as the interval between the baseline and follow-up angiogram exceeded 12 months, and the clinically indicated angiogram was performed according to the research protocol. Two hundred and forty-five of the 300 randomized subjects had entry and follow-up quantitative arteriography that met study specifications.

Computer-assisted quantitation

The quantitative coronary angiographic system employed in this study was developed at Stanford Medical Center to measure coronary vessels on 35-mm cineangiograms. Its design, accuracy, precision, and intra- and inter-observer variability have been reported[5]. The system has two cine film digitizers that simultaneously process paired coronary arteriograms for evaluation of serial changes in coronary arteries. A pair of video monitors for each projector allow the operator real-time viewing of the film for frame selection.

Comparable segments on baseline and follow-up angiograms were digitized. Single-plane coronary quantitation was used. The operator manually defined approximate edges and an automatic edge-finding algorithm defined matching segment lengths and the margins for measurement of mean and minimum diameters. The operator was blinded as to the subjects' randomization assignment. For each quantitation segment, the minimum diameter was measured.

Angiographic assessment of progression, regression and new lesion formation

Individual diseased segments were categorized as progressing, regressing or unchanged on the basis of whether the minimum diameter of diseased segments changed by more than a specified threshold of 0.2 mm. For the purposes of comparing risk reduction vs usual-care responses to the risk intervention, patients were categorized according to whether any progressing or regressing diseased segment was present *without* a segment performing in the opposite direction[1]. Progression was equivalent in both usual-care and risk-reduction groups; however, regressing subjects were twice as likely to be in the risk-reduction group as in the usual-care group (risk-reduction: 20.2% vs usual-care: 10.3%).

A patient was considered as progressing or regressing in this report based on occurrence of *any* lesion progression or *any* regression. The threshold of change between any two angiograms had been set in the main effects paper at 0.2 mm based on a three-fold multiple of the within-procedure measurement variability (standard deviation = 0.033 mm) multiplied by a factor of two, to account for between-procedure variation[6]. This threshold of 0.2 mm change has been retained in this report to define *regressing* segments.

A more restrictive threshold of 0.4 mm was used in this report to define *progression*. The differing threshold between regression and progression reflects the observation that the vast majority of segments with coronary disease tend to progress with time, particularly in a study of four years duration, creating a substantial imbalance in the number of progressing lesions. Moreover, the risk-reduction subjects had a significantly smaller standard deviation, i.e. spread in the distribution of segmental changes in minimum diameter than did usual-care subjects (risk-reduction: -0.021 ± 0.078; usual-care: 0.051 ± 0.125) (1). Thus, the wider spread of usual-care subject changes in minimum diameter compared with risk-reduction subjects, introduces a bias that diminishes the relative proportion of regressors in risk-reduction subjects vis-a-vis usual-care subjects. This effect is magnified by the fact that the mean disease progression of risk-reduction subjects was half that of usual-care subjects. For these reasons, a different threshold for progression and regression was considered appropriate. Total occlusion was included as progression only if the site had been considered at study entry to be a qualifying lesion.

New lesions were assessed by two experienced angiographers (blinded to patient randomization assignment) who visually assessed each segment that had an interval reduction in minimum diameter, i.e. progression, exceeding 0.2 mm within a segment previously considered free of visually apparent coronary disease[7]. Using simultaneous side-by-side cine projectors, identical projections of the baseline and follow-up angiograms were compared visually. Visual assessment for interval coronary segment change was based on both static images and dynamic display at variable rates to confirm or refute serial change. Results of the visual assessment were recorded as three possible outcomes: no apparent change, definite new lesion, or prior disease present with progression. This definition of new lesion differs from that used in other studies, by excluding progression of minor pre-existing lesions, e.g. < 20%, from inclusion as new lesions in order to avoid redundant counting of stenosis progression.

Statistical analysis

For within-group comparisons from baseline to on-study, one-sample *t*-tests were used. The significance of differences in the proportion of subjects with different angiographic outcomes based on their randomization assignment or drug treatment group was determined by Chi-square. The significance of differences in lipid risk factors or angiographic measures between the usual-care and risk-reduction groups or between groups with or without progression, regression or new lesions was determined by two-sample *t*-tests. Significance was set $p < 0.05$.

Table 14.1.   Percentage of patients taking lipid-altering medications and response of lipid-related risk factors.

Lipid lowering drug category	Taking drug during any on-study year	Taking drug for 2 y beyond midstudy	n	LDL-C mmol/L [mg/dl]			HDL-C mmol/L [mg/dl]		
				Baseline	On-study	Change	Baseline	On-study	Change
All UC subjects	30.7	24.4	127	4.03 [156]	3.88 [150]	−0.15 [−6]	1.09 [42]	1.16 [45]	0.07 [3]
All RR subjects	93.2	87.2	118	4.06 [157]	3.1 [120]	−0.96 [−37]	1.01 [39]	1.32 [51]	0.31 [12]
All subjects: (UC and RR)	60.8	54.7	245	4.06 [157]	3.52 [136]	−0.54 [−21]	1.14 [44]	1.24 [48]	0.1 [4]
All subjects taking drug for two years beyond midstudy									
BAS*	47.8	36.7	90	4.29 [166]	3.18† [123]	−1.11 [−43]	1.19 [46]	1.37 [53]	0.18 [7]
Niacin*	34.3	19.2	47	4.4 [170]	3.34† [129]	−1.06 [−41]	1.14 [44]	1.37 [53]	0.23 [9]
Gemfibrozil*	20.8	8.6	21	3.78 [146]	3.36† [130]	−0.42 [−16]	0.93 [36]	0.98 [38]	0.05 [2]
Lovastatin*	22.9	14.3	35	4.32 [167]	3.34† [129]	−0.98 [−38]	1.11 [43]	1.22 [47]	0.11 [4]
Any lipid drug*	60.8	54.7	134	4.22 [163]	3.31† [128]	−0.91 [−35]	1.14 [44]	1.29 [50]	0.15 [6]
No lipid drug	39.2	45.3	110	3.83 [148]	3.75 [145]	−0.08 [−3]	1.11 [43]	1.16 [45]	0.05 [2]

*Note: Many subjects were taking more than one-hypolipidemic drug; †Significantly different from subjects not taking the specified drug; UC = usual care; RR = risk reduction; BAS = bile acid sequestrant.

Results

Lipid-lowering drugs were taken at some time during the four-year study duration by 93.2% of risk-reduction and 30.7% of usual-care SCRIP subjects (Table 14.1). Because of a one-year lag in subjects achieving lipid-reduction goals and the late availability of lovastatin, lipid drug use was considered most relevant to the study outcome if taken consistently during both of the last two years of the study. Lipid-altering drugs were taken by 87.2% of risk-reduction subjects compared with 24.4% of usual-care subjects according to this criteria. Bile acid sequestrants were taken for two years beyond mid-study by 37% of subjects (risk-reduction: 67% vs usual-care: 9.4%); niacin was taken by 19% of subjects (risk-reduction: 29% vs usual-care: 10%); Gemfibrozil by 8.6% (risk-reduction: 15% vs usual care: 3%) and lovastatin by 14% (risk-reduction: 22% vs usual care: 7%). For all SCRIP participants (usual-care and risk-reduction), 54.7% were taking one or another hypolipidaemic drug during their third and fourth year of study participation.

The responses of blood lipids to drugs are shown in Table 14.1 for usual-care

Table 14.1   (continued)

	T-C/HDL		Triglycerides mmol/L [mg/dl]			Fasting insulin pmol/L [µmol/l]			Fasting glucose [mmol/L [mg/dl]		
Baseline	On-study	Change	Baseline	On-study	Change	Baseline	On-study	Change	Baseline	On-study	Change
			1.75	1.76	0.01	123	126	3	5.79	6.16	0.37
5.6	5.3	−0.3	[155]	[156]	[1]	[17.1]	[17.6]	[3]	[104]	[111]	[7]
			1.77	1.42	−0.35	130	101	29	5.79	5.62	−0.17
5.4	4.1	−1.3	[157]	[126]	[−31]	[18.1]	[14.1]	[−29]	[104]	[101]	[−3]
			1.73	1.59	−0.14	117	105	−12	5.77	5.88	0.11
5.5	4.7	−0.8	[153]	[141]	[−12]	[16.3]	[14.7]	[−1.6]	[104]	[106]	[2]
			1.67	1.38	−0.29	102	78	−24	5.6	5.38	−0.22
5.4	4	−1.4	[148]	[122]	[−26]	[14.2]	[10.9]	[−3.3]	[101]	[97]	[−4]
			1.94	1.63	−0.31	104	103	−1	6.11	5.77	−0.34
5.8	4.3	−1.5	[172]	[144]	[−28]	[14.5]	[14.4]	[−0.1]	[110]	[104]	[−6]
			2.8	1.9	−0.9	135	109	−26	5.77	6.22	0.45
6.5	5.3	−1.2	[248]	[168]	[−80]	[18.8]	[15.2]	[−3.6]	[104]	[112]	[8]
			2.19	1.8	−0.39	174	121	−53	6.27	6.16	−0.11
6.1	4.6	−1.5	[194]	[159]	[−35]	[24.2]	[16.9]	[−7.3]	[113]	[111]	[−2]
			1.83	1.52	−0.31	121	96	−25	5.88	5.72	−0.16
5.6	4.4	−1.2	[162]	[135]	[−27]	[16.9]	[13.4]	[−3.5]	[106]	[103]	[−3]
			1.61	1.68	0.07	113	117	4	5.66	6.11	0.45
5.3	5.1	−0.2	[143]	[149]	[6]	[15.7]	[16.3]	[0.6]	[102]	[110]	[8]

and risk-reduction subjects and for those taking or not taking lipid-altering drugs. Many subjects were taking more than one drug. The on-study lipid levels achieved by risk-reduction subjects were generally more favourable than those of combined usual-care and risk-reduction subjects, reflecting the more intensive treatment of risk-reduction subjects by using higher doses and greater use of drug combinations. Subjects receiving bile acid sequestrants, niacin or lovastatin had elevated baseline LDL-C levels and responded with a 23–25% reduction. All drugs lowered fasting insulin. Subjects receiving gemfibrozil had substantially higher baseline triglyceride levels, which fell by 33% in response to the drug. Niacin had the greatest beneficial effect on HDL-C (18% increase) and gemfibrozil caused a rise in fasting glucose (7.7% increase).

The minimum diameter of diseased segments declined by 0.096 mm in the 119 risk-reduction subjects who had four-year follow-up angiography compared with a 0.180-mm decline in 127 usual-care subjects ($p = 0.02$; Table 14.2). The four-year change in minimum diameter is shown for each category of sustained drug use during the last half of the study. For all drug categories except gemfibrozil,

Table 14.2.   Four-year change in minimum diameter of diseased segments.

			Change (%)	*p*
All subjects	**UC**	**RR**		
n	127	119		
Mean	−0.18	−0.096	−47	0.02
SD	0.292	0.184		
All subjects taking drugs for last two	**No**			
years of the study	**drug**	**Drug**		
BAS*				
n	155	90		
mean	−0.16	−0.1	−37	0.09
SD	0.293	0.245		
Niacin				
n	198	47		
Mean	−0.151	−0.082	−46	0.1
SD	0.283	0.247		
Gemfibrozil				
n	224	21		
Mean	−0.136	−0.165	21	0.68
SD	0.274	0.312		
Lovastatin				
n	210	35		
Mean	−0.145	−0.097	−33	0.18
SD	0.29	0.175		
Any lipid-altering drug				
n	111	134		
Mean	−0.171	−0.111	−35	0.09
SD	0.289	0.264		

BAS = bile acid sequestrant.

there was a substantial decline in the rate of coronary disease progression (bile acid sequestrants: −37%; niacin: −46%; gemfibrozil: −21%; lovastatin: −33% and any hypolipidaemic drug: −35%). However, neither use of individual drugs nor use of any lipid-lowering drug led to statistically significant differences.

Patients were categorized according to whether any diseased segment showed progression exceeding 0.4 mm or regression exceeding 0.2 mm over four years (Table 14.3 and Figure 14.1). Progressing segment(s) were found in 25% of risk-reduction subjects compared with 48% of usual-care subjects ($p=0.0003$). Regressing segment(s) were found in 31% of both risk-reduction and usual-care subjects (NS). Subjects using any lipid-altering medication had a 29% progression rate compared with 47% for subjects not taking any lipid-lowering drug ($p=0.005$). Use of a bile acid sequestrant was associated with a 28% stenosis progression rate compared with a 43% rate in non-users ($p=0.028$).

New lesions developed in 23.3% of risk-reduction subjects compared with 31.3% in usual-care subjects ($p=0.16$; Figure 14.1)[7]. However, new lesion development was significantly reduced in those subjects taking one or more

Table 14.3. Four-year changes in pre-existing lesions and development of new lesions by drug treatment.

				p^*
All subjects	Total	UC	RR	
n	245	127	119	
Any progression (%)	91	48	25	0.0003
Any regression (%)	77	31	32	0.89
New lesion (%)	66	31	22	0.1
All subjects taking drugs for two years beyond midstudy		**No drug**	**Drug**	
BAS				
n	245	155	90	
Any progression (%)	91	43	28	0.028
Any regression (%)	77	30	33	0.62
New lesion (%)	66	32	19	0.03
Niacin				
n	245	198	47	
Any progression (%)	91	40	26	0.09
Any regression (%)	77	33	26	0.33
New lesion (%)	66	28	21	0.33
Gemfibrozil				
n	245	224	21	
Any progression (%)	91	37	38	1
Any regression (%)	77	32	24	0.43
New lesion (%)	66	28	19	0.39
Lovastatin				
n	245	210	35	
Any progression (%)	91	39	29	0.34
Any regression (%)	77	31	31	1
New lesion (%)	66	28	23	0.56
Any lipid-altering drug				
n	245	111	134	
Any progression (%)	91	47	29	0.005
Any regression (%)	77	32	31	0.76
New lesion (%)	66	36	19	0.003

$^*p$ by chi-square. Note: subjects may show both progression and regression based on changes in individual segments.

lipid-altering drugs compared with non-drug users ($p=0.003$; Table 14.3). SCRIP subjects taking bile acid sequestrants had a significantly lower percentage of new lesions compared with individuals not taking this medication ($p=0.03$). Other drug categories showed directionally similar but not statistically significant results. To some extent, statistical significance in these analyses reflects the number of subjects taking a drug, which was largest for the bile acid sequestrants (90 subjects, compared with 47 taking niacin, 21 taking gemfibrozil and 35 taking lovastatin).

Table 14.4 subdivides all SCRIP subjects with follow-up angiography into

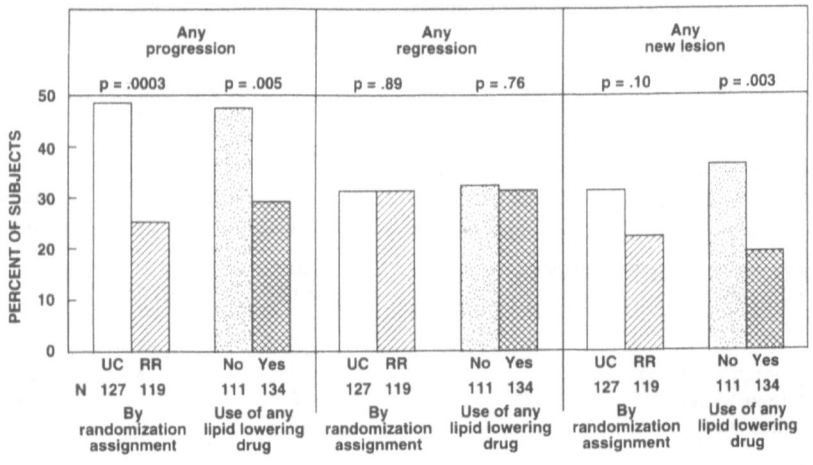

Figure 14.1.   Four year prevalence of any progression and any regression of pre-existing lesions and development of new lesions are presented in three panels. The main study comparison between usual-care and risk-reduction subjects is shown by the left-hand pair of bars in each panel. The results in subjects taking lipid-altering medications are compared with those not taking drugs (irrespective of randomization group) by the right-hand bars in each panel.

quintiles of blood lipids and related risk factors. Each quintile is characterized by the mean level of the quintile. Each quintile represents 49 of the 245 subjects. The four-year change in the minimum diameter of diseased segments is listed for each quintile. The p values are derived from correlation analysis. Fasting blood sugar and serum insulin were significantly associated with four-year declines in minimum lumen diameter (Table 14.4 and Figure 14.2). There were similar trends towards associations of changes in minimum diameter with triglyceride levels and with the ratio of total cholesterol to HDL-cholesterol (Figure 14.2).

The percentages of SCRIP subjects showing progression, regression and new lesion development by quintiles of blood lipids and related risk factors are listed in Table 14.5. No statistically strong associations with quintiles of serum lipid levels emerged. There were several trends towards a decline in new lesion development in subjects with the highest HDL-C levels ($p=0.08$) and an increase in new lesions in subjects in the highest quintiles of LDL-C ($p=0.14$).

Discussion

A comparison of the primary treatment strategies shows risk-reduction subjects had a 47% reduction in the rate of decline in minimum lesion diameter ($p=0.02$), a 48% reduction in subjects with progressing lesions ($p=0.0003$), a 29% reduction in subjects with new lesions ($p=0.16$) and no difference in the number of subjects with regressing lesions.

SCRIP participants taking any lipid-altering drug beyond the study midpoint

Table 14.4. Rate of progression of coronary disease by quintiles of risk factors.

Quintile	LDL-C On-study blood level mmol/L [mg/dl]	LDL-C Four-year change in min. diam. of diseased segments	HDL-C On-study blood level mmol/L [mg/dl]	HDL-C Four-year change in min. diam. of diseased segments	T-C/HDL-C On-study blood level	T-C/HDL-C Four-year change in min. diam. of diseased segments	TG On-study blood level mmol/L [mg/dl]	TG Four-year change in min. diam. of diseased segments	Serum insulin On-study blood level pmol/L [μU/ml]	Serum insulin Four-year change in min. diam. of diseased segments	FBS On-study blood level mmol/L [mg/dl]	FBS Four-year change in min. diam. of diseased segments
Lowest 1	2.62 [101]	-0.158	0.85 [33]	-0.096	3	-0.126	0.79 [70]	-0.071	49 [6.8]	-0.098	4.66 [84]	-0.094
2	3.03 [117]	-0.082	1 [40]	-0.216	3.8	-0.11	1 [97]	-0.119	66 [9.2]	-0.13	5.16 [93]	-0.063
3	3.44 [133]	-0.101	1.16 [45]	-0.137	4.6	-0.116	1.39 [123]	-0.142	83 [11.5]	-0.148	5.55 [100]	-0.197
4	3.83 [148]	-0.118	1.34 [52]	-0.133	5.4	-0.148	1.77 [157]	-0.152	110 [15.3]	-0.124	5.94 [107]	-0.146
Highest 5	4.65 [180]	-0.23	1.76 [68]	-0.103	6.8	-0.187	2.91 [258]	-0.148	226 [31.5]	-0.177	8.22	-0.211
p*	0.18		0.39		0.08		0.09		0.05		0.002	

*By Pearson correlation coefficient (quintiles considered directionally related to outcome).

Table 14.5.   Four-year changes in pre-existing lesions and development of new lesions by on-study lipid-related risk factor.

Quintile	LDL-C			HDL-C			T-C/HDL-C		
	Subjects with any progression (%)	Subjects with any regression (%)	Subjects with any new lesion (%)	Subjects with any progression (%)	Subjects with any regression (%)	Subjects with any new lesion (%)	Subjects with any progression (%)	Subjects with any regression (%)	Subjects with any new lesion (%)
Lowest 1	37	31	20	40	38	30	31	33	29
2	35	31	31	44	27	31	36	32	10
3	31	31	22	37	31	31	30	26	22
4	43	49	24	47	29	24	44	29	44
Highest 5	42	17	37	19	33	18	46	37	29
p*	0.66	0.82	0.14	0.03	0.52	0.08	0.13	0.73	0.13

*By *t*-test comparing blood levels in subjects with vs without progression, regression or new lesion.

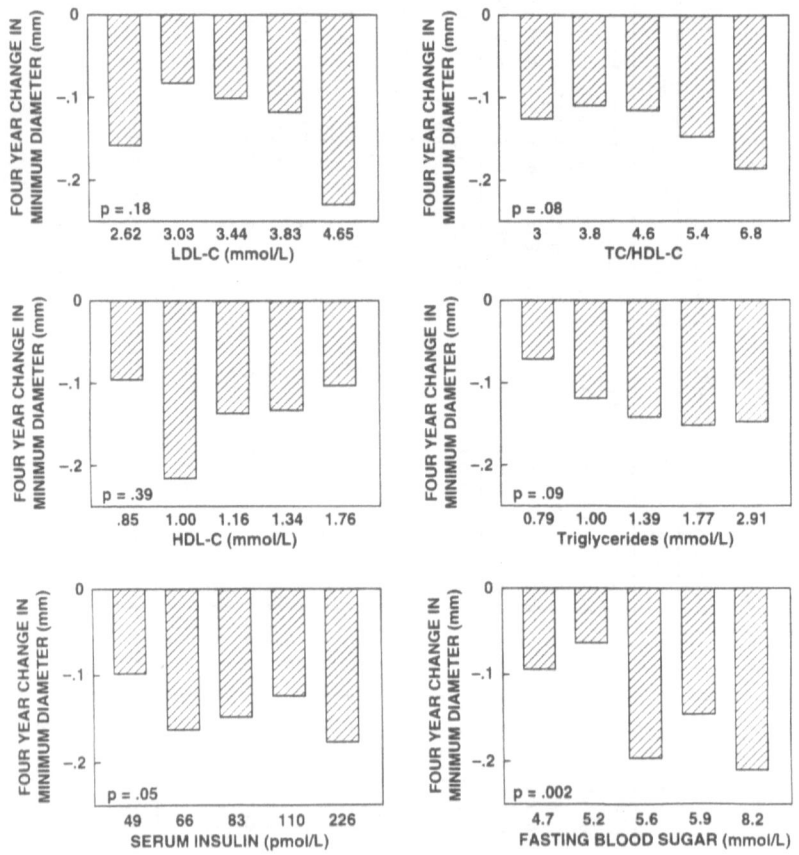

Figure 14.2.   The rate of change in the minimum diameter of diseased coronary segments is plotted against the mean blood level of each risk factor quintile (245 subjects subdivided into 49 subjects in each quintile).

Table 14.5.   (continued)

Triglycerides			Fasting insulin			Fasting glucose		
Subjects with any progression (%)	Subjects with any regression (%)	Subjects with any new lesion (%)	Subjects with any progression (%)	Subjects with any regression (%)	Subjects with any new lesion (%)	Subjects with any progression (%)	Subjects with any regression (%)	Subjects with any new lesion (%)
37	37	22	38	42	32	2	36	19
35	33	29	33	23	19	29	37	24
39	29	27	40	27	25	47	28	26
39	27	29	31	29	20	48	33	37
37	33	29	47	36	36	41	24	26
0.29	0.39	0.64	0.38	0.88	0.84	0.06	0.87	0.76

had a 35% lower rate of change in lesion minimum diameter ($p = 0.09$), a 38% reduction in progressing lesions ($p = 0.005$) and a 47% reduction in the number of new lesions ($p = 0.003$). Those SCRIP participants taking a bile acid sequestrant during the last half of the study, showed a trend towards less narrowing of the minimum lesion diameter ($p = 0.09$), less stenosis progression by categorical definition ($p = 0.028$) and fewer new lesions ($p = 0.03$).

These results are consistent with the results of multiple angiographic trials reported to date. Most have been monotherapy studies focused on drugs with a beneficial effect on LDL-cholesterol. Many studies have imposed varying degrees of age or gender limitation or restricted study entry to those with LDL-cholesterol levels above a certain threshold consistent with current therapeutic guidelines. SCRIP differed from some previous studies by its absence of any lipid entry criteria, intensive multiple risk intervention strategy, inclusion of male and female subjects up to age 75, careful exclusion of bypassed or instrumented arteries, calibration based on cylindrical metal band at catheter tip and longer duration (4 years).

Study limitations

Drug therapy was one component of an intensive, individualized multiple risk intervention that was focused on the risk-reduction subjects. This retrospective analysis is based on actual drug treatment received by the entire study population, irrespective of randomization assignment. However, it is likely that subjects in the usual-care group who received drugs from their local physicians may not have received the same level of close monitoring, dose adjustments and multiple drug use as the risk-reduction subjects.

The fact that there was a 47% reduction in the rate of lumen narrowing in the risk-reduction compared with the usual-care subjects and this difference was not matched by any of the drug-treatment groups may result from several causes. The number of subjects taking any particular lipid-altering drug was based on the individuals' lipid profile diminishing the statistical power to identify a unique contribution of one or another drug. In a multifactor study, in which both drug and life-style interventions were intensively pursued, it is difficult to identify any particular risk intervention that accounts for most of the observed effect on coronary dimensions. This benefit to risk-reduction subjects, almost certainly reflects a substantial contribution that a low-fat low-cholesterol diet, weight reduction, enhanced physical activity and lowered blood pressure made irrespective of lipid changes resulting from drug treatment.

The multivariate regression analysis results described in the main effects publication[1] identified change in max mets achieved on exercise testing and Framingham risk score as the most significant correlates of angiographic outcome. The latter includes LDL-C, HDL-C, blood pressure and weight as components of the score. An additional limitation of a by-drug analysis is that subjects taking hypolipidaemic medications had a more adverse lipid profile at study entry than subjects who were not given drugs. These subjects might be more likely to have a beneficial response to drug treatment. In general, subjects taking any lipid-altering drug continuously beyond the study midpoint had a statistically important reduction in lesion progression and new lesion development as well as a greater proportion of regressing segments.

It should be emphasized that definitions of progression, regression and new lesion development differ from study to study. The use of a threshold to trichotomize lesion change as progression, regression or no change is somewhat arbitrary and results in measurement error (variance) substantially influencing the proportion of subjects in each category. Even more problematic is the manner in which a study participant is categorized as a 'progressor' or 'regressor'. Because an individual subject may have multiple segments, varying combinations of lesion progression and regression result. In the SCRIP main effects publication, subjects were categorized as progressors or regressors, only if no segment changed in the opposite direction. The threshold to define lesion change over four years was set at 0.2 mm. In the analyses carried out in this report, we included subjects as progressing or regressing based on the change in any single lesion. This is based on recent unpublished observations of our own and of others, that the intraclass (i.e. within subject) correlation of lesion change is very low at approximately 0.1. Lesions seem to respond independently of each other to the study interventions.

In addition, on average, stenoses tend to worsen over a span of four years. A more stringent threshold of 0.4 mm change was used to define lesion progression in this paper, reflecting the fact that progression is the natural state of coronary atherosclerosis. Use of a very sensitive threshold to define progression has the awkward effect of including most lesions and patients as progressing and thus, a usual care vs risk reduction comparison duplicates the statistically sounder analysis that uses the measurement of minimum lesion diameter as a continuous outcome variable. We chose, in this report, to analyse drug and lipid correlates using a more rigorous threshold for progression in order to detect what might be a more meaningful angiographic surrogate.

It is also likely that specific risk factors and associated drug therapies may differentially affect changes in existing lesions and development of new lesions. Progression of pre-existing lesions has a different pathophysiology from regression of lesions. This reflects differing factors leading to increases in atheroma mass (thrombus accretion, macrophage migration, calcification, lipid imbibition and scarring) compared with factors associated with regression (changes in concentration of various lipid phases as resorbtion from atheroma occurs and diminution of inflammation). The development of new atheroma is the result of a complex interaction of factors, including local intimal injury, release of cytokines, circulating atherogenic lipoproteins and the balance between local tissue growth promoters and inhibitors.

References

1. Haskell WL, Alderman EL, Fair JM, et al. Effects of intensive multiple risk factor reduction on coronary atherosclerosis and clinical cardiac events in men and women with coronary artery disease: The Stanford Coronary Risk Intervention Project (SCRIP). Circulation. 1994;89:975–90.
2. Trinder P. Determination of glucose in blood using glucose oxidase with an alternative oxygen acceptor. Ann Clin Biochem. 1969;6:24–7.
3. Hales CN, Randle PJ. Immunoassay of insulin with insulin antibody precipitate. Biochem J. 1963;88:137–46.
4. Leung WH, Demopulos PA, Alderman EL, Sanders W, Stadius ML. Evaluation of catheters and metallic catheter markers as calibration standard for measurement of coronary dimension. Cathet Cardiovasc Diagn. 1990;21:148–53.
5. Leung WH, Sanders W, Alderman EL. Coronary artery quantitation and data management system for paired cineangiograms. Cathet Cardiovasc Diagn. 1991;24:121–34.
6. Gao SZ, Alderman EL, Schroeder JS, Hunt SA, Wiederhold V, Stinson EB. Progressive coronary luminal narrowing after cardiac transplantation. Circulation. 1990;82(5 Suppl):IV-269–75.
7. Quinn TG, Alderman EL, McMillan A, Haskell W. Development of new coronary atherosclerotic lesions during a four-year multifactor risk reduction program: The Stanford Coronary Risk Intervention Project (SCRIP). J Am Coll Cardiol. 1994;24:900–8.

15. Canadian coronary atherosclerosis study on the effect of lovastatin on the progression of coronary artery disease (CCAIT): why are results different?

L. CAMPEAU, J. LESPÉRANCE, D. WATERS and the
CCAIT INVESTIGATORS*

Summary

The Canadian Coronary Atherosclerosis Intervention Trial is a multicentre double-blind control study of the effect of 3-hydroxy-3-methylglutaryl coenzyme A reductase inhibitor (lovastatin) on the progression–regression of coronary artery atherosclerosis. It involved 316 men and women who were randomized to either a lipid-lowering diet or the diet and daily lovastatin for a period of 24 months. The changes in coronary artery morphology were assessed by quantitative coronary angiography. It demonstrated significantly less progression of coronary atherosclerosis and fewer new lesions in the drug-treated group. It did not show regression and no clinical benefits were noted. It is suspected that the lack of regression is related primarily to a suboptimal fall in LDL-cholesterol.

Introduction

The design features and results of the Canadian Coronary Artery Atherosclerosis Study (CCAIT) have been published in detail[1,2]. Regression of coronary atherosclerosis was not facilitated by lipid lowering in contrast to other trials. It did show that lovastatin therapy was associated with less progression compared with placebo but only in stenoses ≤50% at baseline unlike several trials that demonstrated a beneficial effect for all lesions irrespective of the severity of the initial narrowing. We suspect that these discordant results may be in part explained on the basis of some distinctive design features. We shall briefly describe the trial and then attempt to evaluate the potential influence of the distinctive methodology on results.

Patients and methods

CCAIT was a multicentre intervention trial to determine whether or not the administration of lovastatin (a 3-hydroxy-3-methylglutaryl coenzyme A reductase inhibitor) retards the progression and facilitates the regression of coronary atherosclerosis as assessed by quantitative coronary arteriography (QCA). It was a double-blind randomized placebo-controlled trial involving 316

*See Appendix for list of investigators

A.V.G. Bruschke et al. (eds): Lipid-lowering therapy and progression of atherosclerosis, 167–178.
© 1996 Kluwer Academic Publishers.

patients of both sexes (19% were women) aged 27–70 years (mean age 53±8) with or without other coronary artery disease (CAD) risk factors. A history of hypertension was recorded in 37% (excluding diastolic pressure > 120 mmHg in spite of treatment), diabetes in 14% and current smoking in 27%. Almost all had clinical evidence of CAD, 54% with at least one previous infarction and 66% with a history of angina. The lipid inclusion criteria were a total cholesterol between 220 and 300 mg/dl (5.7 and 7.8 mmol/L) and a serum triglyceride level below 500 mg/dl (5.65 mmol/L).

Although the clinical inclusion criteria were representative of the usual population of patients with CAD, the angiographic selection criteria were designed to favour candidates at higher risk for progression in order to reduce the sample size requirement. Based on a retrospective study of 313 patients who had serial symptom-directed coronary arteriography, variables that predicted coronary progression were young age and the number of coronary segments with stenoses between 5% and 75%[3]. In a prospective study using the combination of these two variables, the per-lesion progression rate was 9.8% and the per-patient rate was 43% over 2 years, using a minimum diameter change ≥0.4 mm as the cut-off point for true change[1]. Thus, the angiographic inclusion criteria were based on age and extent score as follows: for candidates <51 years, at least four of a total of 15 pre-selected coronary segments needed at least one stenosis between 5% and 75%, at 51–60 years, five segments were required, and, at 61–70 years, six segments or more. Using this composite age–angiographic selection criterion, the required sample size was calculated at 300 analysable patients. The study population closely reflected CAD patients at large and thus the results would seem probably applicable to a broad population.

Although at least one stenosis ≥50% was not an angiographic prerequisite as in several other trials[4,5], 68% of the candidates had at baseline at least one artery with such a severe lesion. Nonetheless, such lesions were three times less frequent than smaller lesions, 2.1 lesions per patient, compared with 6.1 lesions ≤50% per patient.

All patients had dietary counselling at entry with the goal of adhering to the AHA diet phase I. Most patients received 325 mg of enteric-coated aspirin on alternate days. The most frequent concomitant drugs at baseline noted in 70% of patients was one of the calcium antagonists, a drug which may prevent the development of new lesions and retard the progression of small lesions[6,7]. Concomitant drugs were equally distributed among lovastatin and placebo-treated patients, including aspirin, calcium antagonists, β-blockers, ACE inhibitors and digitalis. In fact, both treatment groups were perfectly well-balanced with respect to all clinical and angiographic characteristics.

A physician otherwise uninvolved with the trial monitored serum LDL-cholesterol (LDL-C) levels and recommended dose changes in order to achieve a target ≤130 mg/dl (3.38 mmol/L) but above 90 mg/dl (2.34 mmol/L). An LDL-C level ≤130 mg/dl was obtained in 69% of the lovastatin-treated patients and in 10% of the placebo patients. The daily amount of lovastatin varied from 20 to 80 mg with an average of 36 mg. If the total cholesterol exceeded 340 mg/dl

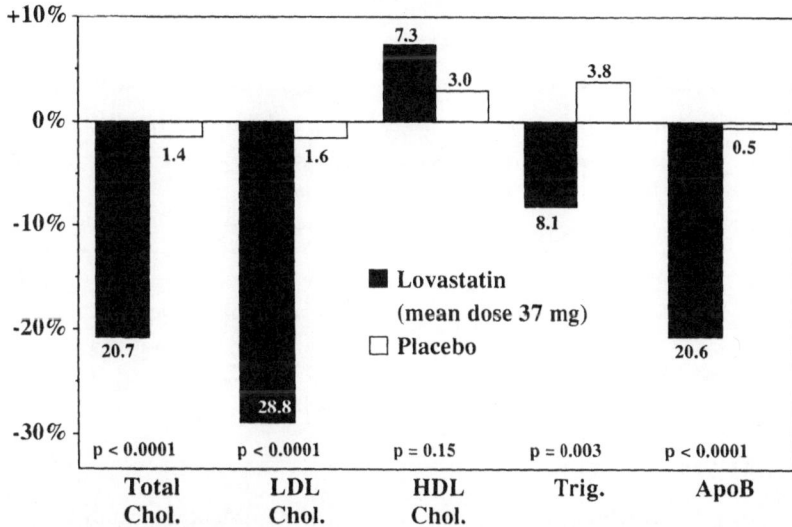

Figure 15.1. Bar graphs showing the changes, from baseline to during-trial, in mean plasma levels of lipids and lipoproteins. Chol. = cholesterol, Trig. = triglyceride.

(8.83 mmol/L) at any of the 8-week-interval lipid measurements, the patient was given special dietary counselling and cholestyramine if no improvement ensued, measures prescribed to only seven patients all in the placebo group. The duration of the trial was 2 years in all but 21 patients were studied earlier because of clinical events.

Results

Effect of treatment on plasma lipids

Significant mean changes were observed in all lipid and lipoprotein plasma levels of patients receiving lovastatin, including a decrease in total cholesterol (C), triglycerides, LDL-C, apolipoprotein B, and a significant increase in HDL-C and apolipoprotein A_1 (Figure 15.1). The mean decrease of LDL-C was $28.8 + 11\%$ and the mean increase in HDL-C was $7.3 + 19\%$. In the placebo group, the mean change during the trial was insignificant, less than 4% for these lipid particles. The intergroup difference, however, was significant only for total C, LDL-C and apolipoprotein B. The changes in lipid and lipoprotein plasma levels at 6-month intervals during the 2-year trial are shown in Figure 15.2 for both groups.

Effect of treatment on angiographic endpoints

The primary endpoint (a continuously variable outcome) was the per-patient average of the changes in the minimum lumen diameter (MLD) of all qualifying lesions. This coronary change score was calculated for each patient by averaging

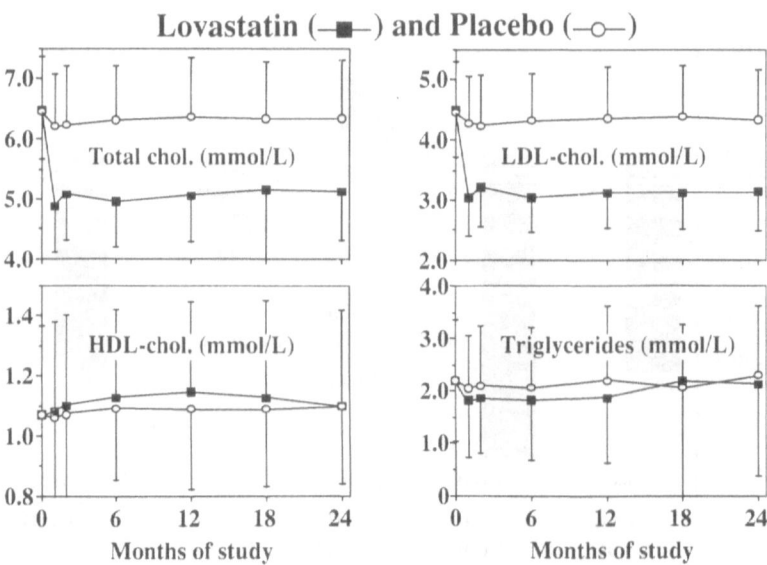

Figure 15.2. Bar graphs showing plasma levels of lipids and lipoproteins at 6-month intervals during the 24-month trial. There was a significant decrease of total cholesterol and LDL-C. No significant change was noted in HDL-C or triglyceride plasma levels.

the change in MLD of qualifying lesions between baseline and follow-up arteriograms. Measurements were obtained using the Cardiovascular Measurement System developed by Reiber et al.[8]. All lesions in segments with a diameter at visual examination ≥1 – 1.5 mm were measured, excluding segments distal to a total occlusion, poorly visualized segments, and segments having a large difference between diameters on the two angiograms compatible with a large difference in vasomotor tone. Only lesions ≥25% diameter by QCA on both films were included whenever coronary change score was concerned. However, all lesions were included in categorical analyses of secondary angiographic endpoints. These dichotomously variable outcomes were as follows:

1. Proportion of patients with progression;
2. Proportion of patients with regression;
3. Proportion of patients with one or more new lesions; and
4. Proportion of patients with one or more new total occlusions.

Progression and regression were respectively defined as narrowing and widening of a coronary segment diameter by ≥0.4 mm or by ≥15% diameter. In a previous study assessing the reproducibility of the cardiovascular measurement system used in this trial, the standard deviation (SD) for repeat measurements of MLD was 0.240 mm for films recorded 1–6 months apart[9]. The comparable SD for diameter stenosis was 8.6%. Changes in MLD of ≥0.4 mm or of ≥15% in diameter were taken to represent true change (close to 2 SD for repeat measurements).

　　The changes in primary angiographic endpoint indicate significantly less progression in the lovastatin-treated patients when all lesions are considered

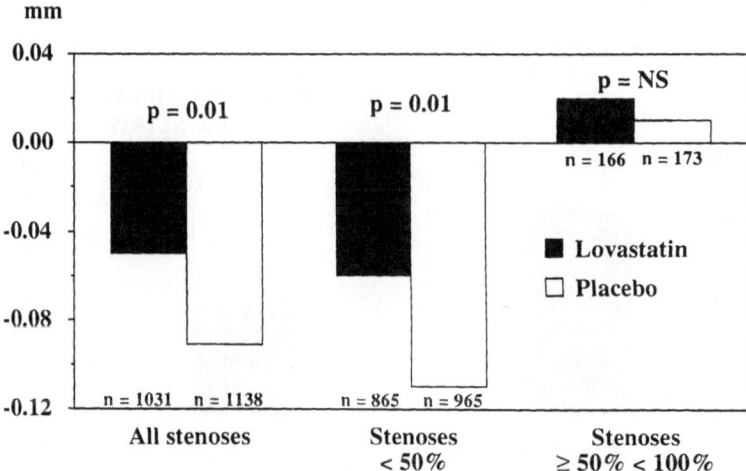

Figure 15.3. Bar graphs comparing the mean per-patient minimum lumen diameter changes in lovastatin and placebo-treated patients for all stenoses, stenoses <50% and stenoses ≥50% and <100%. No significant difference is observed for patients having stenoses ≥50% but significantly less progression is noted in lovastatin-treated patients with stenoses <50%.

whatever their severity (Figure 15.3). In fact, a small negative change in the per-patient mean MLD indicating progression was observed in both groups, but to a significantly greater degree in the placebo patients: -0.09 ± 0.16 vs -0.05 ± 0.13 mm ($p = 0.01$). The per-patient mean MLD change was evaluated separately in patients having stenoses ≥50% and <100%, and in those having less-severe lesions. As also shown in Figure 15.3, a significant difference is observed only between lovastatin and placebo patients having stenosis <50%. Actually, most lesions that progressed were <50% in diameter. Among lesions ≥50% at baseline, only six of the 166 lovastatin lesions and eight of the 173 placebo lesions increased by ≥15%. By contrast, 59 of the 865 lesions <50% in the lovastatin group (6.8%) and 108 of the 965 placebo lesions (11.2%) progressed ($p = 0.01$).

The results of the categorical analyses of the secondary endpoints concerning progression and new lesions are illustrated in Figure 15.4. The proportion of patients with progression only, as well as the proportion of patients with or without associated regression in other coronary segments, was significantly less in the lovastatin group. However, progression to a new total occlusion, which was infrequent (1.7% of qualifying lesions), was similar in both groups. Also, new lesions were less frequent in the lipid-lowering group.

Regression was equally rare in both groups: improvement of stenoses <100% was found in 28 lovastatin and in 20 placebo patients (19% vs 13%). Recanalization of a total occlusion was also uncommon, occurring in only nine patients, seven of whom were in the lovastatin group. Regression or recanalization with or without progression in other segments was observed in 35 of the 146 lovastatin patients, and in 22 of the 153 placebo patients (24% vs 14%, $p = 0.049$).

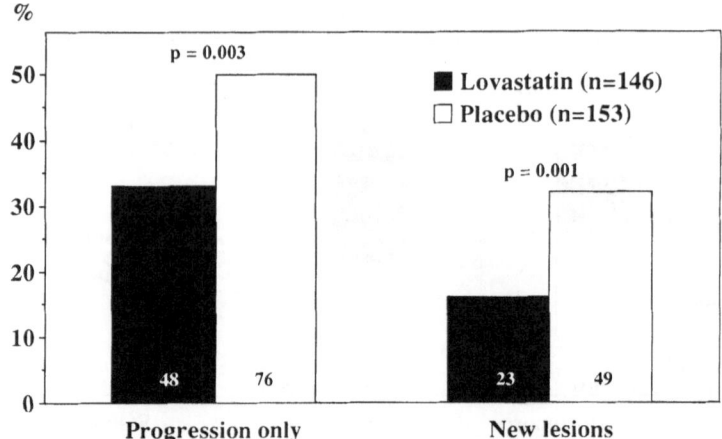

Figure 15.4.   Bar graphs showing results of the study for the categorical analyses of secondary endpoints. The proportions of patients showing progression as well as those having new lesions were significantly smaller in the treated patients compared with the placebo patients.

Effect of treatment in clinical subgroups

The unrestricted clinical inclusion criteria resulted in several clinical subgroups, subgroups of women, of patients with hypertension, of patients with diabetes and smokers. Although the numbers of participants in these subgroups were too small for statistical analysis in most instances, the results were similar in these subgroups as compared with the total study population (Figure 15.5).

Women represented 19% of the total population ($n=54$), one of the highest proportions of women in reported regression–progression trials. The mean coronary change score was -0.05 mm in 25 lovastatin and -0.09 mm in 29 placebo women, as in the entire study population (trend not statistically significant). New lesions developed in only one of the women in the lovastatin group but in 13 in the placebo group (4% vs 45%, $p=0.001$). Also, only seven had progression with lovastatin compared with 17 with placebo (28% vs 59%, $p=0.026$).

There were 72 smokers. The mean coronary score change in smokers given lovastatin as compared with patients on placebo therapy, was significantly smaller, -0.016 mm and -0.07 mm respectively ($p=0.024$), indicating less progression.

Patients with hypertension ($n=109$) and patients with diabetes ($n=39$) had coronary score changes quite similar to that of the total population but the differences were not significant because of the smaller numbers.

Effect of treatment on coronary events during the trial

The incidence of coronary events was not significantly different in both groups, including myocardial infarction, unstable angina and cardiac death. Also, the change in angina class from baseline to end of the study was not different between groups.

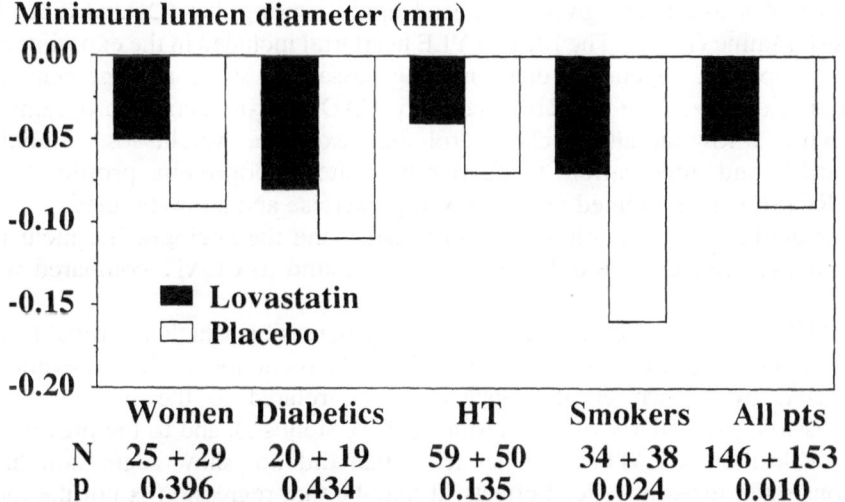

Minimum lumen diameter (mm)

	Women	Diabetics	HT	Smokers	All pts
N	25 + 29	20 + 19	59 + 50	34 + 38	146 + 153
p	0.396	0.434	0.135	0.024	0.010

Figure 15.5. Bar graphs showing the mean coronary change score in lovastatin and placebo patients of clinical subgroups. The relationship of results between treated and control patients was similar to that of the total study population, but the differences are not significant because of the small numbers except for smokers. HT = hypertension.

Discussion

There are three striking differences between this trial and reported lipid-lowering trials:

1. Lack of regression;
2. No slowing of progression of stenosis ≥50%;
3. No obvious clinical benefit during the trial.

Discordant results among clinical trials may be related to differences in methodology, more specifically in the selection of patients, the type and modalities of the intervention, the choice of the endpoints and their measurements, and finally the analysis of the results.

CCAIT was compared with the following 10 lipid-lowering trials in which coronary morphology changes were measured by QCA: FATS[4], LIFESTYLE[10], SCOR[11], CLAS[12], STARS[13], EXERCISE[14], MARS[5], SCRIP[15], MAAS[16] and PLAC I[17,18].

The fenofibrate study[19] was not considered because of the inappropriate control group (patients selected retrospectively after symptom-directed angiographic examination).

The interventions in seven of these trials consisted of a lipid-lowering diet, and drug therapy, including bile acid sequestrants, niacin and CoA reductase inhibitors, given alone or in combination (CLAS, FATS, SCOR, STARS, MARS, PLAC I and MAAS). FATS had two separate interventions, colestipol−niacin C−N) and colestipol−lovastatin (C−L). STARS also had two interventions in addition to a usual-care group: a special lipid-lowering diet (D) and diet plus cholestyramine (D–C). The LIFESTYLE heart trial included in the experimental group a low-fat vegetarian diet, smoking cessation, stress management and regular exercise. The SCRIP trial had CAD risk-reduction programmes involving a low-fat and a cholesterol diet, exercise, weight loss, smoking cessation and medication to favourably alter lipoprotein profiles. The EXERCISE trial combined regular physical exercise and a low-fat diet.

It is doubtful that the clinical characteristics and the angiographic inclusion criteria were related to the discordant results found in CCAIT compared with these trials.

CCAIT showed a definite retardation of progression which is probably the greatest desirable effect of these trials. In fact, the reduction of clinical events as suggested by Brown et al.[20] appears to be related to the prevention of progression, particularly of mild lesions (<50% stenosis), and to the prevention of new lesions. CCAIT and other trials that did not show regression have demonstrated these beneficial effects. It may be that regression is not the most important end result, particularly when one considers the uncertain interpretation of an increase in lumen size: true regression?; remodelling?; thrombus lysis?; recanalization?; or less vasoconstriction?

Nonetheless, we have reviewed the other reported trials in order to find an explanation for the lack of regression in CCAIT, a major difference compared with several trials. We suspect that a plausible cause for the lack of regression was the modest average reduction of LDL-C by only 29% as a result of the therapeutic target set at 130 mg/dl or less (3.38 mmol/L). This particular target was selected on the basis of recommendations at that time of the National Cholesterol Education Program Expert Panel as guidelines for clinical practice in USA[21].

As shown in Table 15.1, eight interventions from six trials were associated with net regression (colestipol–niacin and colestipol–lovastatin, interventions of FATS, LIFESTYLE, SCOR, CLAS, low-fat diet and diet–colestipol interventions of STARS and MARS). Net regression was defined as a significant increase in the coronary artery lumen associated with a significantly greater global change in the treated group as compared with the placebo group. The measurement of the lumen size was one of the following continuous variables: the mean lumen diameter, the minimum lumen diameter (expressed either in mm or in % diameter) and the cross-sectional percent area. Net regression was shown in MARS only for stenoses ≥50%. In the exercise and low-fat diet intervention, the proportions of patients showing no change, progression and regression were significantly different in this three categories analysis, a beneficial effect being in favour of the treated group but there is no evidence of net regression. MAAS report that regression was twice as frequent in patients who received simvastatin than in controls, but without obvious statistical proof to support their claim.

Except for the low-fat diet intervention of STARS, the mean LDL-C plasma level reduction from baseline was between 32% and 46%. On the other hand, in the five trials without evidence of regression, the mean LDL change from

Table 15.1. Mean plasma lipoprotein decrease (%) and during-trial levels with respect to regression.

Trial	LDL-cholesterol		HDL-cholesterol		Regression (net)
	Decrease (%)	During trial (mmol/L)	Increase (%)	During trial (mmol/L)	
FATS					
C–N	32	3.34	41	1.42	Yes
C–L	46	2.77	14	1.06	Yes
LIFESTYLE	38	2.46	–3	0.97	Yes
SCOR	39	4.45	25	1.53	Yes
CLAS	43	2.5	37	1.58	Yes
STARS					
D	16	4.19	0	1.14	Yes
D–C	36	3.37	–4	1.24	Yes
MARS	38	2.41	9	1.18	Yes
EXERCISE	8	3.85	3	0.94	No
SCRIP	23	3.12	12	1.33	No
MAAS	31	3.02	9	1.18	No
PLAC I	26	3.14	8	1.15	No
CCAIT	29	3.15	7	1.12	No

C–N: colestipol–niacin; C–L: colestipol–lovastatin; D: diet; D–C: diet + cholestyramine.

Table 15.2. Relationship of net regression with reduction from baseline of LDL-cholesterol ≥32% in treated groups.

Net regression	Plasma LDL-C reduction ≥32%
Yes (n=8)	n=7
No (n=5)	n=0

Z proportion $p = 0.012$.

baseline was between 23% and 31%. The difference in mean LDL-C fall between these two groups (including the diet-intervention group of STARS) was significant as shown in Table 15.2 ($p=0.01$).

The mean LDL-C during-trial plasma level in CCAIT was 3.15 mmol/L whereas it was below that level in only four of the eight lipid-lowering interventions that were associated with net regression, suggesting that the level at which LDL-C is reduced may play a lesser role than the magnitude of its reduction.

Is the small increase in HDL-C observed in CCAIT (7%) also a contributing factor? It is not clear when one considers that it increased by more than 12% in only four of the eight interventions with regression. In trials without regression, the greatest increase was 12%. The during-trial plasma level does not appear to be relevant, being quite similar in those trials with regression and those without (1.27±0.22 and 1.14±0.14 mmol/L respectively).

As shown in Table 15.3, the difference in the mean extent of LDL-C fall from baseline between the interventions with net regression and those without is

Table 15.3.   Mean change from baseline and during-trial plasma level of lipoproteins in treated groups with and without net regression.

Net regression	LDL-C decrease (%)	On-trial LDL-C level (mmol/L)	HDL-C increase (%)	On-trial HDL-C level (mmol/L)
Yes (n=8)	36.0±9	3.19±0.8	14.9±17.8	1.27±0.22
No (n=5)	23.4±9	3.26±0.3	7.8±3.3	1.14±0.14
p value	0.034	0.9	0.4	0.3

significant, in favour of interventions with regression: 36.0±9 vs 23.4±9 ($p=0.034$). There are no significant differences concerning the during-trial mean LDL-C plasma level, mean extent of rise of HDL-C nor with the during-trial mean HDL-C plasma level.

The modest reduction of LDL-C in CCAIT may also explain the lack of beneficial effect on stenoses ≥50%. In five trials that specifically evaluated the role of lipid lowering on such severe lesions (FATS, LIFESTYLE, STARS, MARS and MAAS), a beneficial effect was noted in all trials, and to a larger degree as compared with lesions <50%. In MARS, no beneficial effect was noted for stenoses <50%. These trials had a reduction of LDL-C varying from 31% to 46% (average 36.4%). In the diet intervention of STARS, where the LDL-C reduction was only 16%, no beneficial effect was observed on severe stenoses whereas it was in the diet plus cholestyramine intervention that had a 36% decrease in LDL-C plasma level. Another explanation for this lack of benefit in stenoses ≥50% in CCAIT is their lower progression rate as compared with smaller stenoses: 4% vs 9% (14/339 vs 169/1880; $p=0.005$). Also, most patients in CCAIT had daily aspirin. Could it be that aspirin had a smaller atherogenic effect in more severe lesions?

The during-trial clinical events are probably associated with progression. Brown et al.[4] observed that, in all 13 patients who had an angiographic examination prior to invasive therapy, clinical deterioration could be related to a lesion that increased in severity. Only five of these 13 lipid-lowering interventions including CCAIT which all showed a beneficial angiographic effect had fewer coronary events during the trial (FATS, STARS, LIFESTYLE, SCRIP and PLAC I).

The POSCH trial, not included in this review because the angiographic results were obtained by visual interpretation, reported, after 10 years of lipid lowering, a significant reduction of myocardial infarction and coronary death[22]. A meta-analysis of clinical outcomes in 14 trials showed significant reduction in total death, cardiac death, non-fatal myocardial infarction and the frequency of interventional therapy in treated compared with control patients[23]. Of interest are studies documenting that patients who were shown to have angiographic progression had more clinical events during the following 3–4 years compared with patients whose coronary arteries had remained unchanged[24,25].

In conclusion, CCAIT showed that modest lipid lowering with monotherapy (lovastatin) retarded progression of coronary atherosclerosis of lesions <50% and prevented the appearance of new lesions. It did not facilitate regression and this is felt to be related primarily to insufficient LDL-C reduction.

The similarity of the response to lovastatin in several clinical subgroups, as compared with the total study population, justifies the application of the results of this trial to the population at large, including both genders and patients with and without diabetes or hypertension, as well as smokers.

References

1. Waters D, Higginson L, Gladstone P, Kimball B, LeMay M, Lespérance J. Design features of a controlled clinical trial to assess the effect of an HMG CoA reductase inhibitor on the progression of coronary artery disease. Control Clin Trials. 1993;14:45–74.
2. Waters D, Higginson L, Gladstone P, et al. Effects of monotherapy with an HMG-CoA reductase inhibitor on the progression of coronary atherosclerosis as assessed by serial quantitative arteriography. The Canadian Coronary Atherosclerosis Intervention Trial. Circulation. 1994;89:959–68.
3. Moise A, Théroux P, Taeymans Y, et al. Clinical and angiographic factors associated with progression of coronary artery disease. J Am Coll Cardiol. 1984;3:659–67.
4. Brown G, Albers JJ, Fisher LD, et al. Regression of coronary artery disease as a result of intensive lipid-lowering therapy in men with high levels of apolipoprotein B. N Engl J Med. 1990;323:1289–98.
5. Blankenhorn DH, Azen SP, Kramsch DM, et al. Coronary angiographic changes with lovastatin therapy. The Monitored Atherosclerosis Regression Study (MARS). Ann Intern Med. 1993; 119:969–76.
6. Lichtlen PR, Hugenholtz PG, Rafflenbeul W, et al. on behalf of the INTACT Group Investigators. Retardation of angiographic progression of coronary artery disease by nifedipine: Results of the International Nifedipine Trial on Antiatherosclerotic Therapy (INTACT). Lancet. 1990;335: 1109–13.
7. Waters D, Lespérance J, Francetich M, et al. A controlled clinical trial to assess the effect of a calcium channel blocker on the progression of coronary atherosclerosis. Circulation. 1990;82: 1940–53.
8. Reiber JHC, van der Zwet PMJ, von Land CD, et al. On-line quantification of coronary angiograms with the DCI system. Medicamundi. 1989;34:89–98.
9. Lespérance J, Waters D. Measuring progression and regression of coronary atherosclerosis in clinical trials: problems and progress. Int J Card Imaging. 1992;8:165–73.
10. Ornish D, Brown SE, Scherwitz LW, et al. Can lifestyle changes reverse coronary heart disease? Lancet. 1990;336:129–33.
11. Kane JP, Malloy MJ, Ports TA, Phillips NR, Diehl JC, Havel RJ. Regression of coronary atherosclerosis during treatment of familial hypercholesterolemia with combined drug regimens. JAMA. 1990;264:3007–12.
12. Blankenhorn DH, Selzer RH, Mack WJ, et al. Evaluation of colestipol/niacin therapy with computer-derived coronary end point measures. A comparison of different measures of treatment effect. Circulation. 1992;86:1701–9.
13. Watts GF, Lewis B, Brunt JNH, et al. Effects on coronary artery disease of lipid-lowering diet, or diet plus cholestyramine, in the St Thomas' Atherosclerosis Regression Study (STARS). Lancet. 1992;339:563–9.
14. Schuler G, Hambrecht R, Schlierf G, et al. Regular physical exercise and low-fat diet. Effects on progression of coronary artery disease. Circulation. 1992;86:1–11.
15. Haskell WL, Alderman EL, Fair JM, et al. Effects of intensive multiple risk factor reduction on coronary atherosclerosis and clinical cardiac events in men and women with coronary artery

disease. The Stanford Coronary Risk Intervention Project (SCRIP). Circulation. 1994;89: 975–90.
16. MAAS Investigators. Effect of simvastatin on coronary atheroma: The Multicentre Anti-Atheroma Study (MAAS) [Published erratum appears in Lancet. 1994;344:762]. Lancet. 1994; 344:633–8.
17. The Pravastatin Multinational Study Group for Cardiac Risk Patients. Effects of pravastatin in patients with serum total cholesterol levels from 5.2 to 7.8 mmol/liter (200 to 300 mg/dl) plus two additional atherosclerotic risk factors. Am J Cardiol. 1993;72:1031–7.
18. Pitt B, Mancini J, Ellis SG, Rosman HS, McGovern ME. for the PLAC I Investigators. Pravastatin limitation of atherosclerosis in the coronary arteries (PLAC I) [abstract]. J Am Coll Cardiol. 1994;23 Suppl:131A.
19. Hahmann HW, Bunte T, Hellwig N, et al. Progression and regression of minor coronary arterial narrowings by quantitative angiography after fenofibrate therapy. Am J Cardiol. 1991;67: 957–61.
20. Brown BG, Zhao X-Q, Sacco DE, Albers JJ. Lipid lowering and plaque regression. Circulation. 1993;87:1781–91.
21. The Expert Panel. Report of the National Cholesterol Education Program expert panel on detection, evaluation, and treatment of high blood cholesterol in adults. Arch Intern Med. 1988;148:36–69.
22. Buchwald H, Varco RL, Matts JP, et al. Effect of partial ileal bypass surgery on mortality and morbidity from coronary heart disease in patients with hypercholesterolemia. N Engl J Med. 1990;323:946–55.
23. Sniderman AD, Ghezzo RH. Meta-analysis of the clinical outcomes of recent quantitative angiographic trials to lower plasma LDL in patients with CAD. Can J Cardiol. 1994;10 (Suppl B):10B–16B.
24. Moise A, Clement B, Saltiel J. Clinical and angiographic correlates and prognostic significance of the coronary extent score. Am J Cardiol. 1988;61:1255–9.
25. Waters D, Craven TE, Lespérance J. Prognostic significance of progression of coronary atherosclerosis. Circulation. 1993;87:1067–75.

Appendix

Clinical centres and principal investigators

Montreal Heart Institute: David Waters, MD; Marilyn Francetich, RN.
University of Ottawa Heart Institute: Lyall Higginson, MD; Michel Le May, MD; Hetty Martin, RN.
The Toronto Hospital Corp: Peter Gladstone, MD; Brian Kimball, MD; Virginia Flintoft, RN.

Quantitative angiographic laboratory (Montreal Heart Institute)

Jacques Lespérance, MD; France Bélanger, RT; Colette Desjardins, RT; Marie-Josée Cloutier, RT; Jean Laurier, B Eng.

16. Impact upon angiographic disease progression following step drug therapy in normolipidaemic patients: results of the Harvard Atherosclerosis Reversibility Project (HARP)

C. M. GIBSON, P. H. STONE, R. C. PASTERNAK and F. M. SACKS
for the Harvard Atherosclerosis Reversibility Project Group

Summary

Although several trials have shown that lipid lowering improves angiographic disease progression in patients with elevated LDL-cholesterol levels, the potential benefit of drug therapy in normocholesterolaemic patients has not been examined in a randomized prospective fashion. Patients with symptomatic coronary artery disease with at least one lesion narrowed by >30% were randomized to either placebo ($n = 39$), or stepped drug therapy using pravastatin, niacin, cholestyramine and gemfibrozil as needed to reach a target total cholesterol of ≤4.1 mmol/L *and* LDL-cholesterol/HDL-cholesterol ≤2.0 ($n = 40$). Baseline lipid values (mmol/L) and the average percent changes between the groups over the 2.5 years of treatment were: total cholesterol 5.48, −28%; LDL-cholesterol 3.55, −41%; HDL-cholesterol 1.07, +13%; and triglycerides 1.88, −26% ($p < 0.001$ for each). By quantitative angiography, the mean baseline minimum lumen diameter for both groups was 1.6±0.7 mm which worsened over a mean of 2.5 years by 0.14±0.42 mm ($p < 0.0001$) in the treatment group and by 0.15±0.41 mm ($p < 0.0001$) in the control group. Baseline percent stenosis for both groups was 47±13% which worsened in the treatment group by 2.1±10.6% ($p = 0.003$) and in the control group by 2.4±10.3 ($p = 0.0004$) (n = 466 lesions in 79 patients). A general linear model with intraclass correlation was used to adjust for any potential correlation among multiple lesions in the same patient, baseline disease severity and the presence of bypass grafts and showed that the adjusted difference between the treatment groups was 0.04 mm in minimum lumen diameter (not significant (NS), 95% confidence interval (CI)=−0.05, 0.12), and 0.0% change in stenosis (NS, 95% CI=−1.6, 1.6). With 80% power, this excludes a benefit of >0.12 mm or >1.6% stenosis, which are differences that have been observed in previous lipid-lowering trials. There was no correlation between baseline lipids or the change in lipids with disease progression. In normocholesterolaemic patients, intensive step drug therapy does not alter the angiographic rate of structural disease progression.

Introduction

Previous trials have shown clinical[1-7] and angiographic benefits[8-16] following intensive lipid lowering. These trials, however, focused on patients with hyper-

A.V.G. Bruschke et al. *(eds): Lipid-lowering therapy and progression of atherosclerosis, 179–191.*
© 1996 *Kluwer Academic Publishers.*

lipidaemia, and unfortunately their results are not broadly applicable to the large group of patients with symptomatic heart disease who have plasma cholesterol and LDL levels that are conventionally considered to be normal[17-19]. While several of these trials have retrospectively examined data pertaining to the non-randomized subset of patients with normolipidaemia[11], there have been no randomized prospective trials examining the potential angiographic benefit of intensive pharmacological therapy in patients with normal cholesterol levels. Thus, the goal of the Harvard Atherosclerosis Reversibility Project (HARP) was to determine in a randomized prospective fashion whether intensive stepped drug therapy would favourably alter angiographic disease progression in normolipidaemic patients (i.e. total cholesterol from 4.65 to 6.47 mmol/L (180–250 mg/dl).

Methods

Patients

The trial has previously been reported elsewhere[20]. Inclusion criteria included the presence of a >30% stenosis of a major coronary artery on cardiac catheterization, a total cholesterol level of 4.65–6.47 mmol/L (180–250 mg/dl), a total cholesterol/HDL ratio of >4.0, and triglycerides <4.0 mmol/L (350 mg/dl), and age 30–75. Qualifying lipid values were based upon the average of the lipid measurements from two visits conducted 1–2 weeks apart. Exclusion criteria included an ejection fraction <40%, insulin-dependent diabetes, current cigarette smoking, and >14 drinks of alcohol per week. Randomization was stratified by medical or surgical treatment (CABG) following catheterization and also by the total cholesterol/HDL ratio (> or ≤6.0). Forty-four patients were randomized to stepped drug therapy and 47 to the control group. Dietary instruction was provided to all patients based upon the guidelines of the National Cholesterol Education Program Step I. A 7-day diet record was collected every 3 months and was analysed using a computerized nutrient data base (Food Processor II, ESHA Research, Salem, Ore).

Step drug therapy algorithm

The goal for pharmacological step therapy was to lower total cholesterol to <4.14 mmol/L (160 mg/dl) and the LDL/HDL ratio to <2.0. Additional drugs were not added if the LDL levels decreased to <2.07 mmol/L (80 mg/dl) irrespective of the LDL/HDL ratio. Initial therapy was pravastatin 40 mg and the following drugs were added in sequence to achieve this goal:

1. Nicotinic acid (Enduracin time-release tablets, Innovite Co., Portland, Ore), 1.5–3.0 g/d,
2. Cholestyramine 8–16 g/d, and
3. Gemfibrozil 600–1200 mg/d.

Lipid levels were measured every six weeks, and, if the goal was not reached, a repeat measurement was obtained within 2 weeks. The patient was advanced to the next step if the average of these two lipid levels did not reach the goal.

Control patients were treated with placebo–pravastatin. If their total cholesterol increased to ≥6.47 mmol/L (250 mg/dl) on two consecutive measurements 6 weeks apart, then intensified dietary instruction was given, followed by drug therapy with cholestyramine, nicotinic acid or lovastatin as needed to lower total cholesterol to <6.47 mmol/L (250 mg/dl). Gemfibrozil was used to treat hyper-triglyceridaemia which did not respond to diet. While patients were blinded to their treatment assignment, study personnel were not blinded given the complexity of the clinical management.

Laboratory values were monitored for adverse effects every 6 weeks. If the SGOT, SGPT, or alkaline phosphatase levels exceeded 3 times the upper limit of normal, or, if the creatine kinase level was confirmed to be > 4 times the baseline level, then the dose of study medication was reduced or discontinued as deemed appropriate.

Lipid measurements

Plasma lipids were measured on fasting fresh plasma and total and HDL-cholesterol measurements were standardized as part of a programme of the National Heart, Lung, and Blood Institute, and the Centers for Disease Control. Cholesterol and triglycerides were measured by enzymatic reagents (Boehringer Mannheim, Indianapolis, Ind.) in whole plasma[21]. HDL-cholesterol was measured in plasma after precipitation of VLDL and LDL by dextran and magnesium chloride[22]. LDL-cholesterol was calculated[23].

Cardiac catheterization and quantitative angiography

The gantry angle and skew, contrast agent, sequence of angiographic views, and the dosing of vasoactive medications were recorded at the time of initial cardiac catheterization and were reproduced at the time of the repeat procedure. On the day before the angiography, patients were treated with the same cardiac medications they were taking at the time of the initial procedure.

Personnel performing quantitative angiography were blinded to both treatment group assignment and the temporal sequence of the films. Quantitative angiography was performed on any lesion with a >20% stenosis by visual inspection. New lesions were defined as lesions which were <20% narrowed initially and narrowed to ≥20% at follow-up and changed by ≥7.8% diameter stenosis (a change previously determined to be significant using this QCA system)[24]. Normal segments without any obstruction >2.0 mm were analysed. Vessels instrumented for PTCA were excluded.

Five end-diastolic frames of the lesion in the view with the narrowest diameter were chosen for analysis. After 3–4-fold optical magnification using a Sony SME-3500 cineviewer, the frames were digitized into a 512×512-pixel array providing a spatial resolution in the image field of approximately 8–10 pixels per mm. The pincushion distortion in each image intensifier used in the study was corrected for using bilinear interpolation. A validated automated algorithm was used to determine the location of the vessel edge as the weighted mean of first and second derivative of a fifth-order polynomial fit to the densitometric profile[25,26].

Statistical methods

The a-priori primary outcome variable for the trial was the change in minimum diameter of coronary artery lesions expressed as a continuous variable analysed on a per-lesion basis. A general linear model with intraclass correlation (GLIMIC) was used to correct for any potential correlation among the multiple segments within a given patient[24,27] as well as to correct for any potential discrepancies in baseline narrowing of the vessels, which has been shown to be a significant predictor of lesion change[28] and for differences between the groups in the proportion of bypassed and unbypassed lesions. The change in percent stenosis was also analysed. Bypassed and unbypassed lesions were included together in the analysis. The data were also analysed on a patient-specific basis using the mean of the changes in diameter of the multiple lesions in each patient. The lesions and patients were also classified categorically as having progressed, regressed or as having not changed based upon a threshold of a 0.27-mm change in diameter or a 7.8% change in percent stenosis[24]. The incidence of sudden cardiac death, fatal and non-fatal myocardial infarction, hospitalization for unstable angina, coronary artery bypass surgery, and coronary angioplasty was determined. All events were confirmed based upon review of hospital records.

Results

Patient population

Forty active treatment patients and 39 control patients (70 men, 9 women) underwent follow-up cardiac catheterization at a mean of 30 ± 5 months (2.5 years). Coronary artery bypass surgery was performed in 31 of the 79 patients prior to randomization. Baseline characteristics were not significantly different between the treatment and control groups except a lower systolic blood pressure and a reduced use of angiotensin converting enzyme inhibitors in the active group (Table 16.1). Changes in blood pressure, body weight and medications other than hypolipidaemic agents were similar in the two groups (Table 16.1).

Lipid changes

The baseline mean total cholesterol level for the entire cohort was 5.47 ± 0.48 mmol/L (212 ± 19 mg/dl), for LDL 3.56 ± 0.54 mmol/L (137 ± 21 mg/dl), for HDL 1.07 ± 0.22 mmol/L (41 ± 9 mg/dl) and for triglycerides 1.88 ± 0.92 mmol/L

Table 16.1.   Baseline and follow-up patient characteristics.

Demographic	Active (n=40)		Control (n=39)	
	Baseline	Follow-up	Baseline	Follow-up
Mean (SD) age (years)	57 (8)	—	59 (9)	—
M/F	36/4	—	34/5	—
Treated hypertension	19	—	20	—
Type 2 diabetes	3	—	5	—
Previous MI	12	—	19	—
Coronary artery surgery	17	—	14	—
Multivessel disease	36	—	33	—
Mean (±SD) weight (kg)	87±15	88±15	81±13	83±13*
Mean (±SD) blood pressure (mmHg)				
Systolic	126±16†	125±13†	136±26	133±15
Diastolic	80±9	79±15	78±12	79±9
β-Blockers	25	16	21	17
Aspirin	37	36	38	35
ACE inhibitors	0†	1†	7	8
Calcium blockers	20	18	18	21

For blood pressure and weight, the follow-up values are means for the entire period of follow-up; for medications, the follow-up values are the number of patients on the medication at the end of follow-up. *$p<0.05$ vs baseline within group; †$p<0.05$ for comparisons of baseline or follow-up means between groups.

(167±82 mg/dl) (Table 16.2). The LDL/HDL ratio of the stepped therapy arm decreased by 47% from 3.4 to 1.8 while, in the control group, it remained constant at 3.3 ($p<0.001$). By 6 weeks after initiation of therapy, significant differences in lipid levels between the two groups were seen. Compared with the control group, the treatment group experienced a 28% reduction in total cholesterol ($p<0.001$), a 41% decrease in LDL ($p<0.001$), a 13% increase in HDL ($p<0.001$), and a 26% reduction in triglycerides ($p<0.01$) (Table 16.2). The goal for total cholesterol of <4.1 mmol/L (160 mg/dl) and LDL/HDL <2.0, or LDL <2.07 mmol/L (80 mg/dl) was reached by 36 of the 40 patients in the active treatment group at a mean follow up of 1.2 years. Addition of nicotinic acid to reach the goal was required in 38 patients, cholestyramine in 24 patients, and gemfibrozil in 12 patients. In the control group, 10 patients did require drug therapy for a persistent total cholesterol >6.47 mmol/L (250 mg/dl); 9 received cholestyramine at a mean dose of 8 g for a mean of 37 weeks, 4 received nicotinic acid 1 g/d for 26 weeks, 1 received lovastatin 10 mg/d for 90 weeks, and 4 received gemfibrozil 900 mg/d for 26 weeks.

Angiographic results

A total of 226 lesions in 40 patients treated with stepped drug therapy, and a total of 240 lesions in 39 control patients were available for analysis. The mean baseline minimum lumen diameter for both groups was 1.6±0.7 mm which

Table 16.2. Plasma lipid levels at baseline and during treatment.

				Weeks in the study				Overall*
	0	6	24	48	72	96	120	
Total cholesterol								
Active	5.53±0.52	4.42±0.67	4.16±0.65	3.59±0.54	4.11±0.75	4.19±0.80	3.96±0.54	4.11±0.47
Control	5.43±0.44	5.58±0.57	5.59±0.62	5.40±0.57	5.56±0.59	5.66±0.65	5.59±0.75	5.56±0.47
% Δ from baseline (active–placebo)		−23%	−28%	−29%	−28%	−29%	−32%	−28%
p		<0.001	<0.001	<0.001	<0.001	<0.001	<0.001	<0.001
LDL-C								
Active	3.62±0.57	2.48±0.59	2.28±0.63	2.02±0.51	2.23±0.68	2.22±0.76	2.17±0.55	2.23±0.42
Control	3.49±0.52	3.62±0.59	3.57±0.63	3.56±0.54	3.62±0.59	3.62±0.55	3.52±0.74	3.59±0.45
% Δ from baseline (active–placebo)		−35%	−39%	−46%	−42%	−43%	−41%	−41%
p		<0.001	<0.001	<0.001	<0.001	<0.001	<0.001	<0.001
HDL-C								
Active	1.08±0.23	1.17±0.31	1.20±0.36	1.22±0.34	1.20±0.36	1.26±0.38	1.18±0.31	1.22±0.33
Control	1.07±0.20	1.07±0.21	1.11±0.24	1.04±0.22	1.05±0.21	1.06±0.21	1.09±0.24	1.07±0.19
% Δ from baseline (active–placebo)		7%	7%	16%	13%	15%	9%	13%
p		0.02	0.06	<0.001	<0.001	<0.001	0.2	<0.001
Triglycerides								
Active	1.84±0.86	1.70±0.86	1.46±0.71	1.52±0.90	1.48±0.83	1.52±0.89	1.26±0.62	1.47±0.61
Control	1.93±0.99	2.00±1.20	1.94±1.16	1.77±0.96	1.94±0.99	2.13±1.26	2.12±1.21	1.95±0.94
% Δ from baseline (active–placebo)		−10%	−21%	−9%	−21%	−28%	−41%	−26%
p		0.09	0.009	0.3	0.01	0.01	0.006	<0.001
n active, control	40,39	40,37	40,38	40,39	39,39	39,40	25,22	40,39

p-value by unpaired t-test on the changes from baseline in the active compared with the control group. %Δ = % change in active − % change in control group.
*Mean for all regularly scheduled visits after the baseline visit. Values expressed as mean±SD.

Table 16.3. Arteriographic changes in the stepped drug therapy group and the control group.

	Minimum diameter			Percent stenosis		
	Baseline	Change	*p*-value	Baseline	Change	*p*-value
Stepped drug therapy						
Lesion-based analysis (*n*=226)	1.65±0.74	−0.14±0.42	<0.0001	48.0±13.8	2.1±10.6	0.003
Patient-based analysis (*n*=40)	1.65±0.43	−0.12±0.24	0.003	47.2±7.3	2.1±5.2	0.02
Control						
Lesion-based analysis (*n*=240)	1.64±0.64	−0.15±0.41	<0.0001	46.6±13.0	2.4±10.3	0.0004
Patient-based analysis (*n*=39)	1.67±0.41	−0.17±0.35	0.005	46.1±8.2	2.4±6.3	0.02

worsened by 0.14 ± 0.42 mm ($p<0.0001$) in the stepped drug therapy group and by 0.15 ± 0.41 mm ($p<0.0001$) in the control group. Baseline percent stenosis for both groups was $47\pm13\%$ which worsened in the stepped drug therapy group by $2.1\pm10.6\%$ ($p=0.003$) and in the control group by $2.4\pm10.3\%$ ($p=0.0004$). A general linear model with intraclass correlation was used to adjust for any potential correlation among the multiple lesions in the same patient, for baseline disease severity as well as the presence or absence of bypass grafting. The adjusted difference in the change in minimum lumen diameter between the treatment groups was 0.04 ± 0.08 mm (NS) and $0.0\pm1.6\%$ stenosis (NS). With 80% power, this excludes a benefit of >0.12 mm or $>1.6\%$ stenosis, which are treatment effects that have been exceeded in previous lipid-lowering trials. The correlations among lesions within the same patient were quite low ($0.05-0.2$) indicating relatively little interdependence among lesions in the rate of disease progression.

For unbypassed lesions, the adjusted difference in the change in minimum lumen diameter between groups was 0.01 ± 0.09 mm (NS), and for percent stenosis was $0.2\pm2.1\%$ (NS). For all bypassed lesions (159 were proximal, 13 were distal to the anastomosis), the adjusted difference in minimum lumen diameter progression between groups was 0.11 ± 0.15 mm (NS), and for percent stenosis was $0.1\pm2.7\%$ (NS).

Similarly, patient-based changes in the coronary artery measurements were not significantly different between the groups (Table 3). The mean changes in the treatment and control groups in minimum diameter were -0.12 ± 0.24 mm and -0.17 ± 0.35 mm, and, in percent stenosis, were $2.1\pm5.2\%$ and $2.4\pm6.3\%$, respectively (within the groups, all $p<0.05$; between the groups, all $p\geq0.5$, i.e. NS). For unbypassed lesions, the mean changes in the treatment and control groups were -0.07 ± 0.21 mm ($p=0.08$) and -0.12 ± 0.37 mm ($p=0.09$), and $1.5\pm5.7\%$ ($p=0.2$) and $2.4\pm6.9\%$ ($p=0.07$), respectively ($p=0.6$, i.e. NS between the groups).

Table 16.4.   Categorical analysis of change in percent stenosis.

	Lesions (% (n))		Patients (% (n))	
	Active	Control	Active	Control
Progression	23 (53)	28 (67)	30 (12)	36 (14)
Regression	14 (31)	14 (33)	12.5 (5)	15 (6)
Mixed	—	—	37.5 (15)	38 (15)
No change	63 (142)	58 (140)	20 (8)	10 (4)

Change defined as ≥7.8 percentage points.

In addition, each lesion was classified as progressing, regressing or not changing based upon the previously defined 7.8% threshold for significant change in percent stenosis (twice the standard deviation of the frame-to-frame variability of the change in percent stenosis)[23]. Each patient was then classified as having progression only, regression only, mixed changes, or no changes. No significant differences were observed between the groups in this categorical analysis (Table 16.4). In the treatment group, 11 vessels (4 unbypassed, 7 bypassed) in 10 patients became occluded compared with 10 vessels (3 unbypassed, 7 bypassed) in 8 control patients (NS). One vessel in each group showed recanalization. Three vessels developed new lesions in the treatment group, and 2 in the control group (NS).

In both univariate models and multivariate models correcting for bypass status and treatment group assignment, there was no correlation between the change in epicardial diameter and either the baseline lipids or the change in lipid levels. Baseline percent stenosis and minimum diameter were both inversely correlated with the subsequent changes ($p < 0.0001$) with mild lesions experiencing more rapid progression than severe lesions. Excluding patients treated with angiotensin converting enzyme inhibitors did not significantly alter the results presented for the entire cohort.

Adverse events

Among control patients, 10 of the 47 randomized patients (21%) experienced 12 events (1 death, 1 congestive heart failure, 2 angioplasties, 1 bypass surgery, and 7 hospitalizations for unstable angina). Among treated patients, 6 of the 44 patients (14%) had 8 events (1 death, 2 non-fatal myocardial infarctions, 1 angioplasty, 1 bypass surgery, and 3 hospitalizations for unstable angina) ($p = 0.19$ between groups).

Discussion

Several trials have now demonstrated that, in hyperlipidaemic patients, atherosclerotic disease progression can be favourably altered by either lipid lowering (drug and dietary therapy)[8-12], exercise[14] or lifestyle modifications[15]. It

Table 16.5. Relationship of baseline LDL to angiographic benefit.

Trial	Baseline LDL	Angiographic benefit
SCOR	283	+
STARS	203	+
	196	+
FATS	196	+
	190	+
POSCH	179	+
CLAS	171	+
Lifestyle	160	+
MARS	166	+/−
SCRIP	157	+/−
HARP	137	−

is unclear, however, that patients with mild hyperlipidaemia derive the same benefits given data from epidemiological studies[18], large-scale clinical trials[29], meta-analyses[30], and retrospective subgroup analyses of angiographic regression trials[11] suggesting that the benefit of lipid lowering is directly proportional to the elevation in baseline lipid values. Accordingly, the goal of the present trial was to determine whether those angiographic benefits observed in hyperlipidaemic patients could also be accrued in the majority of coronary heart disease patients who have total cholesterol and LDL levels that are conventionally considered to be normal[17-19,31,32]. The current study demonstrates that despite aggressive stepped drug therapy to achieve a 41% reduction in LDL, a 28% reduction in total cholesterol and a 13% increase in HDL, there was no impact upon the rate of atherosclerosis progression in normolipidaemic patients.

Table 16.5 underscores the fundamental way in which the HARP trial differs from previous atherosclerosis regression studies. HARP patients had the lowest baseline LDL levels (3.55 mmol/L or 137 mg/dl) of any trial to date (range 3.92–7.32 mmol/L, or 157–283 mg/dl)[10-16]. Interestingly, the two other trials with the closest baseline LDL levels (3.92 mmol/L[15] and 4.24 mmol/L[14]) utilized a combination of several non-pharmacological interventions to produce improvements in luminal diameter that were not correlated with the changes in lipids, but rather with other non-pharmacological aspects of the intervention[14], or adherence to the overall programme[15]. Consistent with the lack of benefit observed in patients with a low baseline LDL in the HARP trial, there was no angiographic benefit for patients whose baseline LDL was below the population median in the CCAIT trial[16].

Within this conventionally 'normal' range of lipid values in the HARP study, there was no correlation between baseline lipids or their change and disease progression. This raises a question as to the relative importance of other risk factors in mediating disease progression within this normal range of lipid values. Indeed, despite a mean cholesterol on entry of 5.5 mmol/L (212 mg/dl), the absence of insulin-dependent diabetes, uncontrolled hypertension, and smoking, 39% of patients in this trial had undergone coronary artery bypass grafting, again raising a question as to the role of unidentified risk factors for atherosclerosis in these normolipidaemic patients that were not modified during the course of the trial.

One question that obviously arises when a study shows no treatment effect is whether the trial was sufficiently powered to demonstrate a relevant difference between the treatment and control groups. Based upon the HARP pilot study and the FATS study, we have previously calculated that atherosclerosis regression trials with sample sizes of 40 patients per treatment arm are adequately powered (80%) to demonstrate the magnitude of treatment effect observed in the FATS study (a 3-percentage point difference between groups for the change in percent stenosis). This is true whether the data are analysed on a per-lesion basis using a general linear model with intraclass correlation[24] or on a per-patient basis[33]. Of note, studies with similar[10,12] or even smaller[15] numbers of patients than in the present trial have demonstrated significant angiographic benefits. Correcting for the presence of bypass grafts, baseline stenosis severity, and the correlation among multiple lesions within the same patient, the present trial was sufficiently sensitive to detect a difference between groups of >0.12 mm or $>1.6\%$ stenosis, which would have permitted the detection of treatment benefits observed in previous regression trials[10-16]. The rate of narrowing in the HARP study was just under 1% stenosis per year, which is consistent with that observed in the control groups of other trials[10,16]. While angiographic follow-up after 2.5 years of lipid lowering may have been sufficient to document improvement in hyperlipidaemic patients, a longer period of treatment may have been required in normo-lipidaemic patients.

The HARP trial did not include any smokers, a subgroup which has been shown to experience four times more atherosclerosis regression in response to lipid lowering compared with non-smokers[16]. Unlike many atherosclerosis regression trials, the HARP trial did enroll patients who had previously or were about to undergo coronary artery bypass grafting. Neither bypassed nor unbypassed lesions experienced a significant benefit from lipid lowering. Given the bidirectional flow that occurs proximal to a bypass graft insertion site, and the relationship that we have previously identified between low shear stress and an increased rate of atherosclerosis progression[34], the adverse impact of disturbed rheology may overshadow the beneficial effects of lipid lowering in *normolipidaemic* patients. In contrast, in bypassed *hyperlipidaemic* patients in the CLAS study, lipid lowering did favourably influence disease progression[11]. The role of local rheology or mechanical factors in influencing disease progression is further supported by the observation that lesions within the same patient progress at nearly independent rates, both when assessed as a continuous variable using a general linear model with intraclass correlation ($r=0.05-0.20$) and when assessed as a categorical variable by the high rate of mixed lesion change (both progression and regression occurring in the same patient). This observation is also true in the FATS dataset[33]. The ways in which local vessel rheology modulates the relationship between lipid lowering and disease regression remain to be fully determined.

In the present trial as well as others[10,16], more severe lesions at baseline tended to regress, and milder lesions tended to progress. The relative role of true atherosclerosis regression and statistical regression to the mean in this phenomenon remains to be determined. It is interesting that the mean severity of lesions in the HARP trial was slightly greater than that of other trials[10-12,14,16] which, based upon the prior observation, would have actually favoured the detection of lesion regression in the HARP trial.

While the HARP trial and other atherosclerosis regression trials have been underpowered to detect an improvement in clinical event rates, it has been assumed that changes in the structural narrowing of arteries are an appropriate surrogate for clinical events. However, if clinical benefit is documented in patient populations with the same risk-factor profile as in the present study, then these clinical benefits may be due to improvements in *dynamic* measures of arterial function (i.e. a reduced incidence of plaque rupture[34] or an improved response to EDRF[35,36]) rather than improvements in *static* measures, such as the structural narrowing of arteries. Large ongoing randomized secondary prevention trials should determine whether aggressive lipid lowering will reduce hard endpoints, such as mortality, in patients with lipid levels that are conventionally considered normal, and hopefully will shed more light on the relationship between arteriographic and clinical endpoints.

Acknowledgements

From the Channing Laboratory and the Cardiovascular Divisions, Departments of Medicine, Brigham and Women's and Beth Israel Hospitals, and Harvard Medical School, Boston, Mass. Supported by grants from the National Heart, Lung and Blood Institute (RO1 HL36392 and NCRR GCRC MO1 RR02635), and with cofunding from Bristol-Myers Squibb.

References

1. The Coronary Drug Project Research Group. Clofibrate and niacin in coronary heart disease. JAMA. 1975;231:360–81.
2. Buchwald H, Varco RL, Matts JP, et al. Effect of partial ileal bypass surgery on mortality and morbidity from coronary heart disease in patients with hypercholesterolemia. N Engl J Med. 1990;323:946–55.
3. Research Committee of the Scottish Society of Physicians. Ischaemic heart disease: a secondary prevention trial using clofibrate. Br Med J. 1971;4:775–84.
4. Carlson LA, Rosenhamer G. Reduction of mortality in the Stockholm Ischaemic Heart Disease Secondary Prevention Study by combined treatment with clofibrate and nicotinic acid. Acta Med Scand. 1988;223:405–18.
5. Leren P. The Oslo diet-heart Study. Eleven-year report. Circulation. 1970;42:935–42.
6. Anonymous. Trial of clofibrate in the treatment of ischaemic heart disease. Five-year study by a group of physicians of the Newcastle Upon Tyne region. Br Med J. 1971;4:767–75.
7. Scandinavian Simvastatin Survival Study Group. Randomised trial of cholesterol lowering in 4444 patients with coronary heart disease: the Scandinavian Simvastatin Survival Study (4S). Lancet. 1994;344:1383–9.

 8. Levy RI, Brensike JF, Epstein SE, et al. The influence of changes in lipid values induced by cholestyramine and diet on progression of coronary artery disease: results of the NHLBI Type II Coronary Intervention Study. Circulation. 1984;69:325–37.
 9. Nikkila EA, Viikinkoski P, Valle M, Frick MH. Prevention of progression of coronary atherosclerosis by treatment of hyperlipidemia: a seven year prospective angiographic study. Br Med J. 1984;289:220–3.
10. Brown BG, Albers JJ, Fisher LD, et al. Regression of coronary artery disease as a result of intensive lipid-lowering therapy in men with high levels of apolipoprotein B. N Engl J Med. 1990;323:1289–98.
11. Blankenhorn DH, Nessim SA, Johnson RL, Sanmarco ME, Azen SP, Cashin-Hemphill L. Beneficial effects of combined colestipol–niacin therapy on coronary atherosclerosis and coronary venous bypass grafts. JAMA. 1987;257:3233–40.
12. Kane JP, Malloy MJ, Ports TA, Phillips NR, Diehl JC, Havel RJ. Regression of coronary atherosclerosis during treatment of familial hypercholesterolemia with combined drug regimens. JAMA. 1990;264:3007–12.
13. Watts GF, Lewis B, Brunt JN, et al. Effects on coronary artery disease of lipid-lowering diet, or diet plus cholestyramine, in the St Thomas' Atherosclerosis Regression Study (STARS). Lancet. 1992;339:563–9.
14. Schuler G, Hambrecht R, Schlierf G, et al. Regular physical exercise and low-fat diet. Effects on progression of coronary artery disease. Circulation. 1992;86:1–11.
15. Ornish D, Brown SE, Scherwitz LW, et al. Can lifestyle changes reverse coronary heart disease? The Lifestyle Heart Trial. Lancet. 1990;336:129–33.
16. Waters D, Higginson L, Gladstone P, et al. Effects of monotherapy with an HMG CoA reductase inhibitor upon the progression of coronary atherosclerosis as assessed by serial quantitative arteriography: The Canadian Coronary Atherosclerosis Intervention Trial (CCAIT). Circulation. 1994;89:959–68.
17. The Bezafibrate Infarction Prevention (BIP) Study Group, Israel. Lipids and lipoproteins in symptomatic coronary heart disease. Distribution, intercorrelations, and significance for risk classification in 6,700 men and 1,500 women. Circulation. 1992;86:839–48.
18. Rose G, Reid DD, Hamilton PJ, McCartney P, Keen H, Jarrett RJ. Myocardial ischemia, risk factors and death from coronary heart disease. Lancet. 1977;1:105–9.
19. Pekkanen J, Linn S, Heiss G, et al. Ten-year mortality from cardiovascular disease in relation to cholesterol level among men with and without preexisting cardiovascular disease. N Engl J Med. 1990;322:1700–7.
20. Sacks FM, Pasternak RC, Gibson CM, Rosner B, Stone PH for the Harvard Atherosclerosis Reversibility Project (HARP) Group. Effect on coronary atherosclerosis of decrease in plasma cholesterol concentrations in normocholesterolaemic patients. Lancet. 1994;344:1182–6.
21. Warnick GR. Enzymatic methods for quantification of lipoprotein lipids. Methods Enzymol. 1986;129:101–23.
22. Bachorik PS, Albers JJ. Precipitation methods for quantification of lipoproteins. Methods Enzymol. 1986;129:78–100.
23. Friedewald WT, Levy RI, Fredrickson DS. Estimation of the concentration of low-density lipoprotein cholesterol in plasma, without use of the preparative ultracentrifuge. Clin Chem. 1972;18:499–502.
24. Gibson CM, Sandor T, Stone PH, Pasternak RC, Rosner B, Sacks FM. Quantitative angiographic and statistical methods to assess serial changes in coronary luminal diameter and implications for atherosclerosis regression trials. Am J Cardiol. 1992;69:1286–90.
25. Spears JR, Sandor T, Als AV, et al. Computerized image analysis for quantitative measurement of vessel diameter from cineangiograms. Circulation. 1983;68:453–61.
26. Sandor T, D'Adamo A, Hanlon WB, Spears JR. High precision quantitative angiography. IEEE Trans Med Imaging. 1987;MI-6:258–65.
27. Rosner B. Multivariate methods in ophthalmology with application to other paired data situations. Biometrics. 1984;40:1025–35.
28. Stone PH, Gibson CM, Pasternak RC, et al. The natural history of coronary atherosclerosis

using quantitative angiography: implications for clinical trials of coronary regression. Am J Cardiol. 1993;71:766–72.

29. Sacks FM, Pfeffer MA, Moye L, et al. Rationale and design of a secondary prevention trial of lowering normal plasma cholesterol levels after acute myocardial infarction: The Cholesterol and Recurrent Event trial (CARE). Am J Cardiol. 1991;68:1436–46.

30. Holme I. An analysis of randomized trials evaluating the effect of cholesterol reduction on total mortality and coronary heart disease incidence. Circulation. 1990;82:1916–24.

31. Ginsburg GS, Safran C, Pasternak RC. Frequency of low serum HDL in hospitalized patients with 'desirable' total cholesterol levels. Am J Cardiol. 1991;68:187–92.

32. Miller M, Seidler A, Kwiterovich PO, Pearson TA. Long-term predictors of subsequent cardiovascular events with coronary artery disease and 'desirable' levels of plasma total cholesterol. Circulation. 1992;86:1165–70.

33. Gibson CM, Rosner B, Hillger L, Fisher LD, Brown BG. A comparison of outcomes and sample sizes using lesion and patient-based analyses of coronary regression data: results of the familial atherosclerosis treatment study (FATS) [abstract]. J Am Coll Cardiol. 1993;21(2 Suppl A):71A.

34. Gibson CM, Diaz L, Kandarpa K, et al. The relationship of vessel wall shear stress to atherosclerosis progression. Arterioscler Thromb. 1993;13:310–15.

35. Richardson PD, Davies MJ, Brown GV. Influence of plaque configuration and stress distribution on fissuring of coronary atherosclerotic plaques. Lancet. 1989;2:941–4.

36. Vita JA, Treasure CB, Nabel EG, et al. The coronary vasomotor response to acetyl-choline relates to risk factors for coronary artery disease. Circulation. 1990;81:491–7.

17. Effect of aggressive versus conventional lipid-lowering treatment on coronary and peripheral atherosclerosis: design and baseline characteristics of the LDL-Apheresis Atherosclerosis Regression Study (LAARS)

A. A. KROON and A. F. H. STALENHOEF

Summary

In this open randomized 2-year study in hypercholesterolaemic men with severe coronary atherosclerosis, the effect of aggressive lipid lowering with LDL-apheresis plus simvastatin will be compared with conventional lipid-lowering treatment with simvastatin alone. Treatments will be compared by means of quantitative coronary angiography and videodensitometric assessment of the coronary perfusion. Secondary, peripheral vascular disease of the carotid artery and the aorto-tibial tract will be followed by ultrasonographic techniques. Changes in endpoints will be related to changes in lipid and lipoprotein levels.

Introduction

The relationship between total cholesterol and LDL-cholesterol (LDL-C) levels and the incidence of coronary artery disease (CAD) and peripheral vascular disease (PVD) is well established[1-5]. Primary and secondary prevention trials, conducted in men with hypercholesterolaemia, have shown that lipid-lowering regimens result in reduction of angiographic lesions and are associated with a decreased incidence of atherosclerosis[6-31]. Most of these trials show slowing or arrest of progression of coronary and femoral atherosclerosis, although studies on the latter are scarce[32]. Currently, intensive lipid lowering in men with established CAD using HMG-CoA reductase inhibitors is the most effective treatment in terms of inducing plaque regression and consequently reducing the number of clinical events[21,22,27,29-31,33]. Quantitative methods for analysing the extent of atherosclerosis from arteriograms have been developed and extensively evaluated[34-37]. The intrinsic limitations of coronary angiography to predict physiological effects of coronary obstruction have been well documented[38]. Therefore, assessment of the functional significance of coronary stenosis seems important. The videodensitometric assessment of coronary perfusion has been shown to be an important functional indicator of the haemodynamic consequences of vascular stenosis[39-41].

Peripheral vascular lesions can be detected non-invasively using ultrasound techniques. The measurement of the intima-media thickness of the carotid artery has been shown to be a reproducible method for the analysis of early vascular lesions[42,43]. However, the combined use of Doppler-derived analysis of blood

A.V.G. Bruschke et al. *(eds): Lipid-lowering therapy and progression of atherosclerosis, 193–202.*
© 1996 *Kluwer Academic Publishers.*

flow velocities in the common femoral artery and the ankle/arm systolic pressure ratio at rest and during reactive hyperaemia has been shown to be a sensitive measure for the assessment of haemodynamically significant stenosis of the lower limb[44-46].

Continuous LDL apheresis, using dextran sulphate cellulose columns, selectively removes apolipoprotein-B-containing lipoproteins from plasma[47,48]. The application of this method of hypolipidaemic treatment may offer opportunities in the prevention of progression, or even inducing regression of coronary atherosclerosis in selected patients with a primary hyperlipidaemia and established CAD[49-51].

The LDL-Apheresis Atherosclerosis Regression Study (LAARS) was designed as an open randomized single-centre study to determine whether aggressive lipid lowering with biweekly LDL-apheresis plus simvastatin, a potent HMG-CoA reductase inhibitor[52,53], exerts a better anti-atherosclerotic effect than conventional lipid lowering with simvastatin alone or in combination with a resin, in primary hypercholesterolaemic men with extensive coronary artery disease[54]. Qualitative and quantitative computer-assisted analyses of coronary angiograms and videodensitometric measurement of coronary perfusion are being employed at the start of the study and after 2 years of treatment. Secondary, ultra-sonographic determination of PVD in the carotid artery and aorto-tibial tract are to be performed at 1-year treatment intervals.

From January 1990 to June 1992, 42 patients, from the Lipid and Cardiology clinics of the University Hospital of Nijmegen, were entered. In this report, we describe the design of the study, the methods of follow-up, and the baseline characteristics of the patients.

Design of the study

Men, aged between 30 and 67 years, who underwent diagnostic coronary angiography for angina pectoris were screened for eligibility. Included were patients with a mean of two successive serum total cholesterol determinations above 8.0 mmol/L or LDL-cholesterol above 5.8 mmol/L, and a mean of two successive fasting serum triglyceride measurements below 5.0 mmol/L on a standard lipid-lowering diet without other lipid-lowering treatments, and extensive coronary atherosclerosis as shown on their coronary angiogram. Specific exclusion criteria are listed in Table 17.1.

To perform the prerandomization evaluations and establish eligibility, three screening visits, spaced by a month were scheduled. The aims of the study and the protocol were explained at visit 1. Instructions about a cholesterol-lowering diet equivalent to the American Heart Association phase I diet were given by a dietician, and all other lipid-lowering treatments were stopped. At visits 2 and 3, blood was drawn for analyses of lipids, (apo)lipoproteins and laboratory safety measures. Exercise tests and assessments of peripheral vascular disease were performed in the meantime, as well as coronary angiography (Figure 17.1). After

Table 17.1.   LAARS exclusion criteria

1. Left ventricular ejection fraction <0.35 (normal=0.55–0.85)
2. Myocardial infarction, PTCA or CABG within previous 3 months
3. Cardiac arrhythmias
4. Impaired hepatic function, or liver function tests with repeated values >30% above the normal range, hepatitis or biliary obstruction
5. Impaired renal function with plasma creatinine ≥150 μmol/L
6. Homozygous familial hypercholesterolaemia
7. Secondary hyperlipidaemias due to any cause
8. Diabetes mellitus or fasting blood glucose ≥8.0 mmol/L
9. Hypertension with diastolic blood pressure ≥100 mmHg
10. Heavy smokers (>10 cigarettes/day)
11. Concurrent use of immunosuppressive drugs or fibrates
12. Severe obesity with body mass index ≥30 kg/m²
13. A history of alcohol or drug abuse

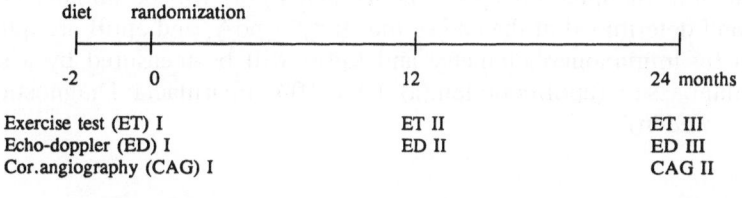

Randomization: LDL-apheresis *plus* medication or medication alone.

Figure 17.1.   Diagram of study design.

visit 3, the final decision with regard to eligibility was taken and written informed consent according to the Declaration of Helsinki was obtained. The patient was allocated at random to either biweekly LDL-apheresis plus simvastatin (40 mg/day) or simvastatin (40 mg/day) alone. Randomization was stratified for total cholesterol and lipoprotein(a) (Lp(a)) levels, age and coronary artery bypass graft status.

LDL-apheresis is performed with an automated system with two small-sized dextran sulphate cellulose columns (MA-01 unit, Kanegafuchi Chemical Industry Co., Japan). A plasma volume of 5000 ml was treated in each patient. The combination of LDL-apheresis and the HMG-CoA reductase inhibitor, simvastatin, can be expected to slow down the post-apheresis rebound in serum cholesterol due to increased cholesterol synthesis, which permits prolongation of the intervals between the apheresis procedures[55,56]. A resin in the highest tolerable doses will be added to the treatment if (pre-apheresis) serum total cholesterol levels in two consecutive months remains above 8.0 mmol/L.

Methods of follow-up

Lipids, lipoproteins and laboratory safety measures

Safety and tolerability of the treatment will be compared by means of medical and laboratory tests. In both groups, lipids, lipoproteins, blood chemistry, haematology, and routine urine analyses will be performed monthly. Apolipoprotein (apo)A1, apoB and Lp(a) will be measured bimonthly. In the apheresis group, lipids and lipoproteins and some extra laboratory safety parameters will be measured biweekly, before and immediately after LDL-apheresis. At each visit the patients are subjected to a brief physical examination and dietary instruction is repeated frequently.

Serum total cholesterol and fasting triglycerides will be determined by enzymatic methods (CHOD-PAP, no. 237574, Boehringer Mannheim GmbH, FTG and Sera-PAK, no. 6639, Miles, Italy, respectively). HDL-C is determined using the polyethylene glycol 6000 precipitation method[57]. LDL-C is calculated by subtraction. Samples for apoA$_1$, apoB, and Lp(a) will be initially stored at $-80°C$, and determined at the end of the study. ApoA$_1$ and apoB are quantified in serum by immunonephelometry and Lp(a) will be measured by a specific radioimmunoassay (apolipoprotein(a) RIA 100, Pharmacia Diagnostics AB, Uppsala, Sweden)[58].

Exercise tests

Replicate bicycle exercise tests (ET) will be performed at baseline, and after 12 months and 24 months. The ET is performed starting with a load of 50 W, and increasing the load every minute by 10 W during continuous ECG monitoring to maximum exercise. Blood pressure and 12-lead ECG registration will be monitored at rest, at maximum exercise, and every minute during the test. Automated calculation of ST-segment depression and slope is used, and data will be corrected for maximal systolic blood pressure – heart rate product.

Coronary angiography

The coronary angiograms will be made at baseline and after 2 years of treatment with the same non-ionic iso-osmolar contrast agent, using the same cine-angiogram techniques (Siemens Bicor and Digitron-3 quantitative measurement software package). No preangiographic vasodilatory agents will be given other than the ones needed to ameliorate catheter-induced vasospasm. The same sequence of projections will be used preferably at the same time of day. A centimetre grid is filmed to adjust for pincushion distortion and the same kind and diameter of catheters will be used and measured with a micrometer after the procedure to maximize quality control. Twelve to 15 coronary segments will be filmed in 2 or 3 projections. Computer-assisted quantitative analysis (CMS) of the paired angiograms will be performed blinded and at the angiography reference laboratory of the University Hospital of Leiden[59,60]. Minimal obstruction diameter will be assessed as a measure for localized atherosclerosis, whereas mean segment diameter will be used as a measure for diffuse changes. Additionally, blinded qualitative analysis (global score) of pairs of angiograms will be performed by a panel of three independent cardiologists. Differences in determination of percent stenosis will be settled by revised general agreement of the whole panel.

Videodensitometric assessment of coronary perfusion

Coronary arteriography will be followed by coronary flow estimation after maximal vasodilation with intracoronary administration of papaverine using digital subtraction techniques (Siemens Digitron-3). Contrast is injected using a power injector. Image acquisition will be performed while holding the breath at maximal inspiration and using the principle of apparent cardiac arrest by achieving synchronization of the X-ray pulses with the paced heart beats as has been described previously[40,41]. At least 5 regions of interest (ROI) will be selected in which measurement of coronary flow should be performed. These ROIs are located adjacent to the three main coronary arteries and an area selected distal to severe stenosis and after bypass grafts. Gamma-fitted time–density curves will be obtained by sampling the average pixel density within a ROI in the consecutive images and corrected by subtraction of the sampled average density in the corresponding background ROI. Data will be normalized for blood pressure values.

Measurement of the intima–media thickness (IMT) of the carotid artery

High resolution B-mode ultrasound examinations of the left and right carotid arteries are performed at baseline, and after 12 and 24 months of treatment, and are stored on videotape. An ACUSON 128XP duplex apparatus equipped with a 7.0-MHz L7384 linear array/5.0-MHz pulsed Doppler transducer combination is used. Measurement of the IMT is based on the distance between ultrasonically defined interfaces of the lumen/intima and media/adventitia. From a fixed latero-lateral angle, the near and far wall of the common carotid artery, bulbus, and internal carotid artery will be scanned. The dilation of the common carotid artery and the flow divider in the carotid artery are used as anatomical landmarks. The blinded off-line quantification of the IMT of the arterial segments is assessed by a semi-automated contour detection program and is performed at the vascular laboratory of Interuniversity Cardiology Institute of the Netherlands (Utrecht).

Doppler spectrum analysis of the femoral artery and ankle/arm blood pressure ratio

These will be performed after a 1-year interval in the vascular laboratory of the University of Nijmegen. Doppler signals are obtained with an 8-MHz bidirectional continuous-wave Doppler apparatus (Medasonics Inc., Mountain View,

Table 17.2.   Baseline characteristics.

	LDL-apheresis	Medication-only
n	21	21
Age (y)	50.2±9.6	53.9±8.7
Weight (kg)	81.5±9.7	80.8±8.6
BMI (kg/m^2)	26.6±2.0	26.2±2.0
Blood pressure		
Systolic (mmHg)	129.3±17.3	126.3±18.1
Diastolic (mmHg)	78.2±8.9	76.5±9.0
Smoking	3	4
Infarction	16	18
CABG	10	10
PTCA	2	5
Hypertension	2	5
Stroke	1	3
Claudication	3	5

Values indicate numbers or means±SD.

CA). Reactive hyperaemia is induced by thigh cuff compression for 5 minutes at a pressure of at least 50 mmHg above the systolic arterial thigh pressure and Doppler spectra will be obtained approximately 15 s after relief of the thigh compression. Doppler signals are processed by a real-time spectrum analyser (Radionics SA8000; Scarborough, Ontario, Canada) and subsequently fed into a Digital MNC 11/23 computer on the basis of electrocardiographic triggering for off-line analysis. Maximum-frequency waveforms are calculated from the spectra by local convolution algorithm. To describe the shape of the waveforms, several parameters will be calculated[61]. Based on a combination of six of these Doppler parameters, the presence of haemodynamically significant aorto-iliac pathology can be assessed accurately[46]. The same Doppler probe is used to determine the ankle/arm pressure index. Haemodynamically significant vascular disease is defined as an ankle/arm pressure index at rest <0.90 and/or a decrease of the pressure index during reactive hyperemia ≥0.20.

Baseline characteristics

In both treatment groups, 21 men were enrolled and some baseline characteristics are shown in Table 17.2. All patients had severe coronary atherosclerosis: a previous history of myocardial infarction was present in 16 vs 18 men in the apheresis and the medication group, respectively, and CABG had been performed in 10 men in both groups. In the apheresis group 17 of 21, and in the medication group 19 of 21 men, had 3-vessel CAD, whereas the other patients had 2-vessel disease. Haemodynamically significant lesions in the aorto-tibial tract were found in 4 and 5 men, and carotid artery segments with a mean IMT >1.0 mm were found in 29% and 22.8% in the apheresis and medication groups, respectively. Baseline cholesterol levels were very high, and predominant elevation of apoB-containing lipoproteins was found (Table 17.3).

Table 17.3. Baseline lipids and lipoproteins.

	LDL-apheresis	Medication-only
	(mmol/L)	(mmol/L)
Total cholesterol		
Mean±SD	9.72±1.84	9.85±2.21
Range	7.9–14.3	7.8–16.6
Triglycerides		
Mean±SD	2.50±1.23	2.65±1.44
Range	0.83–5.93	0.66–5.29
HDL-cholesterol		
Mean±SD	0.95±0.19	0.93±0.21
Range	0.60–1.45	0.64–1.33
LDL-cholesterol		
Mean±SD	7.72±1.96	7.85±2.36
Range	5.73–12.62	5.44–14.55
	(g/L)	(g/L)
Apolipoprotein A_1		
Mean±SD	1.43±0.30	1.46±0.38
Range	0.97–2.18	0.84–2.33
Apolipoprotein B		
Mean±SD	2.59±0.48	2.60±0.63
Range	1.70–3.50	1.40–4.20
	(mg/dl)	(mg/dl)
Lipoprotein(a)		
Mean±SD	57.0±63.4	38.4±39.4
Median	30.0	20.4
Range	2.9–254.1	1.7–138.6

Conclusion

LAARS will evaluate whether aggressive lipid lowering with LDL-apheresis in men with primary hypercholesterolaemia and extensive coronary artery disease will exert better retardation of the progression of atherosclerosis or even regression of coronary and peripheral atherosclerosis in comparison to conventional treatment. This study may help to answer the question of whether extreme lipid lowering is indicated in this particular group of patients.

References

1. Pooling Project Research Group. Relationship of blood pressure, serum cholesterol, smoking habit, relative weight and ECG abnormalities to incidence of major coronary events: final report of the pooling project. J Chronic Dis. 1978;31:201–306.
2. Stamler J, Wentworth D, Neaton JD. Is relationship between serum cholesterol and risk of premature death from coronary heart disease continuous and graded? Findings in 356,222 primary screenees of the Multiple Risk Factor Intervention Trial (MRFIT). JAMA. 1986;256:2823–8.
3. Pomrehn P, Duncan B, Weissfeld L, et al. The association of dyslipoproteinemia with

symptoms and signs of peripheral arterial disease. The Lipid Research Clinics Program Prevalence Study. Circulation. 1986;73(1 Pt 2):II00–7.

4. Ruhn G, Erikson U, Olsson AG. Prevalence of femoral atherosclerosis in asymptomatic men with hyperlipoproteinaemia. J Intern Med. 1989;225:317–23.

5. Bergstrand L, Olsson AG, Erikson U, et al. The relation of coronary and peripheral arterial disease to the severity of femoral atherosclerosis in hypercholesterolaemia. J Intern Med. 1994;236:367–75.

6. Committee of Principal Investigators, WHO Clofibrate Trial. A co-operative trial in the primary prevention of ischaemic heart disease using clofibrate. Report from the Committee of Principal Investigators. Br Heart J. 1978;40:1069–118.

7. Kuo PT, Hayase K, Kostis JB, Moreyra AE. Use of combined diet and colestipol in long-term (7–7½ years) treatment of patients with type II hyperlipoproteinemia. Circulation. 1979; 59:199–211.

8. Nash DT, Gensini G, Esente P. Effect of lipid-lowering therapy on the progression of coronary atherosclerosis assessed by scheduled repetitive coronary arteriography. Int J Cardiol. 1982; 2:43–55.

9. Duffield RG, Lewis B, Miller NE, Jamieson CW, Brunt JN, Colchester AC. Treatment of hyperlipidaemia retards progression of symptomatic femoral atherosclerosis. A randomized controlled trial. Lancet. 1983;2:639–42.

10. Nikkila EA, Viikinkoski P, Valle M, Frick MH. Prevention of progression of coronary atherosclerosis by treatment of hyperlipidaemia: a seven year prospective angiographic study. Br Med J (Clin Res Ed). 1984;289:220–3.

11a. Lipid Research Clinics Program. The Lipid Research Clinics Coronary Primary Prevention Trials results. I. Reduction in incidence of coronary heart disease. JAMA. 1984;251:351–64.

11b. Lipid Research Clinics Program. The Lipid Research Clinics Coronary Primary Prevention Trial results. II. The relationship of reduction in incidence of coronary heart disease to cholesterol lowering. JAMA. 1984;251:365–74.

12. Levy RI, Brensike JF, Epstein SE, et al. The influence of changes in lipid values induced by cholestyramine and diet on progression of coronary artery disease: results of NHLBI Type II Coronary Intervention Study. Circulation. 1984;69:325–37.

13. Arntzenius AC, Kromhout D, Barth JD, et al. Diet, lipoproteins, and the progression of coronary atherosclerosis. The Leiden Intervention Trial. N Engl J Med. 1985;312:80–11.

14. Shea S, Sciacca RR, Esser P, Han J, Nichols AB. Progression of coronary atherosclerotic disease assessed by cinevideodensitometry: relation to clinical risk factors. J Am Coll Cardiol. 1986;8:1325–31.

15. Frick MH, Elo O, Haapa K, et al. Helsinki Heart Study: primary-prevention trial with gemfibrozil in middle-aged men with dyslipidemia. Safety of treatment, changes in risk factors, and incidence of coronary heart disease. N Engl J Med. 1987;317:1237–45.

16. Blankenhorn DH, Nessim SA, Johnson RL, Sanmarco ME, Azen SP, Cashin-Hemphill L. Beneficial effects of combined colestipol–niacin therapy on coronary atherosclerosis and coronary venous bypass grafts [published erratum appears in JAMA. 1988;259:2698]. JAMA. 1987;257:3233–40.

17. Rossouw JE, Lewis B, Rifkind BM. The value of lowering cholesterol after myocardial infarction [Review]. N Engl J Med. 1990;323:1112–19.

18. Buchwald H, Varco RL, Matts JP, et al. Effect of partial ileal bypass surgery on mortality and morbidity from coronary heart disease in patients with hypercholesterolaemia. Report of the Program on the Surgical Control of the Hyperlipidemias (POSCH). N Engl J Med. 1990; 323:946–55.

19. Olsson AG, Ruhn G, Erikson U. The effect of serum lipid regulation on the development of femoral atherosclerosis in hyperlipidaemia: a non-randomized controlled study. J Intern Med. 1990;227:381–90.

20. Ornish D, Brown SE, Scherwitz LW, et al. Can lifestyle changes reverse coronary heart disease? The Lifestyle Heart Trial. Lancet. 1990;336:129–33.

21. Brown G, Albers JJ, Fisher LD, et al. Regression of coronary artery disease as a result of

intensive lipid-lowering therapy in men with high levels of apolipoprotein B. N Engl J Med. 1990;323:1289–98.

22. Kane JP, Malloy MJ, Ports TA, Phillips NR, Diehl JC, Havel RJ. Regression of coronary atherosclerosis during treatment of familial hypercholesterolemia with combined drug regimens. JAMA. 1990;264:3007–12.

23. Cashin-Hemphill L, Mack WJ, Pogoda JM, Sanmarco ME, Azen SP, Blankenhorn DH. Beneficial effects of colestipol–niacin on coronary atherosclerosis. A 4-year follow-up. JAMA. 1990;264:3013–17.

24. Blankenhorn DH, Azen SP, Crawford DW, et al. Effects of colestipol–niacin therapy on human femoral atherosclerosis. Circulation. 1991;83(2):438–47.

25. Watts GF, Lewis B, Brunt JN, et al. Effects on coronary artery disease of lipid-lowering diet, or diet plus cholestyramine, in the St Thomas' Atherosclerosis Regression Study (STARS). Lancet. 1992;339:563–9.

26. Schuler G, Hambrecht R, Schlierf G, et al. Regular physical exercise and low-fat diet. Effects on progression of coronary artery disease. Circulation. 1992;86:1–11.

27. Blankenhorn DH, Azen SP, Kramsch DM, et al. Coronary angiographic changes with lovastatin therapy. The Monitored Atherosclerosis Regression Study (MARS). The MARS Research Group. Ann Intern Med. 1993;119:969–76.

28. Haskell WL, Alderman EL, Fair JM, et al. Effects of intensive multiple risk factor reduction on coronary atherosclerosis and clinical cardiac events in men and women with coronary artery disease. The Stanford Coronary Risk Intervention Project (SCRIP). Circulation. 1994;89:975–90.

29. Waters D, Higginson L, Gladstone P, et al. Effects of monotherapy with an HMG-CoA reductase inhibitor on the progression of coronary atherosclerosis as assessed by serial quantitative arteriography. The Canadian Coronary Atherosclerosis Intervention Trial. Circulation. 1994;89:959–68.

30. MAAS Investigators. Effect of simvastatin on coronary atheroma: the Multicentre Anti-Atheroma Study (MAAS) (published erratum appears in Lancet. 1994;344:762). Lancet. 1994;344:633–8.

31. Scandinavian Simvastatin Survival Study Group. Randomised trial of cholesterol lowering in 4444 patients with coronary heart disease: the Scandinavian Simvastatin Survival Study (4S). Lancet. 1994;344:1383–9.

32. Vos J, de Feyter PJ, Simoons ML, Tijssen JG, Deckers JW. Retardation and arrest of progression or regression of coronary artery disease: a review [Review]. Prog Cardiovasc Dis. 1993;35:435–54.

33. Brown BG, Zhao XQ, Sacco DE, Albers JJ. Lipid lowering and plaque regression. New insights into prevention of plaque disruption and clinical events in coronary disease [Review]. Circulation. 1993;87:1781–91.

34. Crawford DW, Brooks SH, Selzer RH, Barndt R Jr, Beckenbach ES, Blankenhorn DH. Computer densitometry for angiographic assessment of arterial cholesterol content and gross pathology in human atherosclerosis. J Lab Clin Med. 1977;89:378–92.

35. Brown BG, Bolson EL, Dodge HT. Quantitative computer techniques for analyzing coronary arteriograms [Review]. Prog Cardiovasc Dis. 1986;28:403–18.

36. Kooijman CJ, Reiber JH, Gerbrands JJ, et al. Computer-aided quantitation of the severity of coronary obstructions from single view cineangiograms. Proc SPIE. 1982;375:59–64.

37. Reiber JH, Serruys PW, Kooijman CJ, et al. Assessment of short-, medium-, and long-term variations in arterial dimensions from computer-assisted quantitation of coronary cineangiograms. Circulation. 1985;71:280–8.

38. Hong MK, Mintz GS, Popma JJ, et al. Limitations of angiography for analyzing coronary atherosclerosis progression or regression. Ann Intern Med. 1994;121:348–54.

39. Pijls NH, Uijen GJ, Hoevelaken A, et al. Mean transit time for the assessment of myocardial perfusion by videodensitometry. Circulation. 1990;81:1331–40.

40. Pijls NH, Aengevaeren WR, Uijen GJ, et al. Concept of maximal flow ratio for immediate evaluation of percutaneous transluminal coronary angioplasty result by videodensitometry. Circulation. 1991;83:854–65.

41. Pijls NH, Uijen GJ, Pijnenburg T, et al. Reproducibility of mean transit time for maximal myocardial flow assessment by videodensitometry. Int J Card Imaging. 1990/91;6:101–8.
42. Salonen R, Salonen JT. Determinants of carotid intima-media thickness: a population-based ultrasonography study in eastern Finnish men. J Intern Med. 1991;229:225–31.
43. Bots ML. Wall thickness of the carotid artery as an indicator of generalized atherosclerosis: the Rotterdam study [Dissertation]. Rotterdam, Erasmus University, 1993.
44. Fronek A, Coel M, Bernstein EF. The importance of combined multisegmental pressure and Doppler flow velocity studies in the diagnosis of peripheral arterial occlusive disease. Surgery. 1978;84:840–7.
45. Lepantalo M, Lindfors O, Pekkola P. The ankle/arm systolic blood pressure ratio as a screening test for arterial insufficiency in the lower limb. Ann Chir Gynaecol. 1983;72:57–61.
46. van Asten WN, Beijneveld WJ, Pieters BR, van Lier HJ, Wijn PF, Skotnicki SH. Assessment of aortoiliac obstructive disease by Doppler spectrum analysis of blood flow velocities in the common femoral artery at rest and during reactive hyperemia. Surgery. 1991;109:633–9.
47. Yokoyama S, Hayashi R, Satani M, Yamamoto A. Selective removal of low density lipoprotein by plasmapheresis in familial hypercholesterolemia. Arteriosclerosis. 1985;5:613–22.
48. Mabuchi H, Michishita I, Takeda M, et al. A new low density lipoprotein apheresis system using two dextran sulfate cellulose columns in an automated column regenerating unit (LDL continuous apheresis). Atherosclerosis. 1987;68:19–25.
49. Koga N, Iwata Y. Pathological and angiographic regression of coronary atherosclerosis by LDL-apheresis in a patient with familial hypercholesterolemia. Atherosclerosis. 1991;90:9–21.
50. Yamamoto A. Regression of atherosclerosis in humans by lowering serum cholesterol. [Review]. Atherosclerosis. 1991;89:1–10.
51. Gordon BR, Kelsey SF, Bilheimer DW, et al. Treatment of refractory familial hyper-cholesterolemia by low-density lipoprotein apheresis using an automated dextran sulfate cellulose adsorption system. The Liposorber Study Group. Am J Cardiol. 1992;70:1010–6.
52. Stalenhoef AF, Mol MJ, Stuyt PM. Efficacy and tolerability of simvastatin (MK-733) [Review]. Am J Med. 1989;87(4A):39S–43S.
53. Walker JF. Simvastatin: the clinical profile. Am J Med. 1989;87(4A):44S–46S.
54. Superko HR, Krauss RM. Coronary artery disease regression. Convincing evidence for the benefit of aggressive lipoprotein management [Review]. Circulation. 1994;90:1056–69.
55. Mabuchi H, Fujita H, Michishita I, et al. Effects of CS-514 (eptastatin), an inhibitor of 3-hydroxy-3-methylglutaryl coenzyme A (HMG-CoA) reductase, on serum lipid and apolipo-protein levels in heterozygous familial hypercholesterolemic patients treated by low density lipoprotein (LDL)-apheresis. Atherosclerosis. 1988;72:183–8.
56. Pfohl M, Naoumova RP, Klass C, et al. Acute and chronic effects on cholesterol biosynthesis of LDL-apheresis with or without concomitant HMG-CoA reductase inhibitor therapy. J Lipid Res. 1994;35:1946–55.
57. Demacker PN, Hijmans AG, Vos-Janssen HE, van't Laar A, Jansen AP. A study of the use of polyethylene glycol in estimating cholesterol in high-density lipoprotein. Clin Chem. 1980; 26:1775–9.
58. Lopes-Virella MF, Virella G, Evans G, Malenkos SB, Colwell JA. Immunonephelometric assay of human apolipoprotein AI. Clin Chem. 1980;26:1205–8.
59. Reiber JH, Kooijman CJ, Slager CJ, et al. Computer assisted analysis of the severity of obstructions from coronary cineangiograms: a methodological review. Automedica. 1984; 5:219–38.
60. Reiber JH, Kooijman CJ, Slager CJ, et al. Coronary artery dimensions from cineangiograms: methodology and validation of a computer assisted analysis procedure. IEEE Trans Med Imaging. 1984;3:131–41.
61. Fronek A, Coel M, Berstein EF. Quantitative ultrasonographic studies of lower extremity flow velocities in health and disease. Circulation. 1976;53:957–60.

18. The NHLBI Post-Coronary Artery Bypass Graft Clinical Trial (Post-CABG): angiographic outcomes

L. CAMPEAU, G. KNATTERUD, C. WHITE, M. DOMANSKI,
N. L. GELLER, Y. ROSENBERG and the Post-CABG Clinical Trial
Investigators*

Summary

The Post-Coronary Artery Bypass Graft Clinical Trial (Post-CABG) is a multi-centre randomized double-blind controlled study in 1351 patients 1–11 years after coronary artery bypass graft surgery. The principal objective of this study is to assess the effects on late saphenous vein graft status of lipid lowering and low-intensity oral anticoagulation. The factorial design had two interventions with two treatment arms each: LDL-cholesterol lowering at two plasma levels, low (mean of 85 mg/dl, 2.2 mmol/L) and moderately low (mean of 140 mg/dl, 3.6 mmol/L) using the HMG-CoA reductase inhibitor lovastatin and, if needed, cholestyramine, and low-dose (1–4 mg daily) warfarin to achieve an international normalized ratio (INR) between 1.5 and 2 vs warfarin–placebo. These patients had 1–5 patent vein grafts at entry (mean ± SD = 2.4 ± 1). Follow-up angiography for quantitative analysis, after 4–5 years of treatment was completed in June 1995. The primary angiographic outcome is the per-patient proportion of grafts having substantial worsening (≥ 0.6 mm reduction in lumen diameter). Secondary analysis outcome measurements include, among others, the average mean and minimum diameter changes per patient and the proportion of grafts per patient with substantial regression. Secondary objectives deal with assessment of changes in internal mammary artery grafts and in unbypassed native coronary vessels.

Introduction

The purpose of this chapter is to describe the angiographic outcomes chosen for the NHLBI (USA) Post-Coronary Artery Bypass Graft (Post-CABG) Clinical Trial. The Post-CABG Clinical Trial is a multicentre randomized double-blind controlled clinical trial to study the effects of lipid lowering and oral anti-coagulation during a 4–5-year period on saphenous vein grafts (SVGs) placed 1–11 years prior to study entry. The hypothesis being tested is whether these drug interventions, alone or in combination, diminish the occurrence of obstructive changes and total occlusion caused by atherosclerosis and thrombosis.

Secondary objectives concern the effects on internal mammary artery (IMA)

*See Appendix for list of Investigators

A.V.G. Bruschke et al. *(eds): Lipid-lowering therapy and progression of atherosclerosis, 203–213.*
© 1996 *Kluwer Academic Publishers.*

grafts status and non-bypassed native vessels. The changes in grafts and in native vessels will be assessed by quantitative angiography using the cardiovascular angiography analysis system developed by Reiber et al.[1]. The effect on combined clinical endpoints, including coronary death, non-fatal myocardial infarction, revascularization procedures and stroke will also be assessed.

Post-CABG is one of the first clinical trials that aims to study the effects of drug interventions on SVGs years after surgery, based on quantitative coronary angiography (QCA) assessment. The CLAS lipid lowering clinical trial[2] was carried out in post-bypass patients. Both grafts and native vessels were included in the original primary angiographic outcome, based on visual angiography interpretation of 'global change score'. Later, changes in grafts were analysed separately by QCA[3]. The REGRESS study evaluates the effect of lipid lowering on SVGs, in addition to the native vessels (Van Boven, 1993, unpublished observations).

Description and rationale of drug interventions

The rationale for lipid-lowering intervention in SVGs is based on correlations between dyslipidaemias and late SVG changes found at pathological examination of grafts from reoperated patients and also obtained at postmortem[4-6]. Similar correlations were documented between plasma lipid and plasma lipoprotein changes and late graft changes documented at control angiography[7,8]. These late graft modifications were shown to be associated with atherosclerosis and thrombosis. Clots were found in 75–80% of grafts, frequently without atherosclerosis in contrast to the native coronary vessels where clots are almost always a complication of the atherosclerotic process[9].

Because of this high prevalence of graft thrombosis, with and without atherosclerosis, a 2×2 factorial design was selected to evaluate lipid lowering and anticoagulation therapy.

The NHLBI National Cholesterol Education Program (NCEP) expert panel on detection, evaluation and treatment of high blood cholesterol in adults recommended in the autumn of 1987 that patients with documented coronary artery disease receive dietary counselling and drug therapy if LDL-cholesterol (LDL-C) plasma levels remain above 160 mg/dl[10].

Because of this recommendation, the original protocol which included a control group on usual care was changed to evaluate two groups of lipid lowering therapy with lovastatin: one group with plasma LDL-C lowering to achieve low levels (mean 85 mg/dl, 2.2 mmol/L) and a second group with lowering to achieve moderate levels (mean 140 mg/dl, 3.6 mmol/L). Large international longitudinal prospective surveys of cholesterol plasma levels and CHD death suggested that countries where the mean level was very low had lower death rates than countries having higher levels[11,12]. Also, large cohort follow-up studies have shown that the risk of coronary events and cardiac death is related to total cholesterol and LDL-C plasma levels starting at very low levels with no clear threshold[13,14].

Furthermore, CLAS[2] had reported that 24% of patients randomly assigned to colestipol and niacin therapy, who had a mean LDL-C plasma level during the trial of 97 mg/dl (2.5 mmol/L), developed adverse changes in their grafts, suggesting that further lowering of LDL-C might be beneficial.

In the Post-CABG trial, participants randomly assigned to the low LDL level group receive, in addition to diet counselling, lovastatin 40–80 mg daily, and, if needed, cholestyramine 8 g daily. Participants randomly assigned to the moderate LDL-C level have diet counselling as well and only lovastatin 2.5–5 mg daily, and, in some, cholestyramine placebo to preserve masking of treatment assignment. In order to achieve such lipid lowering targets and respect the NCEP guidelines, only subjects having an LDL-C between 130 and 175 mg/dl (3.4 and 4.5 mmol/L) after diet were included.

The other treatment included in this clinical trial is low-intensity oral anticoagulation vs placebo. Low-dose warfarin has been reported to be no less effective and safer than standard anticoagulant therapy[15–17]. The effect of low-dose warfarin may be through mechanisms other than its increase in prothrombin time, for example its effect on Factor VIIc, and fibrinogen levels[18]. It was thought that the combination of aspirin and low-dose oral anticoagulation might be more beneficial and less hazardous than full anticoagulation. The candidates who had fulfilled the clinical and angiographic inclusion criteria were randomly assigned to daily warfarin 1–4 mg to achieve an INR between 1.5 and 2, or to warfarin placebo. In addition, all patients were encouraged to take aspirin, 80 mg per day, in keeping with the recommendations of NHLBI Consensus conference based on favourable reports about the beneficial role of aspirin on both primary and secondary prevention of coronary atherosclerosis, possibly related to its antithrombotic and antiatherogenic effects[19]. Both lipid-lowering and oral warfarin-placebo interventions were administered in a double-blind fashion.

Characteristics of the study population

A total of 1351 individuals were randomly assigned to the four treatment groups. There were 1249 men and 102 women, age 36–75 years old (61.1 ±7.3 years). In order to be eligible, male patients had to have at least two patent SVGs without stenosis >75%, or one SVG and one IMA graft that were patent at the time of screening angiography. Women were to have at least one patent SVG with or without a patent IMA graft. Enrolment began in March 1989 and ended in August 1991.

The lipid inclusion criteria were: LDL-C plasma level between 130 mg/dl (3.4 mmol/L) and 175 mg/dl (4.5 mmol/L), as well as a triglyceride level <300 mg/dl (3.5 mmol/L) after institution of study diet. Patients with severe effort angina, heart failure or an ejection fraction <25% were not eligible. Moderate to severe hypertension, diabetes mellitus, significant kidney or liver disease, and other life-threatening diseases were also exclusion criteria. Of the 1650 patients who had fulfilled the clinical lipid and angiographic eligibility criteria, 1351 were recruited for this 4–5-year trial. Follow-up angiography began in December 1993 and was completed in June 1995.

Angiographic outcome measures

The angiographic outcome measures will be based on evaluation of the baseline angiogram and the follow-up angiogram obtained 4–5 years after entry, to be read side by side as a pair. Analysis of all grafts will be based on three segments plus the proximal and distal anastomotic sites; some of the outcome measures used for analyses of grafts will also be applied to analyses of segments (including the anastomotic sites). If a graft is completely occluded on the follow-up angiogram, all segments of the graft will be classified as having a mean minimum diameter of 0 mm except for the proximal segments of continuation and Y grafts which may remain open up to the coronary anastomosis of the occluded segment.

Graft disease as documented by coronary cineangiography presents complex morphological changes. For example, narrowings may be discrete or diffuse, concentric or eccentric, and mild to severe. Severity of lumen narrowing and the extent of the obstructive disease along the graft length are both important. Furthermore, the sites of changes are unpredictable: a stenotic area may remain unchanged whereas a normal segment may develop a severe stenosis. No one angiographic endpoint covers all these characteristics. In spite of the complexity of graft disease, it was decided that it would be preferable to select a single primary outcome rather than two co-equal endpoints. Two co-equal endpoints have the disadvantages of requiring adjustments in the critical *p*-values to keep the alpha level fixed, and they may show discordant results.

The primary angiographic outcome in most progression–regression studies of coronary artery atherosclerosis was based on a continuous variable expressing the change in the mean lumen diameter[20], or the minimum lumen diameter[21–24]. These lumen diameter changes have been expressed in mm or in percent diameter stenosis. The mean minimum diameter is theoretically a summary of the extent of the disease along the entire length of the vessel. It does not assess well the severity of the obstructive process: for instance, the same mean diameter measurement may be related to three 30% focal narrowings in a graft or to a single 90% stenosis. On the other hand, the minimum lumen diameter is a precise measure of the severity of the vessel narrowing which is of paramount importance to the clinician. Both variables have the advantage of evaluating total change, both progression and regression simultaneously by adding ± changes (decreased lumen diameter equals progression and increased lumen size indicates regression).

The change in these continuous measurements (mean or minimum lumen diameter) are obtained from all qualified coronary segments and are averaged for each patient. A mean coronary change score per patient is calculated for each arm of the intervention. The difference within groups of this per-patient coronary change score, as reported in those progression–regression trials on coronary artery atherosclerosis, is very small, varying between 0.002 and 0.11 mm, or between 1 and 3% in diameter stenosis. This per-patient analysis of a continuous variable is precise and comprehensive, but is not well appreciated by the clinician since the within-group differences are small even though they may be statistically significant.

Angiographic outcomes derived from these continuously variable measurements reflect the change in the atherosclerotic disease without considering its biological and clinical significance. On the contrary, categorical analysis of an endpoint expressed as the proportion of either patients, or coronary segments or grafts having substantial worsening or improvement is more meaningful to the clinician once the definition of substantial change is agreed upon. The primary angiographic outcome chosen for this clinical trial is based on a categorical variable which we expect will reflect the changes in graft lumen of potential future clinical relevance (new or worsening of existing graft disease).

Selected primary angiographic endpoint

The primary angiographic outcome selected for this trial was the following: the proportion of major SVGs per patient with substantial reduction of the lumen diameter measured at the site with the greatest change in each graft between baseline and follow-up angiograms.

Only major saphenous vein grafts at baseline will be included in the primary outcome analyses. Grafts are defined as major and minor on the basis of their usual length, a major graft being sufficiently long to be divided in three segments whereas a minor graft is too short for this purpose. Some of the secondary outcomes will consider graft segments in an attempt to evaluate the extent of the changes along the graft length. Major SVGs are:

1.   All single coronary anastomosis grafts,
2.   Segment proximal to the first coronary anastomosis of continuation or sequential grafts, and
3.   The main trunk and the longest limb of Y grafts, considered as a single graft (when both limbs are of equal length, one limb is randomly selected).

Minor grafts are all other segments of grafts with multiple coronary anastomoses, and they will be included in repeated analyses of secondary outcome measures.

Substantial worsening is defined by a decrease of the lumen diameter by 0.6 mm or more. This cut-off of 0.6 mm represents three times the standard deviation of repeat measurements of the minimum diameter which is estimated at 0.2 mm. In CLAS, 0.4 mm was selected as true change (variability×2), one of the Post-CABG trial participating institutions has reported a variability in graft diameter measurements of 0.2 mm[25]. If the results of a reproducibility study which is now being carried out in grafts of Post-CABG patients from the participating clinical centres indicates that the variability is greater or less than 0.2 mm, the proposed criterion of 0.6 mm for substantial worsening will be redefined.

The site with the greatest change is not necessarily the site of the narrowest diameter at baseline or at follow-up. As illustrated in Figure 18.1, four possibilities were considered concerning measurement of the diameter changes:

1.   Site of minimum lumen diameter (MLD) at baseline as compared with the equivalent site at follow-up angiogram,

(a)

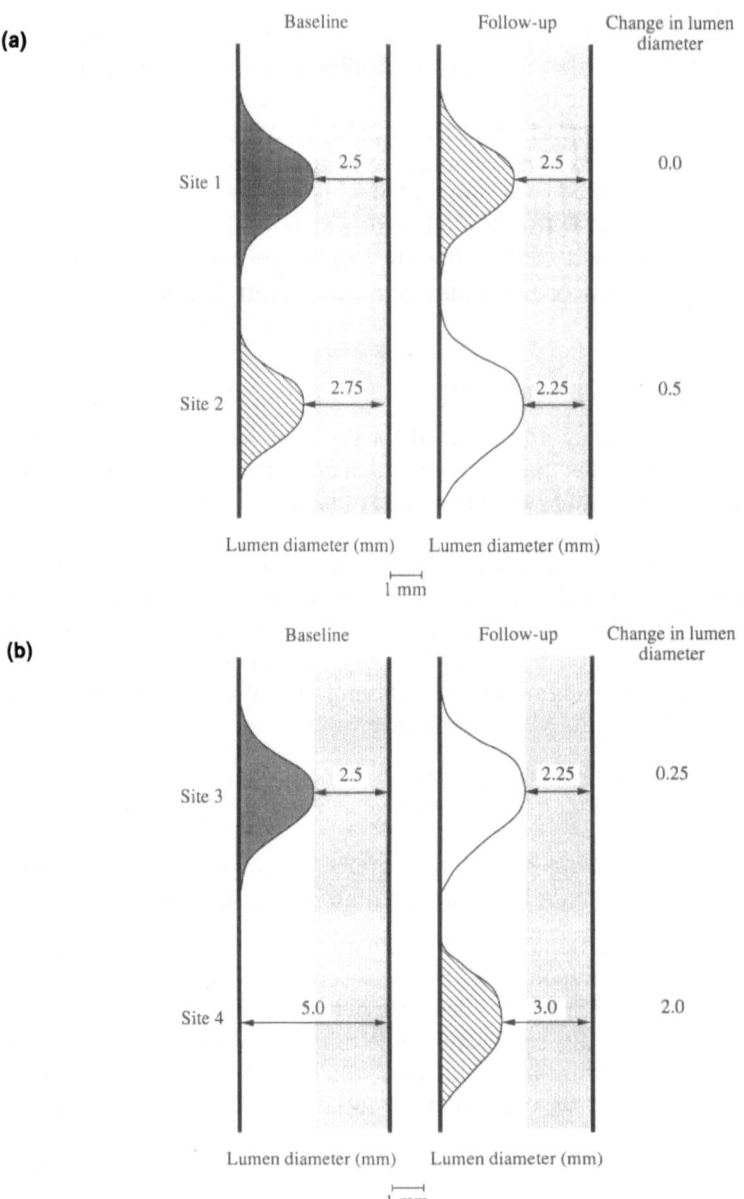

Figure 18.1. Schematic representation of the angiographic view of grafts at baseline and follow-up illustrating the various sites where the change in lumen diameter may be measured. (**A**) Site 1: No change between minimum lumen diameter (MLD) at baseline and equivalent site at follow-up (dark area represents the most severe stenosis at baseline). Site 2: The change between MLD at follow-up at the site of the most severe narrowing (opened area) and the lumen diameter at an equivalent site at baseline is only 0.5 mm, thus not a substantial change, being <0.6 mm. In fact, the MLD at follow-up may not be at the site of the MLD at baseline. (**B**) Site 3: The change between MLD at follow-up and MLD at baseline is only 0.25 mm and is not considered substantial (<0.6 mm).

continued

2. Site of MLD at follow-up as compared with the same anatomical site at baseline,
3. Site of the MLD at baseline, as compared with the MLD at follow-up.
4. Site of the greatest change irrespective of the MLD sites at baseline and follow-up.

The fourth option was chosen for the primary endpoint and the others were included in designated secondary outcomes. The site of greatest change was selected because it may recognize substantial change which can be missed with the first three methods of diameter change measurement. The site of greatest change may also be any one of the three other sites. Lesions showing the greatest change may frequently be new lesions. In this series at baseline, 34% of the grafts had focal narrowing $\geq 25\%$, at a mean of 4 years after grafting. We suspect that new lesions may be as frequent as progression of old lesions at follow-up.

This primary outcome is a categorical variable (proportion of grafts with significant worsening), but it is based on multiple continuous measurements and the patient remains the unit of comparison. It takes into consideration the within-patient variation in the number of grafts, and thus permits an equal contribution of all grafts. It has the capacity to indicate important morphological change in a way which is clinically meaningful.

However, this primary outcome considers only progression and it does not address regression. When this research protocol was established, the suggestion that regression of coronary atherosclerosis could be facilitated by lipid-lowering drugs in man came from CLAS[2]. Their analysis combined graft and native coronary vessels so that the evidence for regression in SVGs was not clear. It was then decided that regression of graft stenosis would be assessed by secondary angiographic endpoints.

Selected secondary angiographic outcomes

The analyses of the secondary outcome measures will be carried out separately for major and minor SVGs and repeated to include both major and minor SVGs.

Concerning progression

1. The per-patient proportion of grafts that show new *total* occlusion at follow-up.

Figure 18.1. Continued. In this example which may occur frequently, both MLD at baseline and at follow-up are at the same site. Site 4: The diameter change between a new focal narrowing at follow-up (hatched area) and the normal segment at baseline, in spite of a lumen diameter larger than the MLD at follow-up, is substantial (>0.6 mm). It reflects the greatest change (2 mm as compared with 0.25 mm at Site 3, 0.5 mm at site 2 and 0.0 mm at Site 1). The graft blood flow is influenced by the MLD (tunnel effect as presented by the shaded area along the graft length), and its reduction may have haemodynamic and clinical repercussions. New lesions associated with a lumen diameter larger than the MLD do not have such consequences, but instead they reflect the change in quantity of atherosclerotic disease

This outcome is the most severe angiographic outcome and has the most potential haemodynamic and clinical repercussions. It may study, in particular, the effect of the anticoagulation therapy.

2. The per patient proportion of grafts with substantial worsening of disease *or occlusion* at the site of minimum lumen diameter at baseline and follow-up.

    This outcome reflects roughly the change in blood flow capacity of the graft at follow-up as compared with baseline (Figure 18.1). It has a haemo-dynamic importance; but angiography is meant to assess morphological changes and only indirectly and imperfectly does it assess its haemodynamic consequences.

3. The proportion of patients with one or more grafts with substantial worsening *and/or total occlusion*.

4. The per-patient proportion of grafts with substantial worsening of disease in two or more segments at the site of greatest change.

    This outcome adds information about the extent of the disease along the graft length.

5. The per-patient proportion of graft segments with substantial worsening and/or occlusion

    This outcome is a summary of the extent of disease worsening.

6. *The per-patient proportion of grafts with substantial worsening at the site of minimum diameter at follow-up.*

7. The per-patient proportion of grafts with one or more new lesions. New lesions are expected to occur frequently after the fifth postoperative year[26]. *It is defined as a narrowing which has become apparent at visual inspection at follow-up, and with a difference ≥0.6 mm between diameters of this lesion and its equivalent site at baseline.*

Concerning regression

1. The per-patient proportion of grafts with substantial regression of disease, defined as increase in the lumen diameter of 0.6 mm or more at any site of the graft.

    Although regression has seldom been described in SVGs, it is expected to be as frequent if not more frequent than regression of stenoses in the native vessels because the lesions in grafts are recent and their content is lipid rich.

2. The per-patient proportion of graft segments with substantial regression.

    This outcome is a summary of the extent of disease regression.

Concerning progression and regression

1. The per-patient change in the mean minimum diameter of all grafts: (a) expressed in absolute measurement (mm) and (b) as percent diameter stenosis.

This outcome has the disadvantage of resulting in very small numerical differences that are less meaningful to the clinician.

2. Average minimum lumen diameters of two major grafts (selected at random).

   This outcome is a simple way to display results but does not utilize all available information for a given patient.

3. The per-patient change in the average mean lumen diameter of all grafts.

   This outcome expresses the change in the extent of the disease along the entire length of the graft. However, it is not a sensitive method of assessing the degree of obstructive changes.

Other analyses

Additional analyses will include subgroup analyses, for example by classifying patients according to the status of grafts at baseline and at follow-up: no focal narrowing at visual inspection (lumen reduction $\leq 0.6\,mm$), mild lesions ($< 50\%$), moderate lesions (50 to $< 75\%$) and severe lesions ($\geq 75\%$).

Some analyses will be based on a summary measure of the changes in all grafts for individual patients on the basis of whether the grafts primarily show progression, regression or no change.

Conclusion

The Post-CABG trial will provide a very rich data set on the detailed changes of saphenous vein grafts over a 4–5-year period. It is hoped that this trial will provide definitive answers concerning the quantitative angiographic changes resulting from very low vs moderate lipid-lowering and oral anticoagulation vs placebo. Follow-up angiography has been completed in June 1995. Results will be reported in early 1996.

References

1. Reiber JHC, Kooijman CJ, Slager CJ, et al. Coronary artery dimensions from cineangiograms: methodology and validation of a computer-assisted analysis procedure. IEEE Trans Med Imaging. 1984;3:131–40.
2. Blankenhorn DH, Nessim SA, Johnson RL, Sanmarco ME, Azen SP, Cashin-Hemphill L. Beneficial effects of combined colestipol–niacin therapy on coronary atherosclerosis and coronary venous bypass grafts. JAMA. 1987;257:3233–40.
3. Blankenhorn DH, Selzer RH, Mack WJ, et al. Evaluation of colestipol/niacin therapy with computer-derived coronary endpoint measures. Circulation. 1992;86:1701–9.
4. Neitzel GF, Barboriak JJ, Pintar K, Qureshi I. Atherosclerosis in aortocoronary bypass grafts. Morphologic study and risk factor analysis 6 to 12 years after surgery. Arteriosclerosis. 1986; 6:594–600.
5. Atkinson JB, Forman MB, Vaughn WK, Robinowitz M, McAllister HA, Virmani R. Morphologic changes in long-term saphenous vein bypass grafts. Chest.1985;88:341–8.
6. Lie JT, Lawrie GM, Morris GC. Aortocoronary bypass saphenous vein graft atherosclerosis.

Anatomic study of 99 vein grafts from normal and hyperlipoproteinemic patients up to 75 months postoperatively. Am J Cardiol. 1977;40:906–14.

7. Palac RT, Meadows WR, Hwang MH, Loeb HS, Pifarre R, Gunnar RM. Risk factors related to progressive narrowing in aortocoronary vein grafts studied 1 and 5 years after surgery. Circulation. 1982;66(Suppl):I40–4.

8. Campeau L, Enjalbert M, Lespérance J, et al. The relation of risk factors to the development of atherosclerosis in saphenous-vein bypass grafts and the progression of disease in the native circulation. N Engl J Med. 1984;311:1329–32.

9. Solymoss BC, Nadeau P, Millette D, Campeau L. Late thrombosis of saphenous vein coronary bypass grafts related to risk factors. Circulation. 1988;78(Suppl):I140–3.

10. The Expert Panel. Report of the National Cholesterol Education Program Expert Panel on Detection, Evaluation and Treatment of High Blood Cholesterol in Adults. Arch Intern Med. 1988;148:36–69.

11. Keys A. Coronary heart disease. Atherosclerosis. 1975;22:149–92.

12. Pyörälä K. Interpopulation correlations between serum cholesterol level and the occurrence of coronary heart disease. Eur Heart J. 1987;8(Suppl E):23–30.

13. Martin MJ, Hulley SB, Browner WS, Kuller LH, Wentworth D. Serum cholesterol, blood pressure, and mortality: Implications from a cohort of 361 662 men. Lancet. 1986;2:933–6.

14. Castelli WP, Garrison RJ, Wilson PWF, et al. Incidence of coronary heart disease and lipo-protein cholesterol levels: The Framingham Study. JAMA. 1986;256:2835–8.

15. Meade TW, Wilkes HC, Stirling Y, Brennan PJ, Kelleher C, Browne W. Randomized controlled trial of low dose warfarin in the primary prevention of ischaemic heart disease in men at high risk: design and pilot study. Eur Heart J. 1988;9:836–43.

16. Turpie AGG, Gunstensen J, Hirsch J, Nelson H, Gent M. Randomised comparison of two intensities of oral anticoagulant therapy after tissue heart valve replacement. Lancet. 1988;1:1242–5.

17. Poller L, McKernan A, Thomson JM, Elstein M, Hirsch PJ, Jones JB. Fixed minidose warfarin: A new approach to prophylaxis against venous thrombosis after major surgery. Br Med J. 1987;295:1309–12.

18. Meade TW, Brozovic M, Chakrabarti RR, et al. Haemostatic function and ischaemic heart disease: Principal results of the Northwick Park heart study. Lancet. 1986;2:533–7.

19. Hennekens CH, Peto R, Hutchison CB. An overview of the British and American aspirin studies. N Engl J Med. 1988;318:923–4.

20. Watts GF, Lewis B, Brunt JNH, et al. Effects on coronary artery disease of lipid-lowering diet, or diet plus cholestyramine, in the St Thomas' Atherosclerosis Regression Study (STARS). Lancet. 1993;339:563–9.

21. Brown G, Albers JJ, Fisher LD, et al. Regression of coronary artery disease as a result of intensive lipid-lowering therapy in men with high levels of apolipoprotein B. N Engl J Med. 1990;323:1289–98.

22. Ornish D, Brown SE, Scherwitz LW, et al. Can lifestyle changes reverse coronary heart disease? Lancet. 1990;336:129–33.

23. Blankenhorn DH, Azen SP, Kramsch DM, et al. Coronary angiographic changes with lovastatin therapy. The Monitored Atherosclerosis Regression Study (MARS). Ann Intern Med. 1993;119:969–76.

24. Waters D, Higginson L, Gladstone P, et al. Effects of monotherapy with an HMG-CoA reductase inhibitor on the progression of coronary atherosclerosis as assessed by serial quanti-tative arteriography. Circulation. 1994;89:959–68.

25. Lespérance J, Campeau L, Laurier J, et al. Reproducibility (true change) of coronary artery saphenous vein graft measurements using quantitative angiography [abstract]. Atherosclerosis. 1994;109:298.

26. Campeau L, Enjalbert M, Lespérance J, Vaislic C, Grondin CM, Bourassa MG. Atherosclerosis and late closure of aortocoronary saphenous vein grafts: sequential angiographic studies at 2 weeks, 1 year, 5 to 7 years, and 10 to 12 years after surgery. Circulation. 1983;68(Suppl):III1–7. Kane JP, Malloy MJ, Ports TA, Phillips NR, Diehl JC, Havel RJ. Regression of coronary

atherosclerosis during treatment of familial hypercholesterolemia with combined drug regimens. JAMA. 1990;264:3007–12.

Appendix

NGHLBI Post-CABG Clinical Trial Participating Units and Principal Officers

Study chairman: Lucien Campeau, MD, Montreal Heart Institute (University of Montreal), Montreal, Canada; Bernadine Healy, MD, Cleveland Clinic Foundation, November 1987–June 1991.

NHLBI project officers: Michael Domanski, MD, Yves Rosenberg, MD, and Nancy Geller, PhD (study initiated in 1986 by Salim Yusuf, MD and Jeffrey Probstfield, MD).

Coordinating centre: Maryland Medical Research Institute, Baltimore, MD: Genell Knatterud, PhD, Michael Terrin, MD, Fran LoPresti, MS, Sharon Fick.

Angiography reading centre: University of Minnesota, Minneapolis, MN: Carl White, MD.

Apolipoprotein core laboratory: Oklahoma Medical Research Foundation, OK: Peter Alaupovic, MD.

Haematology core laboratory: Loyola University Medical Center, IL: Jeanine Walenga, PhD.

Data and safety monitoring board: Chairman: Richard Carleton, MD, Pawtucket, RI; Kent Baily, PhD; Baruch Brody, MD: John Cairns, MD; Curt Furberg, MD, PhD; Valentin Fuster, MD; Claude Grondin, MD; C. David Jenkins, PhD; John LaRosa, MD; Paul Meier, PhD.

Participating clinical centres and principal investigators:
Baylor College of Medicine (Methodist and VA Hospitals), Houston, TX: J. Alan Herd, MD; Kelly Maresh, RN; Patti Shackelford, RN.
Cedars–Sinai Medical Center, Los Angeles, CA: James S. Forrester, MD; Richard Gray, MD; Ann Hickey, MD; Marge Raymond, RN.
Cleveland Clinic Foundation, Cleveland, OH: Byron Hoogwerf, MD; William Stewart, MD; Laurie Harris, RN; Fran Yanak, RN.
Montreal Heart Institute (University of Montreal), Montreal, Canada: Lucien Campeau, MD; Claude Goulet, MD; Suzy Foucher, RN; Suzanne Bujold, RN.
University of Minnesota Hospitals, Minneapolis, MN: Donald Hunninghake, MD; Erving London, RN; Kay Gardner, RN; (Minneapolis Heart Institute), Irvin Goldenberg, MD; Connie Baumgard, RN.

Epilogue

H. J. J. WELLENS and A. V. G. BRUSCHKE

The studies reported in this book almost unanimously demonstrate that, in patients with symptomatic coronary atherosclerosis, lipid lowering retards progression of the disease process and may even lead to regression. As suggested by most angiographic trials, in particular by REGRESS[1], this is accompanied by a favourable effect on morbidity and mortality. A beneficial clinical effect was also convincingly demonstrated by the 4S study[2] which was designed to determine the clinical effects of lipid lowering in patients with coronary atherosclerosis and moderately elevated serum cholesterol levels (5.5–8.0 mml/L).

As indicated in Table 1, many questions are as yet unresolved. Although during recent years significant progress has been made in our understanding of the pathophysiology of atherosclerosis, we still have insufficient insight into the mechanisms that govern progression and regression. Our diagnostic tools are inadequate to assess what happens following lipid-lowering intervention in different layers of the arterial wall or what the effects are at cellular level. Quantitative angiography only informs us about the size of the lumen and configuration of the inner lining of the vessels. Intravascular ultrasound studies may provide additional information; however, at present this information is still relatively crude and it is practically impossible to depict the entire coronary artery system by ultrasound and subsequently to assess accurately changes over time. Likewise, functional parameters of coronary flow (e.g. coronary flow reserve) or endothelial function (e.g. acetylcholine tests) may provide valuable additional information but cannot resolve the major shortcomings in our diagnostic armamentarium. In future, hopefully, it may be possible to obtain more information about the composition of atherosclerotic lesions by techniques that are currently under investigation, such as catheter spectroscopy. However, the results of these investigations have yet to be awaited.

One of the major questions for clinical practice is, 'Who should be treated by lipid-lowering drugs?' There is now ample evidence that a broad range of patients with coronary artery disease profits from lipid-lowering. Interestingly, as shown in REGRESS, patients with 'normal' or slightly elevated serum cholesterol appear to benefit from lipid lowering just as much as patients with higher (by current standards 'abnormal') cholesterol levels. We hypothesize that this may be due to two factors. In the first place, it is possible that newer lipid-lowering drugs (in particular the HMG-CoA reductase inhibitors) have, in addition to cholesterol lowering, a direct effect on atherosclerotic lesions. In the

A.V.G. Bruschke et al. (eds): Lipid-lowering therapy and progression of atherosclerosis, 215–217.
© 1996 *Kluwer Academic Publishers.*

Table 1.   Some questions related to lipid lowering in secondary prevention.

1.	Mechanisms of progression and regression of atherosclerotic disease?
2.	Who should be treated?
3.	Are there biochemical markers to identify patients who will benefit most?
4.	What is the role of genetic factors?
5.	What is the influence of female gender and hormonal factors?
6.	Is there an optimal serum lipid level and, if so, is this the same for all patients?
7.	Are the factors that govern progression and regression the same in different arterial territories?
8.	Are there long-term side-effects of lipid-lowering drugs?

second place, we should realize that these results have been observed in secondary prevention studies, in other words in patients who by definition have a propensity towards development of the disease. In patients with normal serum cholesterol, this suggests an increased susceptibility of the vessel wall for serum lipids. This also indicates that the results of secondary prevention trials should not be extrapolated to primary prevention strategies.

Relatively little is known about the role of factors like age, race, gender and other genetic factors in the context of the efficacy of lipid lowering. In women, the situation is further complicated in that the influence of hormonal changes on the evolution of the atherosclerotic process is still poorly understood. In this perspective, it is extremely important that the role of lipid lowering in postmenopausal women be clarified and compared with hormone replacement as adjunctive or sole therapy.

To complicate matters further, it is not clear how the vessels in different arterial territories respond to lipid lowering. Studies using B-mode ultrasound have shown a beneficial effect of lipid lowering in the carotid and femoral arteries. However, in an ultrasound substudy of REGRESS, it appeared that per patient there was no good correlation between peripheral and coronary arteries in lipid-lowering effect[3]. These questions can only be resolved by long-term (costly!) studies in combination with good co-ordination between basic sciences and specialties dealing with the vascular supply of different territories. This stresses the necessity of further developing the new field of vascular medicine.

Another interesting question concerns the best approach to achieve lipid lowering. This relates again to the question of whether only the serum lipid levels are important or whether certain drugs have additional beneficial effects. If there are differences between various approaches, these are probably small and difficult to demonstrate in clinical trials. It is also possible that there is no single best approach but that there are individual variations as is probably the case in the presence of certain lipid metabolism abnormalities. In this context, potential side-effects of drugs should also be considered. Although the side-effects of short-term use of modern lipid-lowering drugs (in particular HMG-CoA reductase inhibitors) appears reassuring, little is known about long-term (e.g. >5 years) side-effects and post-marketing surveillance of these drugs should be stressed. Also, more information is needed about cost–benefit profiles.

Naturally, the importance of lipid lowering should not detract from the importance of reduction of other risk factors, such as cessation of smoking, control of hypertension, maintenance of normoglycaemia in the diabetic patient, physical activity, control of obesity, small-to-moderate alcohol intake, etc.

If at present it is not feasible or desirable to treat all patients with coronary atherosclerosis, the guidelines formulated by the National Cholesterol Educational Program[4] may be useful, although, in Europe at least, many physicians are still hesitant to follow these strict recommendations. On the other hand, one may argue that, perhaps for the patient with coronary artery disease, the rule applies: 'The lower the serum cholesterol the better'. Hopefully, in the future, biochemical and genetic markers will become available to help identify patients who will benefit most from lipid lowering interventions. At present, it seems reasonable in decision making not to rely solely on lipid levels but to take other prognostic indicators (symptoms, ECG, exercise testing, coronary angiography etc.) into account too. If by these parameters a patient belongs to a low-risk category, the disadvantages of lipid-lowering intervention may outweigh the potential benefit.

However, it must be emphasized that the questions which remain to be solved should not detract from what is so clearly demonstrated in this volume, namely, that we currently have at our disposal several possibilities to lower effectively serum lipids, to reduce progression of coronary atherosclerosis, and to reduce the occurrence of ischaemic events in a wide range of patients with coronary atherosclerosis.

References

1. Jukema JW, Bruschke AVG, Van Boven AJ, et al. Effects of lipid lowering by pravastatin on progression and regression of coronary artery disease in symptomatic men with normal to moderately elevated serum cholesterol levels. The Regression Growth Evaluation Statin Study (REGRESS). Circulation. 1995;91:2528–40.
2. Scandinavian Simvastatin Survival Study Group. Randomized trial of cholesterol lowering in 4444 patients with coronary heart disease. The Scandinavian Simvastatin Survival Study (4S). Lancet. 1994;344:1383–9.
3. De Groot E, Jukema JW, Van Boven AJ, et al. on behalf of the REGRESS Study Group. The effect of pravastatin on progression and regression of coronary atherosclerosis and vessel wall changes in carotid and femoral arteries. Am J Cardiol. 1995;76:40C–46C.
4. Grundey SM. National cholesterol education program: second report of the expert panel on detection, evaluation, and treatment of high blood cholesterol in adults. Circulation. 1994; 89:1329–445.

Index

A.V.G. Bruschke et al. *(eds): Lipid-lowering therapy and progression of atherosclerosis, 219–221.*
© 1996 *Kluwer Academic Publishers.*

Developments in Cardiovascular Medicine

1. Ch.T. Lancée (ed.): *Echocardiology.* 1979   ISBN 90-247-2209-8
2. J. Baan, A.C. Arntzenius and E.L. Yellin (eds.): *Cardiac Dynamics.* 1980
                                                     ISBN 90-247-2212-8
3. H.J.Th. Thalen and C.C. Meere (eds.): *Fundamentals of Cardiac Pacing.* 1979
                                                     ISBN 90-247-2245-4
4. H.E. Kulbertus and H.J.J. Wellens (eds.): *Sudden Death.* 1980   ISBN 90-247-2290-X
5. L.S. Dreifus and A.N. Brest (eds.): *Clinical Applications of Cardiovascular Drugs.*
   1980   ISBN 90-247-2295-0
6. M.P. Spencer and J.M. Reid: *Cerebrovascular Evaluation with Doppler Ultrasound.*
   With contributions by E.C. Brockenbrough, R.S. Reneman, G.I. Thomas and D.L.
   Davis. 1981   ISBN 90-247-2384-1
7. D.P. Zipes, J.C. Bailey and V. Elharrar (eds.): *The Slow Inward Current and Cardiac
   Arrhythmias.* 1980   ISBN 90-247-2380-9
8. H. Kesteloot and J.V. Joossens (eds.): *Epidemiology of Arterial Blood Pressure.* 1980
                                                     ISBN 90-247-2386-8
9. F.J.Th. Wackers (ed.): *Thallium-201 and Technetium-99m-Pyrophosphate. Myocardial Imaging in the Coronary Care Unit.* 1980   ISBN 90-247-2396-5
10. A. Maseri, C. Marchesi, S. Chierchia and M.G. Trivella (eds.): *Coronary Care Units.*
    Proceedings of a European Seminar (1978). 1981   ISBN 90-247-2456-2
11. J. Morganroth, E.N. Moore, L.S. Dreifus and E.L. Michelson (eds.): *The Evaluation of
    New Antiarrhythmic Drugs.* Proceedings of the First Symposium on New Drugs and
    Devices, held in Philadelphia, Pa., U.S.A. (1980). 1981   ISBN 90-247-2474-0
12. P. Alboni: *Intraventricular Conduction Disturbances.* 1981   ISBN 90-247-2483-X
13. H. Rijsterborgh (ed.): *Echocardiology.* 1981   ISBN 90-247-2491-0
14. G.S. Wagner (ed.): *Myocardial Infarction.* Measurement and Intervention. 1982
                                                     ISBN 90-247-2513-5
15. R.S. Meltzer and J. Roelandt (eds.): *Contrast Echocardiography.* 1982
                                                     ISBN 90-247-2531-3
16. A. Amery, R. Fagard, P. Lijnen and J. Staessen (eds.): *Hypertensive Cardiovascular
    Disease.* Pathophysiology and Treatment. 1982   IBSN 90-247-2534-8
17. L.N. Bouman and H.J. Jongsma (eds.): *Cardiac Rate and Rhythm.* Physiological,
    Morphological and Developmental Aspects. 1982   ISBN 90-247-2626-3
18. J. Morganroth and E.N. Moore (eds.): *The Evaluation of Beta Blocker and Calcium
    Antagonist Drugs.* Proceedings of the 2nd Symposium on New Drugs and Devices,
    held in Philadelphia, Pa., U.S.A. (1981). 1982   ISBN 90-247-2642-5
19. M.B. Rosenbaum and M.V. Elizari (eds.): *Frontiers of Cardiac Electrophysiology.*
    1983   ISBN 90-247-2663-8
20. J. Roelandt and P.G. Hugenholtz (eds.): *Long-term Ambulatory Electrocardiography.*
    1982   ISBN 90-247-2664-6
21. A.A.J. Adgey (ed.): *Acute Phase of Ischemic Heart Disease and Myocardial Infarc-
    tion.* 1982   ISBN 90-247-2675-1
22. P. Hanrath, W. Bleifeld and J. Souquet (eds.): *Cardiovascular Diagnosis by Ultra-
    sound.* Transesophageal, Computerized, Contrast, Doppler Echocardiography. 1982
                                                     ISBN 90-247-2692-1
23. J. Roelandt (ed.): *The Practice of M-Mode and Two-dimensional Echocardiography.*
    1983   ISBN 90-247-2745-6
24. J. Meyer, P. Schweizer and R. Erbel (eds.): *Advances in Noninvasive Cardiology.*
    Ultrasound, Computed Tomography, Radioisotopes, Digital Angiography. 1983
                                                     ISBN 0-89838-576-8
25. J. Morganroth and E.N. Moore (eds.): *Sudden Cardiac Death and Congestive Heart
    Failure.* Diagnosis and Treatment. Proceedings of the 3rd Symposium on New Drugs
    and Devices, held in Philadelphia, Pa., U.S.A. (1982). 1983   ISBN 0-89838-580-6
26. H.M. Perry Jr. (ed.): *Lifelong Management of Hypertension.* 1983
                                                     ISBN 0-89838-582-2
27. E.A. Jaffe (ed.): *Biology of Endothelial Cells.* 1984   ISBN 0-89838-587-3

Developments in Cardiovascular Medicine

28. B. Surawicz, C.P. Reddy and E.N. Prystowsky (eds.): *Tachycardias.* 1984
ISBN 0-89838-588-1
29. M.P. Spencer (ed.): *Cardiac Doppler Diagnosis.* Proceedings of a Symposium, held in Clearwater, Fla., U.S.A. (1983). 1983 ISBN 0-89838-591-1
30. H. Villarreal and M.P. Sambhi (eds.): *Topics in Pathophysiology of Hypertension.* 1984 ISBN 0-89838-595-4
31. F.H. Messerli (ed.): *Cardiovascular Disease in the Elderly.* 1984
Revised edition, 1988: see below under Volume 76
32. M.L. Simoons and J.H.C. Reiber (eds.): *Nuclear Imaging in Clinical Cardiology.* 1984 ISBN 0-89838-599-7
33. H.E.D.J. ter Keurs and J.J. Schipperheyn (eds.): *Cardiac Left Ventricular Hypertrophy.* 1983 ISBN 0-89838-612-8
34. N. Sperelakis (ed.): *Physiology and Pathology of the Heart.* 1984
Revised edition, 1988: see below under Volume 90
35. F.H. Messerli (ed.): *Kidney in Essential Hypertension.* Proceedings of a Course, held in New Orleans, La., U.S.A. (1983). 1984 ISBN 0-89838-616-0
36. M.P. Sambhi (ed.): *Fundamental Fault in Hypertension.* 1984 ISBN 0-89838-638-1
37. C. Marchesi (ed.): *Ambulatory Monitoring.* Cardiovascular System and Allied Applications. Proceedings of a Workshop, held in Pisa, Italy (1983). 1984
ISBN 0-89838-642-X
38. W. Kupper, R.N. MacAlpin and W. Bleifeld (eds.): *Coronary Tone in Ischemic Heart Disease.* 1984 ISBN 0-89838-646-2
39. N. Sperelakis and J.B. Caulfield (eds.): *Calcium Antagonists.* Mechanism of Action on Cardiac Muscle and Vascular Smooth Muscle. Proceedings of the 5th Annual Meeting of the American Section of the I.S.H.R., held in Hilton Head, S.C., U.S.A. (1983). 1984 ISBN 0-89838-655-1
40. Th. Godfraind, A.G. Herman and D. Wellens (eds.): *Calcium Entry Blockers in Cardiovascular and Cerebral Dysfunctions.* 1984 ISBN 0-89838-658-6
41. J. Morganroth and E.N. Moore (eds.): *Interventions in the Acute Phase of Myocardial Infarction.* Proceedings of the 4th Symposium on New Drugs and Devices, held in Philadelphia, Pa., U.S.A. (1983). 1984 ISBN 0-89838-659-4
42. F.L. Abel and W.H. Newman (eds.): *Functional Aspects of the Normal, Hypertrophied and Failing Heart.* Proceedings of the 5th Annual Meeting of the American Section of the I.S.H.R., held in Hilton Head, S.C., U.S.A. (1983). 1984
ISBN 0-89838-665-9
43. S. Sideman and R. Beyar (eds.): [3-D] *Simulation and Imaging of the Cardiac System.* State of the Heart. Proceedings of the International Henry Goldberg Workshop, held in Haifa, Israel (1984). 1985 ISBN 0-89838-687-X
44. E. van der Wall and K.I. Lie (eds.): *Recent Views on Hypertrophic Cardiomyopathy.* Proceedings of a Symposium, held in Groningen, The Netherlands (1984). 1985
ISBN 0-89838-694-2
45. R.E. Beamish, P.K. Singal and N.S. Dhalla (eds.), *Stress and Heart Disease.* Proceedings of a International Symposium, held in Winnipeg, Canada, 1984 (Vol. 1). 1985 ISBN 0-89838-709-4
46. R.E. Beamish, V. Panagia and N.S. Dhalla (eds.): *Pathogenesis of Stress-induced Heart Disease.* Proceedings of a International Symposium, held in Winnipeg, Canada, 1984 (Vol. 2). 1985 ISBN 0-89838-710-8
47. J. Morganroth and E.N. Moore (eds.): *Cardiac Arrhythmias.* New Therapeutic Drugs and Devices. Proceedings of the 5th Symposium on New Drugs and Devices, held in Philadelphia, Pa., U.S.A. (1984). 1985 ISBN 0-89838-716-7
48. P. Mathes (ed.): *Secondary Prevention in Coronary Artery Disease and Myocardial Infarction.* 1985 ISBN 0-89838-736-1
49. H.L. Stone and W.B. Weglicki (eds.): *Pathobiology of Cardiovascular Injury.* Proceedings of the 6th Annual Meeting of the American Section of the I.S.H.R., held in Oklahoma City, Okla., U.S.A. (1984). 1985 ISBN 0-89838-743-4

Developments in Cardiovascular Medicine

50. J. Meyer, R. Erbel and H.J. Rupprecht (eds.): *Improvement of Myocardial Perfusion.* Thrombolysis, Angioplasty, Bypass Surgery. Proceedings of a Symposium, held in Mainz, F.R.G. (1984). 1985   ISBN 0-89838-748-5
51. J.H.C. Reiber, P.W. Serruys and C.J. Slager (eds.): *Quantitative Coronary and Left Ventricular Cineangiography.* Methodology and Clinical Applications. 1986   ISBN 0-89838-760-4
52. R.H. Fagard and I.E. Bekaert (eds.): *Sports Cardiology.* Exercise in Health and Cardiovascular Disease. Proceedings from an International Conference, held in Knokke, Belgium (1985). 1986   ISBN 0-89838-782-5
53. J.H.C. Reiber and P.W. Serruys (eds.): *State of the Art in Quantitative Cornary Arteriography.* 1986   ISBN 0-89838-804-X
54. J. Roelandt (ed.): *Color Doppler Flow Imaging and Other Advances in Doppler Echocardiography.* 1986   ISBN 0-89838-806-6
55. E.E. van der Wall (ed.): *Noninvasive Imaging of Cardiac Metabolism.* Single Photon Scintigraphy, Positron Emission Tomography and Nuclear Magnetic Resonance. 1987   ISBN 0-89838-812-0
56. J. Liebman, R. Plonsey and Y. Rudy (eds.): *Pediatric and Fundamental Electrocardiography.* 1987   ISBN 0-89838-815-5
57. H.H. Hilger, V. Hombach and W.J. Rashkind (eds.), *Invasive Cardiovascular Therapy.* Proceedings of an International Symposium, held in Cologne, F.R.G. (1985). 1987   ISBN 0-89838-818-X
58. P.W. Serruys and G.T. Meester (eds.): *Coronary Angioplasty.* A Controlled Model for Ischemia. 1986   ISBN 0-89838-819-8
59. J.E. Tooke and L.H. Smaje (eds.): *Clinical Investigation of the Microcirculation.* Proceedings of an International Meeting, held in London, U.K. (1985). 1987   ISBN 0-89838-833-3
60. R.Th. van Dam and A. van Oosterom (eds.): *Electrocardiographic Body Surface Mapping.* Proceedings of the 3rd International Symposium on B.S.M., held in Nijmegen, The Netherlands (1985). 1986   ISBN 0-89838-834-1
61. M.P. Spencer (ed.): *Ultrasonic Diagnosis of Cerebrovascular Disease.* Doppler Techniques and Pulse Echo Imaging. 1987   ISBN 0-89838-836-8
62. M.J. Legato (ed.): *The Stressed Heart.* 1987   ISBN 0-89838-849-X
63. M.E. Safar (ed.): *Arterial and Venous Systems in Essential Hypertension.* With Assistance of G.M. London, A.Ch. Simon and Y.A. Weiss. 1987   ISBN 0-89838-857-0
64. J. Roelandt (ed.): *Digital Techniques in Echocardiography.* 1987   ISBN 0-89838-861-9
65. N.S. Dhalla, P.K. Singal and R.E. Beamish (eds.): *Pathology of Heart Disease.* Proceedings of the 8th Annual Meeting of the American Section of the I.S.H.R., held in Winnipeg, Canada, 1986 (Vol. 1). 1987   ISBN 0-89838-864-3
66. N.S. Dhalla, G.N. Pierce and R.E. Beamish (eds.): *Heart Function and Metabolism.* Proceedings of the 8th Annual Meeting of the American Section of the I.S.H.R., held in Winnipeg, Canada, 1986 (Vol. 2). 1987   ISBN 0-89838-865-1
67. N.S. Dhalla, I.R. Innes and R.E. Beamish (eds.): *Myocardial Ischemia.* Proceedings of a Satellite Symposium of the 30th International Physiological Congress, held in Winnipeg, Canada (1986). 1987   ISBN 0-89838-866-X
68. R.E. Beamish, V. Panagia and N.S. Dhalla (eds.): *Pharmacological Aspects of Heart Disease.* Proceedings of an International Symposium, held in Winnipeg, Canada (1986). 1987   ISBN 0-89838-867-8
69. H.E.D.J. ter Keurs and J.V. Tyberg (eds.): *Mechanics of the Circulation.* Proceedings of a Satellite Symposium of the 30th International Physiological Congress, held in Banff, Alberta, Canada (1986). 1987   ISBN 0-89838-870-8
70. S. Sideman and R. Beyar (eds.): *Activation, Metabolism and Perfusion of the Heart.* Simulation and Experimental Models. Proceedings of the 3rd Henry Goldberg Workshop, held in Piscataway, N.J., U.S.A. (1986). 1987   ISBN 0-89838-871-6

Developments in Cardiovascular Medicine

71. E. Aliot and R. Lazzara (eds.): *Ventricular Tachycardias*. From Mechanism to Therapy. 1987   ISBN 0-89838-881-3
72. A. Schneeweiss and G. Schettler: *Cardiovascular Drug Therapoy in the Elderly*. 1988
                                                                          ISBN 0-89838-883-X
73. J.V. Chapman and A. Sgalambro (eds.): *Basic Concepts in Doppler Echocardiography*. Methods of Clinical Applications based on a Multi-modality Doppler Approach. 1987   ISBN 0-89838-888-0
74. S. Chien, J. Dormandy, E. Ernst and A. Matrai (eds.): *Clinical Hemorheology*. Applications in Cardiovascular and Hematological Disease, Diabetes, Surgery and Gynecology. 1987   ISBN 0-89838-807-4
75. J. Morganroth and E.N. Moore (eds.): *Congestive Heart Failure*. Proceedings of the 7th Annual Symposium on New Drugs and Devices, held in Philadelphia, Pa., U.S.A. (1986). 1987   ISBN 0-89838-955-0
76. F.H. Messerli (ed.): *Cardiovascular Disease in the Elderly*. 2nd ed. 1988
                                                                          ISBN 0-89838-962-3
77. P.H. Heintzen and J.H. Bürsch (eds.): *Progress in Digital Angiocardiography*. 1988
                                                                          ISBN 0-89838-965-8
78. M.M. Scheinman (ed.): *Catheter Ablation of Cardiac Arrhythmias*. Basic Bioelectrical Effects and Clinical Indications. 1988   ISBN 0-89838-967-4
79. J.A.E. Spaan, A.V.G. Bruschke and A.C. Gittenberger-De Groot (eds.): *Coronary Circulation*. From Basic Mechanisms to Clinical Implications. 1987
                                                                          ISBN 0-89838-978-X
80. C. Visser, G. Kan and R.S. Meltzer (eds.): *Echocardiography in Coronary Artery Disease*. 1988   ISBN 0-89838-979-8
81. A. Bayés de Luna, A. Betriu and G. Permanyer (eds.): *Therapeutics in Cardiology*. 1988   ISBN 0-89838-981-X
82. D.M. Mirvis (ed.): *Body Surface Electrocardiographic Mapping*. 1988
                                                                          ISBN 0-89838-983-6
83. M.A. Konstam and J.M. Isner (eds.): *The Right Ventricle*. 1988   ISBN 0-89838-987-9
84. C.T. Kappagoda and P.V. Greenwood (eds.): *Long-term Management of Patients after Myocardial Infarction*. 1988   ISBN 0-89838-352-8
85. W.H. Gaasch and H.J. Levine (eds.): *Chronic Aortic Regurgitation*. 1988
                                                                          ISBN 0-89838-364-1
86. P.K. Singal (ed.): *Oxygen Radicals in the Pathophysiology of Heart Disease*. 1988
                                                                          ISBN 0-89838-375-7
87. J.H.C. Reiber and P.W. Serruys (eds.): *New Developments in Quantitative Coronary Arteriography*. 1988   ISBN 0-89838-377-3
88. J. Morganroth and E.N. Moore (eds.): *Silent Myocardial Ischemia*. Proceedings of the 8th Annual Symposium on New Drugs and Devices (1987). 1988
                                                                          ISBN 0-89838-380-3
89. H.E.D.J. ter Keurs and M.I.M. Noble (eds.): *Starling's Law of the Heart Revisted*. 1988   ISBN 0-89838-382-X
90. N. Sperelakis (ed.): *Physiology and Pathophysiology of the Heart*. Rev. ed. 1988
                                          3rd, revised edition, 1994: see below under Volume 151
91. J.W. de Jong (ed.): *Myocardial Energy Metabolism*. 1988   ISBN 0-89838-394-3
92. V. Hombach, H.H. Hilger and H.L. Kennedy (eds.): *Electrocardiography and Cardiac Drug Therapy*. Proceedings of an International Symposium, held in Cologne, F.R.G. (1987). 1988   ISBN 0-89838-395-1
93. H. Iwata, J.B. Lombardini and T. Segawa (eds.): *Taurine and the Heart*. 1988
                                                                          ISBN 0-89838-396-X
94. M.R. Rosen and Y. Palti (eds.): *Lethal Arrhythmias Resulting from Myocardial Ischemia and Infarction*. Proceedings of the 2nd Rappaport Symposium, held in Haifa, Israel (1988). 1988   ISBN 0-89838-401-X
95. M. Iwase and I. Sotobata: *Clinical Echocardiography*. With a Foreword by M.P. Spencer. 1989   ISBN 0-7923-0004-1

Developments in Cardiovascular Medicine

96. I. Cikes (ed.): *Echocardiography in Cardiac Interventions.* 1989
ISBN 0-7923-0088-2
97. E. Rapaport (ed.): *Early Interventions in Acute Myocardial Infarction.* 1989
ISBN 0-7923-0175-7
98. M.E. Safar and F. Fouad-Tarazi (eds.): *The Heart in Hypertension.* A Tribute to Robert C. Tarazi (1925-1986). 1989 ISBN 0-7923-0197-8
99. S. Meerbaum and R. Meltzer (eds.): *Myocardial Contrast Two-dimensional Echocardiography.* 1989 ISBN 0-7923-0205-2
100. J. Morganroth and E.N. Moore (eds.): *Risk/Benefit Analysis for the Use and Approval of Thrombolytic, Antiarrhythmic, and Hypolipidemic Agents.* Proceedings of the 9th Annual Symposium on New Drugs and Devices (1988). 1989 ISBN 0-7923-0294-X
101. P.W. Serruys, R. Simon and K.J. Beatt (eds.): *PTCA - An Investigational Tool and a Non-operative Treatment of Acute Ischemia.* 1990 ISBN 0-7923-0346-6
102. I.S. Anand, P.I. Wahi and N.S. Dhalla (eds.): *Pathophysiology and Pharmacology of Heart Disease.* 1989 ISBN 0-7923-0367-9
103. G.S. Abela (ed.): *Lasers in Cardiovascular Medicine and Surgery.* Fundamentals and Technique. 1990 ISBN 0-7923-0440-3
104. H.M. Piper (ed.): *Pathophysiology of Severe Ischemic Myocardial Injury.* 1990
ISBN 0-7923-0459-4
105. S.M. Teague (ed.): *Stress Doppler Echocardiography.* 1990 ISBN 0-7923-0499-3
106. P.R. Saxena, D.I. Wallis, W. Wouters and P. Bevan (eds.): *Cardiovascular Pharmacology of 5-Hydroxytryptamine.* Prospective Therapeutic Applications. 1990
ISBN 0-7923-0502-7
107. A.P. Shepherd and P.A. Öberg (eds.): *Laser-Doppler Blood Flowmetry.* 1990
ISBN 0-7923-0508-6
108. J. Soler-Soler, G. Permanyer-Miralda and J. Sagristà-Sauleda (eds.): *Pericardial Disease.* New Insights and Old Dilemmas. 1990 ISBN 0-7923-0510-8
109. J.P.M. Hamer: *Practical Echocardiography in the Adult.* With Doppler and Color-Doppler Flow Imaging. 1990 ISBN 0-7923-0670-8
110. A. Bayés de Luna, P. Brugada, J. Cosin Aguilar and F. Navarro Lopez (eds.): *Sudden Cardiac Death.* 1991 ISBN 0-7923-0716-X
111. E. Andries and R. Stroobandt (eds.): *Hemodynamics in Daily Practice.* 1991
ISBN 0-7923-0725-9
112. J. Morganroth and E.N. Moore (eds.): *Use and Approval of Antihypertensive Agents and Surrogate Endpoints for the Approval of Drugs affecting Antiarrhythmic Heart Failure and Hypolipidemia.* Proceedings of the 10th Annual Symposium on New Drugs and Devices (1989). 1990 ISBN 0-7923-0756-9
113. S. Iliceto, P. Rizzon and J.R.T.C. Roelandt (eds.): *Ultrasound in Coronary Artery Disease.* Present Role and Future Perspectives. 1990 ISBN 0-7923-0784-4
114. J.V. Chapman and G.R. Sutherland (eds.): *The Noninvasive Evaluation of Hemodynamics in Congenital Heart Disease.* Doppler Ultrasound Applications in the Adult and Pediatric Patient with Congenital Heart Disease. 1990
ISBN 0-7923-0836-0
115. G.T. Meester and F. Pinciroli (eds.): *Databases for Cardiology.* 1991
ISBN 0-7923-0886-7
116. B. Korecky and N.S. Dhalla (eds.): *Subcellular Basis of Contractile Failure.* 1990
ISBN 0-7923-0890-5
117. J.H.C. Reiber and P.W. Serruys (eds.): *Quantitative Coronary Arteriography.* 1991
ISBN 0-7923-0913-8
118. E. van der Wall and A. de Roos (eds.): *Magnetic Resonance Imaging in Coronary Artery Disease.* 1991 ISBN 0-7923-0940-5
119. V. Hombach, M. Kochs and A.J. Camm (eds.): *Interventional Techniques in Cardiovascular Medicine.* 1991 ISBN 0-7923-0956-1
120. R. Vos: *Drugs Looking for Diseases.* Innovative Drug Research and the Development of the Beta Blockers and the Calcium Antagonists. 1991 ISBN 0-7923-0968-5

Developments in Cardiovascular Medicine

121. S. Sideman, R. Beyar and A.G. Kleber (eds.): *Cardiac Electrophysiology, Circulation, and Transport*. Proceedings of the 7th Henry Goldberg Workshop (Berne, Switzerland, 1990). 1991   ISBN 0-7923-1145-0
122. D.M. Bers: *Excitation-Contraction Coupling and Cardiac Contractile Force*. 1991
                                                                    ISBN 0-7923-1186-8
123. A.-M. Salmasi and A.N. Nicolaides (eds.): *Occult Atherosclerotic Disease*. Diagnosis, Assessment and Management. 1991   ISBN 0-7923-1188-4
124. J.A.E. Spaan: *Coronary Blood Flow*. Mechanics, Distribution, and Control. 1991
                                                                    ISBN 0-7923-1210-4
125. R.W. Stout (ed.): *Diabetes and Atherosclerosis*. 1991   ISBN 0-7923-1310-0
126. A.G. Herman (ed.): *Antithrombotics*. Pathophysiological Rationale for Pharmacological Interventions. 1991   ISBN 0-7923-1413-1
127. N.H.J. Pijls: *Maximal Myocardial Perfusion as a Measure of the Functional Significance of Coronary Arteriogram*. From a Pathoanatomic to a Pathophysiologic Interpretation of the Coronary Arteriogram. 1991   ISBN 0-7923-1430-1
128. J.H.C. Reiber and E.E. v.d. Wall (eds.): *Cardiovascular Nuclear Medicine and MRI*. Quantitation and Clinical Applications. 1992   ISBN 0-7923-1467-0
129. E. Andries, P. Brugada and R. Stroobrandt (eds.): *How to Face 'the Faces' of Cardiac Pacing*. 1992   ISBN 0-7923-1528-6
130. M. Nagano, S. Mochizuki and N.S. Dhalla (eds.): *Cardiovascular Disease in Diabetes*. 1992   ISBN 0-7923-1554-5
131. P.W. Serruys, B.H. Strauss and S.B. King III (eds.): *Restenosis after Intervention with New Mechanical Devices*. 1992   ISBN 0-7923-1555-3
132. P.J. Walter (ed.): *Quality of Life after Open Heart Surgery*. 1992
                                                                    ISBN 0-7923-1580-4
133. E.E. van der Wall, H. Sochor, A. Righetti and M.G. Niemeyer (eds.): *What's new in Cardiac Imaging?* SPECT, PET and MRI. 1992   ISBN 0-7923-1615-0
134. P. Hanrath, R. Uebis and W. Krebs (eds.): *Cardiovascular Imaging by Ultrasound*. 1992   ISBN 0-7923-1755-6
135. F.H. Messerli (ed.): *Cardiovascular Disease in the Elderly*. 3rd ed. 1992
                                                                    ISBN 0-7923-1859-5
136. J. Hess and G.R. Sutherland (eds.): *Congenital Heart Disease in Adolescents and Adults*. 1992   ISBN 0-7923-1862-5
137. J.H.C. Reiber and P.W. Serruys (eds.): *Advances in Quantitative Coronary Arteriography*. 1993   ISBN 0-7923-1863-3
138. A.-M. Salmasi and A.S. Iskandrian (eds.): *Cardiac Output and Regional Flow in Health and Disease*. 1993   ISBN 0-7923-1911-7
139. J.H. Kingma, N.M. van Hemel and K.I. Lie (eds.): *Atrial Fibrillation, a Treatable Disease?* 1992   ISBN 0-7923-2008-5
140. B. Ostadel and N.S. Dhalla (eds.): *Heart Function in Health and Disease*. Proceedings of the Cardiovascular Program (Prague, Czechoslovakia, 1991). 1992
                                                                    ISBN 0-7923-2052-2
141. D. Noble and Y.E. Earm (eds.): *Ionic Channels and Effect of Taurine on the Heart*. Proceedings of an International Symposium (Seoul, Korea , 1992). 1993
                                                                    ISBN 0-7923-2199-5
142. H.M. Piper and C.J. Preusse (eds.): *Ischemia-reperfusion in Cardiac Surgery*. 1993
                                                                    ISBN 0-7923-2241-X
143. J. Roelandt, E.J. Gussenhoven and N. Bom (eds.): *Intravascular Ultrasound*. 1993
                                                                    ISBN 0-7923-2301-7
144. M.E. Safar and M.F. O'Rourke (eds.): *The Arterial System in Hypertension*. 1993
                                                                    ISBN 0-7923-2343-2
145. P.W. Serruys, D.P. Foley and P.J. de Feyter (eds.): *Quantitative Coronary Angiography in Clinical Practice*. With a Foreword by Spencer B. King III. 1994
                                                                    ISBN 0-7923-2368-8

Developments in Cardiovascular Medicine

Developments in Cardiovascular Medicine

173. C.A. Nienaber and U. Sechtem (eds.): *Imaging and Intervention in Cardiology.* 1996
      ISBN 0-7923-3649-6
174. G. Assmann (ed.): *HDL Deficiency and Atherosclerosis.* 1995   ISBN 0-7923-8888-7
175. N.M. van Hemel, F.H.M. Wittkampf and H. Ector (eds.): *The Pacemaker Clinic of the 90's.* Essentials in Brady-Pacing. 1995   ISBN 0-7923-3688-7
176. N. Wilke (ed.): *Advanced Cardiovascular MRI of the Heart and Great Vessels.* 1995
      ISBN 0-7923-3720-4
177. M. LeWinter, H. Suga and M.W. Watkins (eds.): *Cardiac Energetics: From Emax to Pressure-volume Area.* 1995   ISBN 0-7923-3721-2
178. R.J. Siegel (ed.): *Ultrasound Angioplasty.* 1995   ISBN 0-7923-3722-0
179. D.M. Yellon and G.J. Gross (eds.): *Myocardial Protection and the K_{ATP} Channel.* 1995   ISBN 0-7923-3791-3
180. A.V.G. Bruschke, J.H.C. Reiber, K.I. Lie and H.J.J. Wellens (eds.): *Lipid Lowering Therapy and Progression of Coronary Atherosclerosis.* 1995   ISBN 0-7923-3807-3
181. A.-S.A. Abd-Eyattah and A.S. Wechsler (eds.): *Purines and Myocardial Protection.* 1995   ISBN 0-7923-3831-6

Previous volumes are still available

KLUWER ACADEMIC PUBLISHERS – DORDRECHT / BOSTON / LONDON